Methods in Neuronal Modeling

Computational Neuroscience

Terrence J. Sejnowski and Tomaso A. Poggio, editors

Methods in Neuronal Modeling: From Synapses to Networks, edited by Christof Koch and Idan Segev, 1989

Methods in Neuronal Modeling
From Synapses to Networks

edited by Christof Koch and Idan Segev

A Bradford Book

The MIT Press

Cambridge, Massachusetts, and London, England

Second Printing, 1990

This book was set in LaT$_{\text{E}}$X
by Candace Hochenedel
and printed and bound in the United States of America.

Library of Congress Cataloging-in-Publication Data

Methods in neuronal modeling.

(Computational neuroscience)
"A Bradford book."
Bibliography: p.
Includes index.
1. Neural circuitry—Computer simulation. 2. Nervous system—Computer simulation. 3. Neurons—Computer simulation. I. Koch, Christof. II. Segev, Idan. III. Series.
QP363.3.M47 1988   599'.0188   88–8279
ISBN 0–262–11133–0

Throughout all his existence man has been striving to hear the music of the spheres, and has seemed to himself once and again to catch some phrase of it, or even a hint of the whole form of it. Yet he can never be sure that he has truly heard it, nor even that there is any such perfect music at all to be heard. Inevitably so, for if it exists, it is not for him in his littleness.

"Last and First Man"
Olaf Stapledon

Contents

Series Foreword

Computational neuroscience is an approach to understanding the information content of neural signals by modeling the nervous system at many different structural scales, including the biophysical, the circuit, and the systems levels. Computer simulations of neurons and neural networks are complementary to traditional techniques in neuroscience. This book series welcomes contributions that link theoretical studies with experimental approaches to understanding information processing in the nervous system. Areas and topics of particular interest include biophysical mechanisms for computation in neurons, computer simulations of neural circuits, models of learning, representation of sensory information in neural networks, systems models of sensory-motor integration, and computational analysis of problems in biological sensing, motor control, and perception.

Terrence J. Sejnowski
Tomaso Poggio

Preface

How does the brain work? Ever since the hieroglyph for "brain" first appeared in an Egyptian papyrus dated to the 17th century B.C., humans have asked this question. Only in the second part of the twentieth century, however, have quantitative theories dealing with various aspects of the nervous system been proposed. In very general terms, what the brain does is process and use information. In some sense, therefore, the human brain is a kind of computer, whose constituent elements are nerve cells and whose architecture is constrained by the biological nature of its elements and by its evolutionary history. But the critical question is this: What kind of computer is it? What are its principles of operation? How does it process, store, and retrieve information? To fashion theories and models of information processing both in single nerve cells and within large networks of cells, we must be able quantitatively to solve and analyze proposed models. For the essential tasks of simulation and analysis, the digital computer is invaluable, for without the computational power of electronic machines, this new and fledgling area of computational neuroscience would wither away and die.

The field of computational neuroscience does not want for interesting, speculative, insightful, amazing—and possibly even partially correct—theories, it does lack a unified methodology. This book then attempts to fill the need for a how-to-model-your-favorite-nervous-system treatise. In thirteen chapters it discusses techniques for numerically modeling the nervous system, from the level of synapses and membranes to the level of heavily interconnected neurons and connectionist networks. Special emphasis is paid to modern numerical integration methods and to the growing use of parallel computers.

This book evolved in parallel with an annual four-week-long summer course at the Marine Biological Laboratory in Woods Hole, held for the first time during August 1988. The course is entitled "Methods in Computational Neuroscience" and is directed by James Bower and Christof Koch. In lieu of course notes, we used the papers now collected in this volume, and the success of the experiment promoted the publication of the collection. Based on our use of it in the summer course, we suggest that *Methods in Neuronal Modeling* is suitable as a textbook for a one-term advanced undergraduate or graduate course in computational neuroscience, biological information processing, or neural networks, as well as a source book for experimentalists and modelers. It does not, however, start at the very beginning. A basic knowledge of biophysics and neurophysiology, at least a passing familiarity with elementary notions of differential equations and numerical analysis, and knowledge of standard computer programming practices are assumed. Notation has been standardized throughout the entire volume. Some of the more esoteric technical discussions as well as the detailed equations and parameters describing individual models are relegated to appendices following each chapter.

We thank the Office of Naval Research, the Air Force Office of Scientific Research, and the James S. McDonnell Foundation for the funding that made this summer course possible.

We would like to thank Candace Hochenedel, who toiled away day and night to convert the manuscripts submitted by the chapter authors into LaTeX and who looked after the myriad details that go into designing and editing a book. Without her, the book would never have been finished. Thanks also to Lyle Borg-Graham, who provided detailed feedback on an earlier draft of this book, and to Patricia S. Churchland, who helped with the introduction.

Christof Koch, Pasadena
Idan Segev, Jerusalem

Methods in Neuronal Modeling

CHAPTER 1

Introduction

CHRISTOF KOCH and IDAN SEGEV

One of the most exciting endeavors being undertaken in the late twentieth century is the attempt both to understand natural intelligence as well as to build artificial intelligences able in the not too distant future to rival and surpass our own. Although this enterprise is by no means novel, it appears to have entered a qualitative new phase. First, research in neuroscience has accumulated a wealth of experimental data about the brain, ranging from characterizations of the structure of single molecules and ionic channels to imaging brain activity while the brain carries out some cognitive task. Second, our computers have given us the power to simulate and thereby understand some complex systems in great detail. Conjointly, these developments have led to the emergence of a new paradigm, a new approach toward understanding the nervous system, computational neuroscience, with the ultimate goal of explaining how electrical and chemical signals are used in the brain to represent and process information.

To accomplish this goal, computational neuroscience seeks to develop models describing how the nervous system or some part of it carries out certain operations, such as adapting to a long-lasting current stimulus, computing the direction of a moving object, discriminating sound patterns, or learning certain motor skills. In some instances, the models may be very detailed, incorporating as much anatomical and biophysical detail as available. The best known example of such a model is Hodgkin and Huxley's (1952) description of the initiation and propagation of action potentials in the squid giant axon. Unfortunately realistic brain models, as they are referred to (Sejnowski, Koch, and Churchland 1988), are typically so complex as to preclude a detailed mathematical analysis. It is here that the digital computer comes into its own, numerically simulating the behavior of the model in response to various inputs. Computers have therefore emerged as the dominant tool of the computational neuroscientist.

Even with the remarkable increase in computer power during the last decade, modeling networks of neurons that incorporate all the known biophysical details is out of the question. Simplifying assumptions are unavoidable when one is considering the function of parts of a nervous system, such as the visual system of the fly or the mammalian hippocampus. Such models usually postulate very simple threshold units as neurons and reduce the complexity of real synapses with all their dynamics to a single number, the connection strength. What these models lose in specificity, however, they gain in insight and analytical tractability. For instance, the cooperative stereo algorithm of Marr and Poggio (1976) emphasizes the crucial role of constraints in understanding and solving the binocular correspondence problem (at the expense of neglecting the anatomy and physiology of the early visual systems of mammals). Applying the back-propagation learning algorithm to construct the receptive fields of neurons in monkey posterior parietal cortex sensitive to both retinal and eye coordinates (Zipser and Andersen 1988) helps us understand how these neurons decode spatial information. At the single-cell level, examples of such "simplifying brain models" (Sejnowski et al. 1988) are the phase-space models of FitzHugh (1969) and others. They allow us to predict and understand the qualitative features of neuronal firing without requiring detailed knowledge of channel kinetics and distribution.

One frequently hears the criticism that simplifying brain models lack this or the other physiological feature and are thus unbiological and irrelevant for understanding the nervous system. As an instance of such a simplification, consider that current neural network models usually fail to include axonal propagation times for action potentials. This argument, taken to its extreme, implies that we will not be able to understand the brain until we have simulated it at the detailed biophysical level! This is of course impossible for technological reasons; moreover, such a simulation with a vast number of parameters will be as poorly understood as the brain itself. Furthermore, if modeling is a strategy developed precisely because the brain's complexity is an obstacle to understanding the principles governing brain function, then an argument insisting on complete biological fidelity is self-defeating. In physics, simplifying models have been extremely useful in understanding large classes of phenomena. As physics students learn early, models typically sacrifice a realistic construal of the physical system under study on the altar of simplicity, approximation and idealization. Few oscillatory systems in the real world act as ideal harmonic oscillators; yet this concept is extremely powerful for capturing the qualitative behavior of a large number of systems. Moreover, at the macroscopic level theories and models may emerge that do not directly refer to the microscopic variables anymore.

Thus, the hope is that realistic models of cerebral cortex do not need to incorporate explicit information about such minutiae as the various ionic channels. The style of simplifying assumptions could be similar to Boyle's gas law, where no mention is made of the 10^{23} or so molecules making up the gas. In spite of these simplifications, computers are still the *conditio sine qua non* for studying the behavior of the model for all but the most trivial cases.

Computational neuroscience shares this total dependence on computers with a number of other fields, such as hydrodynamics, high energy physics, and meteorology, to name but a few. In fact, over the last decades we have witnessed a profound change in the nature of the scientific enterprise. Traditionally, the course of scientific inquiry has been one of hypothesis and prediction, experimental test and analysis—a process that is repeated over and over again and has led to the spectacular successes of physics and astronomy. The best theories, for instance Maxwell's equations in electrodynamics, have been founded on simple principles that can be relatively simply expressed and solved. However, the major scientific and technological problems facing us today probably do not have theories expressible in easy-to-solve equations. Deriving the properties of the proton from quantum chromodynamics, solving Schrödinger's equation for anything other than the hydrogen molecule, predicting the three-dimensional shape of proteins from their amino-acid sequence or the temperature of earth's atmosphere in the face of increasing carbon dioxide levels or understanding the brain are all instances of theories requiring massive computer power. Thus, the traditional Baconian dyad of theory and experiment must be modified to include *computation*. Computations are required for making predictions as well as for evaluating the data. This new triad of theory, computation, and experiment then leads to a new cycle: mathematical theory, simulation of theory and prediction, experimental test, and analysis. This reliance on computing has led to the emergence of such fields as computational physics, computational chemistry, or even computational molecular biology.[1]

The "computational" in computational neuroscience, however, has a meaning different from large-scale computing, because it derives from the computer metaphor the idea that the brain computes in the sense of representing, processing, and storing information. In fact, if one could

---

[1] The study of chaos has shown, however, some of the principal limitations of this approach, because even quite simple and completely deterministic systems can behave in such a manner that one is unable to predict in any practical sense their exact future behavior.

completely analyze a particular model, say the Hopfield model of associative memory, without the aid of computers, it would still form part of computational neuroscience, because the underlying aim of the model is to make explicit how the brain could store information. Conversely, simulating the detailed physics, hydrodynamics, and anatomy of the eye bulb on a computer would not constitute a model within the realm of computational neuroscience.

But how is any of this different from cybernetics or artificial intelligence? The answer is that computational neuroscience shares with these fields their overall motivation—understanding the nature of complex information-processing systems—however, it differs fundamentally in its approach. Different from cybernetics, it opens the "black box" and studies the nature of the hardware to understand the algorithms carried out by the black box. It differs from artificial intelligence in that it is not interested in how best to solve a particular task, but in understanding how the nervous system solves the task. This is the difference between understanding how humans play chess and designing a machine to beat any human at chess.

A final point of note concerns the relationship between the "top-down" and the "bottom-up" approaches. The majority of models discussed in this book are based more or less directly on experimental data, from the single cell to the network and system level. These models proceed from the detailed study of the biological hardware to its possible involvement in information processing in the widest sense. The alternative to this data-driven approach is a theory-driven top-down approach, in which the question of how the information is processed or how a particular computation could be carried out is addressed first. Once the problem has been characterized at the formal level, a particular algorithm is derived to solve the problem in agreement with the known physiology and anatomy. Whereas the bottom-up paradigm is shared by virtually all neuroscientists, the top-down approach is more typical of artificial intelligence, with its belief that information processing is ultimately independent of the particular nature of the computing hardware. In recent years, the limitations of the two strategies pursued separately by themselves have been realized, and a synthesis of both has come into favor. Thus, understanding how the visual system computes binocular disparity requires a computational analysis of the inverse problem of recovering depth from two spatially displaced two-dimensional images, as well as knowledge of the physiology of disparity-sensitive cells in primate cortex supplemented by perceptual experiments on stereo acuity (Poggio and Poggio 1985).

This collection of papers begins in chapter 2 with an exposition by Wilfrid Rall of linear cable theory as applied to passive and extended dendritic trees of neurons. Rall discusses how the neuron's morphology, membrane properties, and synaptic architecture determine its input/output properties, and how key parameters of the cell, such as its membrane time-constant and its electrotonic length, can be extracted by a set of relatively simple intracellular experiments. This chapter also contains the remarkable application of cable theory that has led to the existence proof of functional dendro-dendritic synapses in the olfactory bulb. A complementary approach is represented in the next two chapters, by Idan Segev, James Fleshman, and Robert Burke and by Walter Yamada, Christof Koch, and Paul Adams. The elegance and at the same time the limitation of Rall's method rely on a number of simplifying assumptions (for example, passive membrane, representing synaptic input as linear current source) to treat the model neuron analytically. In the compartmental approach, the appropriate linear or nonlinear cable equation is discretized in space (and in time), hence the name compartment, and the resulting system of coupled nonlinear difference equations is solved numerically. This enables the modeler to successfully simulate neurons with a simple electrical structure but very complicated dendritic tree (chapter 3), as well as neurons with spatially simple but electrically very complex structures (chapter 4). Chapter 4 also deals extensively with the buffering and the diffusion of intracellular calcium, the key ion underlying a host of intracellular processes such as exocytosis and the induction of neuronal plasticity.

In chapter 5, John Rinzel and Bard Ermentrout explore the dynamic behavior of neurons on the basis of the geometrical phase space treatment. Thus a relatively simple neuronal model produces a rich repertoire of responses, such as repetitive firing, oscillation, and bursting. A similar treatment, borrowed from the theory of dynamic systems, can also be applied to small networks of cells that collectively show bursting and oscillatory behavior. This approach, an instance of a simplifying brain model, is important because it allows us to understand the qualitative properties (for example, threshold behavior, repetitive firing, refractory period) of a large class of dynamical systems without knowing all the relevant biophysical details.

Chapters 2 through 5 should provide the reader with enough background material to model a very wide range of nerve cells, from passively integrating neurons to neurons with intricate electrical and biophysical properties.

Chapters 6 and 7 deal with the analysis of neuronal excitability in small (invertebrate) networks. In these systems of 10, 20, or 30 nerve cells, individual neurons can be identified from animal to animal on the basis of their unique and specific morphologies, patterns of excitability, and synaptic connections with each other and with their environment. Peter Getting reconstructs the network mediating the escape swimming reflex in the marine mollusc *Tritonia diomedea*. On the basis of his extra- and intracellular recordings from this preparation, he handcrafts a number of single compartmental neurons and their connections to fit his data. In chapter 7, David Kleinfeld and Haim Sompolinsky use the formalism developed by John Hopfield—continuous neurons with a sigmoidal nonlinearity whose behavior is governed by the evolution of a "cost" or "energy" functional—to simulate the same system. Although the two implementations differ as to their details, their overall qualitative behavior is similar. Both techniques should appeal to the neuroscientist analyzing small neuronal networks, such as the highly recurrent ones acting as central pattern generators, for instance, in the stomatogastric ganglion of the crayfish and lobster or the flight control system in the cricket.

Chapters 8, 9, and 10 deal with the simulation of networks containing many hundreds if not thousands of cells. Shihab Shamma treats topographically organized sensory networks using a well-explored single-cell representation, the leaky integrate-and-fire model of Bruce Knight. This quasianalytical approach allows one to easily deal with local feedback and feedforward inhibition, as in the case of the *Limulus* visual system or within the mammalian auditory system, the one covered by Shamma. Chapter 9 by Matthew Wilson and James Bower presents the general methodology for simulating neuronal networks with arbitrary patterns of connectivity and complex single cells within the framework of their general purpose neuronal simulation package, GENESIS. The authors discuss this method in relation to the mammalian piriform (olfactory) cortex. The system best studied at the level of theory, psychophysics, and physiology is the mammalian visual system. Thus, Udo Wehmeier, Dawei Dong, Christof Koch, and David Van Essen devote chapter 10 to describing in detail the early visual system in the adult cat, from the regular distribution of ganglion cells in the retina to inhibitory cells in layer IV of the primary visual cortex.

A major fraction of the current excitement in the neural network community has come from the development of powerful learning algorithms, algorithms that can overcome the stifling limitations of the earlier single-layer perceptron, exposed in Marvin Minsky and Seymour

Papert's (1969) famous treatise *Perceptrons.* Sidney Lehky and Terrence Sejnowski discuss in chapter 11 how the "back-propagation" learning algorithms can be applied to real problems in neurobiology, in their case the elucidation of the three-dimensional shape of objects from their shading (shape-from-shading). The promise of this approach is not that it will mimic the processes occuring during development—the manner in which back-propagation works is not very biological—but that it gives the modeler a tool with which to design neurons with very specific properties and then assess to what extent these properties overlap with those of real neurons.

All of these chapters discuss to some extent how to implement the different simulation methods on digital computers (while sparing the reader, however, baroque flow diagrams and endless computer code). Although to most scientists "digital computer" is still synonymous with "serial, digital computer" with a von Neumann architecture, parallel computers with tens, hundreds, or even tens of thousands of processors have arrived in most academic computing centers. Given the analogy between the highly distributed and parallel organization of the nervous system and these concurrent machines, a number of interesting issues arise. In the penultimate chapter 12 by Mark Nelson, Wojtek Furmanski, and James Bower, the efficient use of such machines for simulating single neurons or networks of neurons is discussed, with particular emphasis on the optimal use of all processors (the load-balancing problem).

Faced with the nonstationary nonlinearities of single nerve cells—expressed in their complex anatomy and physiology—and with networks of thousands of such cells connected by delay lines, the dominant method of simulation for the foreseeable future is the general compartmental approach. This entails the numerical solution of nonlinear coupled differential equations with their associated initial and boundary conditions (usually parabolic second-order partial differential equations for single-cell models or first-order ordinary differential equations for simplified neural networks). Chapter 13 by Michael Mascagni treats the topic of the appropriate numerical routine for neuronal modeling. This chapter should be required reading for anybody modeling any neurobiological system on a digital computer! The potential gain when going from the simplest possible forward-Euler method to a more sophisticated second-order, implicit integration scheme can be in one or two orders of magnitude of computing time with only a minimal amount of extra programming.

These simulation methods require not only powerful computers—available to most laboratories—but also the appropriate software. In particular, questions of the proper input and output routines for these large-scale simulation systems become more and more important. Anybody who has ever attempted to write a general simulation package has quickly come to realize that a high-level, symbolic language to define and specify channels, dendrites, and neuronal types (for instance, pyramidal versus stellate cells) is needed. In this manner, very complex neurons or neuronal populations can be constructed using a small number of primitive elements. Sophisticated programs even use graphical icons (for instance, schematic diagrams of synapses or cables) in conjunction with a pointing device such as a mouse to achieve this. At the output end, routines must be designed that can display and evaluate the information contained within hundreds of elements. Such apparent "frills" dramatically reduce the time spent writing, debugging, and understanding large programs. Modern simulation programs such as SPICE (chapter 3), the commercially available SABER designed for analog circuits (chapter 3), the Rochester connectionist simulator, or GENESIS, the neuronal network simulator developed at the California Institute of Technology (chapter 9), all share these features to some extent. We feel that most of these issues are covered in standard computer science texts, and we refrain from discussing them in this book.

One limitation of this book is that it does not discuss experimental approaches and techniques to test theories within computational neuroscience. Such techniques include voltage- and calcium-dependent dyes, the various brain imaging techniques (for example, positron emission tomography, magnetic resonance imaging) and in particular multiunit recording. However, we feel that an in-depth treatment of these techniques and their interplay with computational theories would go beyond the framework of this book (for a brief overview see Sejnowski and Churchland 1989). The chapters in this volume should, nonetheless, provide researchers with enough technical background to start modeling their own nervous system and to understand at the same time the strength and limitations of this new method of investigating brains. Although it is difficult to predict how successful these brain models will be, we certainly appear to be in a golden age on the threshold of understanding our own intelligence.

CHAPTER 2

Cable Theory for Dendritic Neurons

WILFRID RALL

2.1 Background

The designation "cable theory" comes from the derivation and application of the cable equation for calculations essential to the first transatlantic telegraph cable, around 1855, by Professor William Thomson (Lord Kelvin). As a student in Paris, Thomson had mastered the mathematical methods pioneered by Fourier; he knew that his one-dimensional cable equation was formally the same partial differential equation (PDE) that Fourier had used to describe the conduction of heat in a wire or in a ring. In the 1870s, Hermann and Weber derived and applied a different PDE (including three-dimensional space in cylindrical coordinates) to the problem of electric current flow in and around a cylindrical core conductor (model of nerve axon); later, around 1900, Hermann and others explicitly recognized that when this core conductor equation is reduced to one spatial dimension, it becomes equivalent to Kelvin's cable equation. More detail and references to early contributions can be found in Brazier (1959), Taylor (1963), and Rall (1977). Experimental testing with single-fiber preparations in the 1930s (associated with the names of Cole and Curtis, Rushton, Hodgkin, Katz, Tasaki, and others) provided important evidence confirming the relevance of cable theory to nerve axons. Two classic papers, which presented derivations of the cable equation for nerve cylinders and included transient solutions as well as methods for estimating the values of key parameters, are those of Hodgkin and Rushton (1946) and Davis and Lorente de Nó (1947).

The application of cable theory to dendritic neurons began in the late 1950s, when it became necessary to interpret experimental data obtained from individual neurons by means of intracellular microelectrodes located in the neuron soma. Although Coombs, Eccles, and Fatt (1955) did consider current flow to the dendrites in their interpretation of measured input resistance, both they and Frank and Fuortes (1956) neglected the transient cable properties of the dendrites when calculating values for the membrane time constant (τ_m) from their transient data. This neglect resulted not only in erroneously low values for τ_m, but also led to complicated proposals designed to explain how synaptic potentials could decay more slowly than would be expected for a passive exponential decay governed by such low τ_m values. The recognition and correction of these errors and misinterpretations depended on the application of cable theory to dendritic neurons (Rall 1957, 1959, 1960). Valuable functional insights and guidance in the design of experiments followed from these cable theory results and from additional studies designed to explore the effects of different synaptic input distributions over the dendritic surface of a neuron (Rall 1962b, 1964, 1967, 1969, 1977; Jack and Redman 1971; Jack, Noble, and Tsien 1975; also Rall and Shepherd 1968; Rall and Rinzel 1973; Rinzel and Rall 1974; Koch, Poggio, and Torre 1982, 1983; Rall and Segev 1985, 1987).

2.2   Cable Equation

2.2.1   Definitions

The cable equation is a partial differential equation (PDE) that neurophysiologists usually express as

$$\lambda^2(\partial^2 V/\partial x^2) - V - \tau(\partial V/\partial t) = 0 \qquad (2.1)$$

or, in terms of the dimensionless variables, $X = x/\lambda$ and $T = t/\tau$, as

$$\partial^2 V/\partial X^2 - V - \partial V/\partial T = 0 \qquad (2.2)$$

Here V represents the voltage difference across the membrane (interior minus exterior) as a deviation from its resting value (i.e., $V = V_i - V_e - E_r$); x represents distance along the axis of the membrane cylinder, and λ is the length constant of the core conductor (defined by eq. 2.13 or 2.14 below); although both x and λ are expressed in cm or μm, their ratio, $X = x/\lambda$, represents a dimensionless variable that is proportional to distance; also, t represents time, and τ is the membrane time constant (sometimes also expressed as τ_m) of the passive membrane (defined by eq. 2.12 below); although both t and τ are expressed in sec or $msec$, their ratio, $T = t/\tau$, represents a dimensionless variable that is proportional to time.

For a DC steady state, $\partial V/\partial t = 0$; then the cable equation reduces to an ordinary differential equation (ODE) that can be expressed

$$d^2 V/dX^2 - V = 0 \qquad (2.3)$$

Many useful results, such as cable input resistance and steady-state voltage attenuation with distance, can be obtained most simply from solutions of eq. 2.3 for various boundary conditions; see eqs. 2.16–2.30 below.

For AC (sinusoidal) steady states and for the laplace transform domain, the cable equation becomes reduced to a somewhat different ODE, namely,

$$d^2\hat{V}/dX^2 - q^2\hat{V} = 0 \qquad (2.4)$$

where $\hat{V}$ and q are both complex variables (with real and imaginary parts, implying a modulus and a phase angle). For AC steady states, $q^2 = 1 + j\omega\tau$, where $j = \sqrt{-1}$ and ω is the angular frequency $2\pi f$; solutions in this domain can be used to obtain expressions for AC admittance, impedance, and transfer functions (for examples, see appendices of Rall 1960; Rall and Rinzel 1973; Rall and Segev 1985). In the Laplace transform domain, $q^2 = 1 + \tau s$, where the complex variable s (sometimes termed complex frequency) is used to define the relation of $\hat{V}(X,s)$ in the laplace transform domain to $V(X,t)$ in the time domain (for explanations, see the mathematical appendix of Jack et al. 1975, or a textbook on Laplace transforms); solutions in this domain can be used to obtain expressions or numerical algorithms for the solutions to various boundary value problems (Rall 1960; Rinzel and Rall 1974; Rall and Segev 1985; Jack and Redman 1971; Jack et al. 1975; Barrett and Crill 1974; Butz and Cowan 1974; Horwitz 1981, 1983; Koch and Poggio 1985; Holmes 1986).

2.2.2 Assumptions and Derivation for Cable Equation

Nerve axons and dendrites consist of thin tubes of nerve membrane, often idealized as cylinders. They have been referred to as core conductors because both the intracellular cytoplasmic core and the extracellular fluid are ionic media that conduct electric current. What is important conceptually is that for short lengths (i.e., short compared with λ, but many times the cylinder diameter), the resistance to electric current flow across the membrane is much greater than the resistance along the interior core, or along the exterior; this physical fact results in a tendency for the electric current inside the core conductor to flow parallel to the cylinder axis for considerable distance before a significant fraction of this current leaks across the membrane. When this is formulated mathematically, with a focus on only one spatial dimension, one is led to the cable equation.

Here we begin by assuming a uniform cylindrical core conductor of great length. That means uniform membrane properties (resistivity, capacitance, and emf) and a uniform intracellular resistance, r_i, per unit length of the core conductor. One key assumption of one-dimensional cable theory is that the intracellular voltage, V_i, is a function of only two variables, the time, t, and the distance, x, along the axis of the core conductor; a related key assumption is that the gradient of the intracellular potential can be expressed

$$\frac{\partial V_i}{\partial x} = -i_i r_i \qquad (2.5)$$

where i_i represents the intracellular current (core current) taken as positive when flowing to the right, in the direction of increasing values of x, and r_i is the intracellular resistance per unit length noted above. Note that this equation can be obtained from parts A and B of fig. 2.1, by taking the limit of $\Delta V_i / \Delta x$, as Δx approaches zero.

The assumption of a uniform core conductor, or uniform cable, implies that r_i is a constant, independent of x and t; consequently, when eq. 2.5 is differentiated with respect to x, one obtains

$$\partial^2 V_i / \partial x^2 = -r_i (\partial i_i / \partial x) \qquad (2.6)$$

This second derivative of V_i with respect to x can be thought of as a one-dimensional Laplacian of V_i; its relation to the membrane current density is illustrated by parts C and D of fig. 2.1, and described next. (1) If the core current remains unchanged over a length increment, Δx, this means that $\partial i_i / \partial x = 0$, and also the Laplacian of V_i is zero; no current flows in or out across the membrane (along this Δx) because the core current into this core increment equals the core current out. (2) If the core current decreases over the length increment, Δx, this means that $\partial i_i / \partial x$ is negative, and the Laplacian of V_i is positive; in this case more core current flows in from the left than out to the right, implying that current must flow out across the membrane (unless this amount of current is drawn off by an electrode placed in this volume). (3) If the core current increases over the length increment, Δx, this means that $\partial i_i / \partial x$ is positive, and the Laplacian of V_i is negative; in this case more core current flows out to the right than flows in from the left, implying that current must flow in across the membrane (unless this amount of current is supplied by an electrode placed in this volume). In other words, when there is no current supplied by an intracellular electrode, continuity of current requires that the membrane current density, per unit length of cylinder (taken positive outward), be expressed

$$i_m = -\partial i_i / \partial x \qquad (2.7)$$

A.

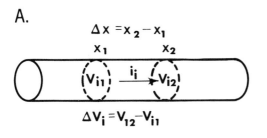

$$\Delta x = x_2 - x_1$$

$$\Delta V_i = V_{i2} - V_{i1}$$

B.

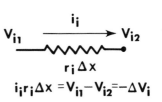

$$i_i r_i \Delta x = V_{i1} - V_{i2} = -\Delta V_i$$

C.

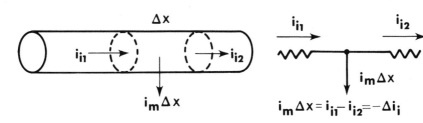

D.

$$i_m \Delta x = i_{i1} - i_{i2} = -\Delta i_i$$

E.

V_i

$i_m \Delta x$

$C_m \Delta x$

$r_m / \Delta x$

E_r

$i_m \Delta x$

V_e

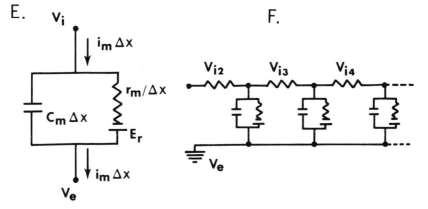

F.

V_{i2} V_{i3} V_{i4}

V_e

Figure 2.1
Diagrams related to cable equation derivation. A and B illustrate core current flow
along core resistance, with focus on the length increment, Δx, and the corresponding
increment in intracellular voltage (see eq. 2.5). C and D illustrate the relation of
membrane current density to change in core current (see eqs. 2.6–2.7). E shows
equivalent electric circuit for membrane (see eq. 2.10). F shows ladder network
providing lumped parameter approximation to a continuous cable. (From Rall 1977.)

Note that this equation can be obtained from parts C and D of fig. 2.1, by taking the limit of $\Delta i_i / \Delta x$, as Δx approaches zero. More general expressions that explicitly include current applied by intracellular and/or extracellular electrodes are given with fig. 17 of Rall (1977).

When eqs. 2.6 and 2.7 are combined, the result can be expressed

$$(1/r_i)(\partial^2 V_i / \partial x^2) = i_m \tag{2.8}$$

Up to this point, no assumptions have been made about the membrane equivalent circuit or about the extracellular voltage distribution. The derivation is made simpler by assuming extracellular isopotentiality (which is quite a good approximation in many cases). The extracellular potential, V_e, is assumed independent of x and t; we assume also that the resting membrane battery, E_r, is independent of x and t. Then, when the variable, $V = V_i - V_e - E_r$, is differentiated with respect to either x or t, the derivatives of V_e and E_r are zero, with the result that the derivatives of V and V_i are equal. Thus V_i in eq. 2.8 can be replaced by V. If we do this and also multiply both sides by r_m, we obtain

$$(r_m/r_i)(\partial^2 V / \partial x^2) = i_m r_m \tag{2.9}$$

We must now make assumptions about the membrane. A uniform passive nerve membrane cylinder has a membrane capacitance per unit length, $c_m = C_m \pi d$ (in F/cm), where C_m is the membrane capacitance per unit area, and πd is the circumference of the circular cross section of the cylinder. This membrane capacitance is electrically in parallel with a membrane conductance per unit length, $g_m = G_m \pi d$ (in S/cm), where G_m is membrane conductance per unit area; the reciprocal, $r_m = (1/g_m) = R_m / \pi d$ (in Ωcm), where R_m is membrane resistance times unit area (in Ωcm^2), is often used in spite of its peculiar dimensions. As shown in the diagram of the membrane equivalent circuit (fig. 2.1E), the membrane conductance lies in series with a battery that corresponds to the resting potential. For this simple membrane model, the membrane current density per unit length, i_m (in A/cm), can be expressed as the sum of the parallel capacitive and conductive currents, as follows:

$$i_m = c_m(\partial V / \partial t) + (V_i - V_e - E_r)/r_m \tag{2.10}$$

or

$$i_m r_m = \tau_m(\partial V / \partial t) + V \tag{2.11}$$

where we have made use of the definition of V and the constancy of V_e and E_r; also, τ_m represents the passive membrane time constant, defined as

$$\tau_m = r_m c_m = R_m C_m \tag{2.12}$$

If we equate eqs. 2.9 and 2.11, the result is the cable equation (2.1), provided that we define λ as

$$\lambda = \sqrt{r_m/r_i} = \sqrt{(R_m/R_i)(d/4)} \tag{2.13}$$

where r_m (in Ωcm) was defined above; also $r_i = R_i/(\pi d^2/4)$ (in Ω/cm), where R_i is the specific intracellular resistivity (in Ωcm) of the cytoplasm, and d is the diameter of the cylinder.

It should be noted that this expression for λ depends on assuming extracellular isopotentiality. A more general definition of λ should be used when there is one-dimensional extracellular current flow through a restricted extracellular resistance, r_e, per unit length (in Ω/cm); then the correct definition of λ is

$$\lambda = \sqrt{r_m/(r_i + r_e)} \tag{2.14}$$

This is appropriate for the thin layer of extracellular fluid that results when a non-myelinated axon is placed in oil (Hodgkin and Rushton 1946; see also eqs. 2.22–2.27 and 3.15–3.22 in Rall 1977). Similar considerations apply also to a population of simultaneously activated core conductors that are closely packed with their axes essentially parallel; then the effective value of r_e per core conductor can be significantly larger than r_i. The relative magnitudes of effective r_e and r_i are important to calculations of extracellular field potentials (see Rall and Shepherd 1968, pp. 887–888; Rall 1970, pp. 558–559; and also Klee and Rall 1977). However, when cable theory is applied to the branches of an individually activated neuron, it is advantageous (and usually justified) to set $r_e = 0$; then eq. 2.14 reduces to 2.13, as it should, because zero extracellular resistivity implies extracellular isopotentiality.

If the value of r_i changes at some value of x (because of a diameter change, or a branch point, or a cytoplasmic inhomogeneity), then r_i does not have a zero derivative with respect to x, and eq. 2.6 is incomplete; it must be replaced by

$$\partial V_i/\partial x^2 = -r_i(\partial i_i/\partial x) - i_i(\partial r_i/\partial x) \tag{2.15}$$

This would complicate the derivation above, implying that the usual cable equation is strictly valid only for uniform stretches of cable. When two adjacent stretches of cable have different properties, they should be regarded as distinct uniform cable segments, each of which satisfies its cable equation along its length. To join these cables mathematically, one must state boundary conditions that provide for continuity of current and voltage. It will be shown below that there exists a family of dendritic branching for which this difficulty disappears because such trees can be transformed to an equivalent cylinder. (It should also be noted that when the one-dimensional Laplacian is used in the analysis of extracellular field potentials, an equation similar to eq. 2.15 [with subscript i replaced by subscript e] is applicable; this means that changes in the effective value of r_e must be taken into account, or spurious sources [or sinks] may be inferred from experimental data.)

2.3 Steady-State Solutions and Properties

2.3.1 General Solution of ODE

For DC steady states obtained with steady applied current or voltage, we use mathematical solutions of the ODE given above as eq. 2.3. This ODE is homogeneous, linear, and of second order, with constant coefficients. It can have only two linearly independent solutions; its general solution is composed of two such linearly independent solutions, with two arbitrary constants. For any specific application, two boundary conditions are needed to determine the values of the arbitrary constants, and thus provide a unique solution of that particular problem.

The general solution of eq. 2.3 is well known, and can be expressed in several alternative but equivalent forms, as follows:

$$V(X) = A_1 e^X + A_2 e^{-X} \tag{2.16}$$

$$V(X) = B_1 \cosh(X) + B_2 \sinh(X) \tag{2.17}$$

$$V(X) = C_1 \cosh(L - X) + C_2 \sinh(L - X) \tag{2.18}$$

where the hyperbolic functions are very useful for certain boundary conditions; also, L is a constant used to express the electrotonic length, $L = \ell/\lambda$, where ℓ is the actual length of a cable. Like the trigonometric cosine, the hyperbolic cosine is an even function that has zero slope and unit magnitude at the origin; it is defined $\cosh(X) = (e^X + e^{-X})/2$. Like the trigonometric sine, the hyperbolic sine is an odd function that has unit slope and zero magnitude at the origin; it is defined $\sinh(X) = (e^X - e^{-X})/2$. The derivative of $\cosh(X)$ with respect to X is $\sinh(X)$, and the derivative of $\sinh(X)$ with respect to X is $\cosh(X)$. The hyperbolic sine, cosine, and tangent are available in standard mathematical tables, in standard computer libraries, and in some inexpensive hand-held calculators. Readers may find it a useful exercise to verify that eqs. 2.16–2.18 are indeed solutions of eq. 2.3; some may also wish to verify the following relations between the different pairs of arbitrary constants:

$$2A_1 = B_1 + B_2 = (C_1 - C_2)e^{-L}$$

$$2A_2 = B_1 - B_2 = (C_1 + C_2)e^{+L}$$

2.3.2 Steady-State Solutions for Different Boundary Conditions

A cable of semi-infinite length extends from $X = 0$ to $X = +\infty$ (this is distinguished from a fully or doubly infinite length that extends also to $-\infty$). Suppose a voltage clamp maintains $V = V_0$ at $X = 0$; that constitutes one boundary condition. Also, suppose this is a uniform cable that may have recording electrodes but has no current or voltage applied anywhere between $X = 0$ and $X = +\infty$; then our second boundary condition can be simply that V remains bounded as X approaches ∞; this implies that $A_1 = 0$ in eq. 2.16. Then the first boundary condition implies that $A_2 = V_0$, and the unique solution of this problem can be expressed simply as

$$V(X) = V_0 e^{-X} = V_0 e^{-x/\lambda} \tag{2.19}$$

This mathematical result expresses the fact that for a semi-infinite length of uniform cable, the steady-state value of V (departure from resting value) decrements exponentially with distance along the cable (see curve E in fig. 2.2). For this semi-infinite case, the length constant, λ, represents the distance over which the voltage decrements to $1/e$ (i.e., $V(x + \lambda)/V(x) = V(X + 1)/V(X) = 1/e$, or about 0.368), and this holds true anywhere along the cable. Given a number of data points, one would plot $\log_e(V/V_0)$ versus x, to fit a straight line whose slope should be $-\lambda$ with respect to x. Although we never actually have a semi-infinite length of axon, it may be noted that when a termination is more than four times λ distant from a point of observation, there is negligible difference from the semi-infinite case.

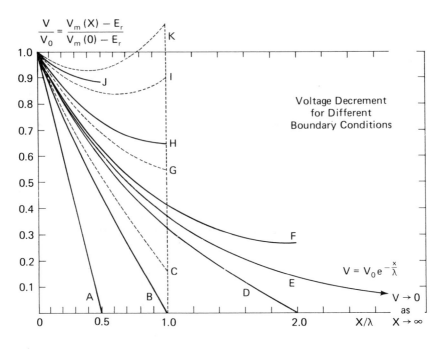

Figure 2.2
Examples of how steady voltage decrement with distance depends on the distal
boundary condition. The applied voltage at $X = 0$ is normalized to 1.0 for all curves.
Curve E shows an exponential decrement (eq. 2.19) for a semi-infinite length. Curves
A, B, and D show steeper decrement (eq. 2.21) obtained when the most distal membrane is clamped to the resting potential, implying that $V = 0$ at $X = L$ for three
different L values, 0.5, 1.0, and 2.0, respectively. Curves F, H, and J show less decrement (eq. 2.20) obtained for a sealed-end boundary condition, $dV/dX = 0$ at $X = L$,
for the same three L values. Curves C and G both correspond to a leaky boundary
condition at $X = 1$; see eq. 2.25 and associated text. Curves I and K both have
a voltage-clamped boundary condition at $X = 1$; see eq. 2.22 and associated text.
(From Rall 1981.)

For finite lengths of cable, we must specify both the length and the terminal boundary condition. The zero slope boundary condition, $dV/dx = 0$ at $x = \ell$, or $dV/dX = 0$ at $X = L$, has been called a sealed end, because the zero slope means zero core current (see eq. 2.5) at the end $(X = L)$, as should be expected when the membrane tube is closed (sealed) with membrane (Rall 1959); engineers call this an open-circuit boundary condition (sometimes also called killed end boundary condition). This boundary condition favors the use of eq. 2.18 because the zero slope at $X = L$ implies that $C_2 = 0$. Then the other boundary condition, usually $V = V_0$ at $X = 0$, implies that $C_1 = V_0/\cosh(L)$, and the unique solution to this problem can be expressed

$$V(X) = \frac{V_0 \cosh(L - X)}{\cosh(L)}, \text{ for } dV/dX = 0 \text{ at } X = L \qquad (2.20)$$

In fig. 2.2, curves F, H, and J illustrate this solution for three different values of L, 2.0, 1.0, and 0.5, respectively; note that the sealed end causes all three of these curves to remain above reference curve E. Intuitively, one can view the sealed end as a dam against onward current flow; then one can predict that as an action potential approaches a sealed end, the membrane current density becomes increased, the spike height increases, and the propagation velocity increases with approach to the terminal (see Goldstein and Rall 1974). It is noted that the approach of an action potential to a sealed end is the same as its approach to a collision with an equal and oppositely propagating action potential; the point of collision satisfies the zero slope condition, $dV/dx = 0$.

On the other hand, curves A, B, and D in fig. 2.2 correspond to a different terminal boundary condition, namely a voltage clamp, $V = 0$ at $X = L$. This boundary condition implies that $C_1 = 0$ in eq. 2.18; if the other boundary condition is $V = V_0$ at $X = 0$, the unique solution is

$$V(X) = \frac{V_0 \sinh(L - X)}{\sinh(L)}, \text{ for clamped } V = 0 \text{ at } X = L \qquad (2.21)$$

which does satisfy the ODE with $V = V_0$ at $X = 0$, and $V = 0$ at $X = L$. Engineers tend to regard $V = 0$ as a short-circuit boundary condition, but here we must make a careful distinction, because we have defined $V = V_i - V_e - E_r$. Thus, $V = 0$ implies that $V_i - V_e = E_r$, meaning that the membrane potential difference, $V_i - V_e$, is clamped to its resting value, E_r. In contrast, an actual short circuit of the membrane (i.e., $V_i = V_e$) must imply $V = -E_r$. For example, if the resting membrane potential difference is -70 mV (interior minus exterior), then a short circuit of the membrane would make $V = +70$ mV.

If the voltage clamp at $X = L$ is set to some other voltage, V_L at $X = L$, we must add to eq. 2.21 a solution that is zero at $X = 0$ and equals V_L at $X = L$; this can be achieved by setting $B_1 = 0$ in eq. 2.17 and setting $B_2 = V_L/\sinh(L)$. By combining this solution with eq. 2.21, we obtain

$$V(X) = \frac{V_0 \sinh(L - X) + V_L \sinh(X)}{\sinh(L)} \tag{2.22}$$

which is the unique solution for the pair of voltage-clamped boundary conditions, $V = V_0$ at $X = 0$, and $V = V_L$ at $X = L$. This solution is illustrated by curves I and K in fig. 2.2, for $L = 1$, with $V_L = 0.9V_0$ for curve I, and $V_L = 1.1V_0$ for curve K; both of these curves exhibit a slope that changes sign because both values of V_L were set above curve H, which has zero slope at $X = L$.

Curves C and G of fig. 2.2 differ from the others; they correspond to a leaky boundary condition at $X = L$. The leakage current is assumed proportional to the value of V at $X = L$, and is expressed as VG_L at $X = L$, where G_L represents the leak conductance at $X = L$. This leak conductance can be larger or smaller than the reference conductance, G_∞, which corresponds to semi-infinite extension of the same cable (curve E). In fig. 2.2, curve C corresponds to $G_L/G_\infty = 4$, while curve G corresponds to $G_L/G_\infty = 1/4$. The solution satisfying such boundary conditions can be expressed

$$V(X)/V_L = \cosh(L - X) + (G_L/G_\infty)\sinh(L - X) \tag{2.23}$$

from which it follows that

$$V_0/V_L = \cosh(L) + (G_L/G_\infty)\sinh(L) \tag{2.24}$$

and that

$$V(X)/V_0 = \frac{\cosh(L - X) + (G_L/G_\infty)\sinh(L - X)}{\cosh(L) + (G_L/G_\infty)\sinh(L)} \tag{2.25}$$

This type of solution has been very useful in the cable analysis of dendritic trees (see below, and also chapter 3).

2.3.3   Input Conductance and Input Resistance

From Ohm's law, the input resistance, R_{in}, at any point of the cable is equal to the ratio of the steady voltage (at that point) to the steady current supplied by the electrode; the input conductance, G_{in}, is the reciprocal of the input resistance. At the origin of a semi-infinite cable the input current can flow in only one direction (to the right is the usual convention); the ratio of this steady current to the steady voltage at the origin is known as G_∞, the reference input conductance for a uniform semi-infinite cable. In the case of a doubly infinite cable (extending to $+\infty$ and to $-\infty$), an equal amount of input current flows in both directions away from an input electrode; thus, for any given steady input voltage, the input current must be twice that for the semi-infinite case, and the input conductance must be twice G_∞. For nonsymmetric cases, where unequal currents flow to left and right, see Rall (1977, pp. 72–74).

When current flows only to the right at $X = 0$, the input current must equal the core current that flows to the right at $X = 0$; this can be expressed

$$I_0 = (1/r_i)(-dV/dx)|_{x=0} = G_\infty(-dV/dX)|_{X=0} \tag{2.26}$$

where the first expression follows from eq. 2.5, while the expression at right is a very useful alternative that is based on the result that follows next. For the semi-infinite case, we refer to eq. 2.19, differentiate with respect to x (or to X, for the last expression), substitute in eq. 2.26, and obtain

$$I_0 = (1/\lambda r_i)V_0 = G_\infty V_0 \tag{2.27}$$

which holds only for the semi-infinite case, while eq. 2.26 holds for other cases like those illustrated in fig. 2.2. Equation 2.27 provides an implicit definition of G_∞; explicit definitions of both R_∞ and G_∞ (for semi-infinite length) can be expressed in several equivalent ways, as follows:

$$R_\infty = V_0/I_0 = \lambda r_i = (r_m r_i)^{1/2} = r_m/\lambda \tag{2.28}$$

$$= (2/\pi)(R_m R_i)^{1/2}(d)^{-3/2} = R_m/(\pi \lambda d) \tag{2.29}$$

and

$$G_\infty = I_0/V_0 = (\lambda r_i)^{-1} = (g_m/r_i)^{1/2} = \lambda g_m \tag{2.30}$$

$$= (\pi/2)(G_m/R_i)^{1/2}(d)^{3/2} = G_m \pi \lambda d \tag{2.31}$$

Useful physical intuition (going back at least to Rushton in the 1930s) may be found in the fact that R_∞ is equal to a λ length of core resistance; also, G_∞ is equal to the parallel membrane conductance for an area of membrane equal to a λ length of the cylinder. However, this should be tempered by the knowledge that the steady-state core current is not constant along this λ length of core; also the membrane current density is not uniform along this λ length of membrane cylinder.

By inspection of the initial slopes of the curves in fig. 2.2, we know which cases have input conductances that are larger or smaller than the reference value provided by G_∞. All of the curves above curve E have initial slopes that are less steep than for the reference case; looking at eqs. 2.26 and 2.27, it follows that their input current values are less than $G_\infty V_0$, and that the input conductance values for these cases are less than G_∞. For example, curves F, H, and J all correspond to sealed ends, for which it is easy to understand that the input conductance must be less than for the reference case. Similarly, all of the curves beneath curve E in fig. 2.2 must correspond to cases with input conductance values greater than G_∞.

For the sealed end boundary condition at $X = L$, we refer to eqs. 2.20 and 2.26 and find that $I_0 = G_\infty V_0 \tanh(L)$. From this it follows that the boundary condition at $X = 0$ can be specified either as the applied current or as the applied voltage, because, in the steady state, each implies the other; this also implies the following expressions for input conductance and resistance at $X = 0$:

$$G_{in} = G_\infty \tanh(L), \text{ for a sealed end at } X = L \qquad (2.32)$$

and

$$R_{in} = R_\infty \coth(L), \text{ for a sealed end at } X = L \qquad (2.33)$$

When we present input conductance expressions for several different cases, we are confronted with the problem of how to distinguish between them; one can use identifying subscripts (e.g., in Rall 1977), or one can use explicit qualifying words, as done here.

In contrast, for a voltage clamp to resting potential ($V = 0$ at $X = L$), we refer to eqs. 2.21 and 2.26 and get $I_0 = G_\infty V_0 \coth(L)$; this implies

$$G_{in} = G_\infty \coth(L), \text{ for clamped } V = 0 \text{ at } X = L \qquad (2.34)$$

and

$$R_{in} = R_\infty \tanh(L), \text{ for clamped } V = 0 \text{ at } X = L \qquad (2.35)$$

For more general voltage clamping, at $X = L$, we refer to eqs. 2.22 and 2.26 to get

$$G_{in}/G_\infty = \coth(L) - \frac{V_L}{V_0 \sinh(L)} \qquad (2.36)$$

for clamped $V = V_L$ at $X = L$, which is relevant to curves I and K of fig. 2.2.

For the leaky boundary condition at $X = L$, we refer to eqs. 2.25 and 2.26 to get

$$G_{in}/G_\infty = \frac{\tanh(L) + G_L/G_\infty}{1 + (G_L/G_\infty)\tanh(L)} \qquad (2.37)$$

for leak current, $G_L V_L$ at $X = L$ and the expression for R_{in}/R_∞ is the inverse of this. It may be noted that one limiting case $(G_L = 0)$ makes eq. 2.37 become equivalent to eq. 2.32, as it should because $G_L = 0$ is like a sealed end; also, the other extreme $(G_L = \infty)$ makes eq. 2.37 become equivalent to eq. 2.34, as it should because $G_L = \infty$ would clamp $V = 0$ at $X = L$. A third special case $(G_L = G_\infty)$ makes G_{in}/G_∞ equal unity; this means that any uniform membrane cylinder of finite length will have the same input conductance as for a semi-infinite length, if it is terminated with a leak conductance equal to G_∞.

Also, eq. 2.37 can apply to the origin $(X = 0)$ of the trunk cylinder of a dendritic tree, provided that G_L corresponds to the sum of the input conductances of the branches that arise from this trunk at $X = L$. Note that here (in eqs. 2.23–2.25 and 2.37, and also in fig. 2.3A, but not in fig. 2.3B, below) we use L to represent the ℓ/λ value of only this trunk; such use should be distinguished from the more frequent use of L to represent the electrotonic length of a dendritic tree. Below we use L_D for dendritic trees that are reducible to an equivalent cylinder, and L_N for some dendritic neurons.

2.4   Dendritic Trees

2.4.1   Steady-State Input Conductance for Dendritic Tree with Arbitrary Branching

A dendritic tree can be idealized by treating all branches as cylinders with uniform membrane properties; these cylinders can have different lengths and diameters and different uniform membrane properties. Extracellular isopotentiality is also assumed. Then the ODE of eq. 2.3

A

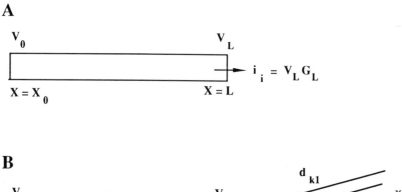

B

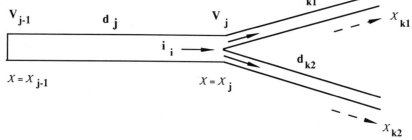

Figure 2.3
Diagrams showing subscript notation used for single cylinder (A) and for branching
(B). Upper diagram (A) shows the notation used in eqs. 2.20–2.25 and 2.32–2.37.
Lower diagram (B) shows the different notation used for a parent cylinder with two
daughter branches used in eqs. 2.38–2.45. (Modified from Rall 1977.)

holds for each of these cylinders; however, the value of λ and of G_∞ can be different in each cylinder. If R_m and R_i are the same for all cylinders, then λ is proportional to $d^{1/2}$, and G_∞ is proportional to $d^{3/2}$. (More generally, the value of R_m might change with diameter or branch order; if this is specified it can be taken into account.) To obtain the mathematical solution for the tree, the two arbitrary constants in the general solution for each branch must be determined from the boundary conditions; these include continuity of V and of core current at every branch point, plus a specification of the boundary condition at the distal end of every terminal branch, plus a specification of the applied voltage or applied current at the electrode location. There are two different procedures for satisfying all of these boundary conditions: one is an iterative method (Rall 1959) that begins with the terminal branches and works back to the electrode location, which is often set at $X = 0$ of the tree trunk; the other method involves solving simultaneously for the $2N$ arbitrary constants in the N general solutions (eqs. 2.16–2.18) for N branches of the dendritic tree. The first method will be sketched here; the second method is a special case of a more general procedure described and used by Holmes (1986).

There are various systems one can use to label every branch of a tree; one useful numerical system is described in chapter 3. Here it is convenient to begin with a parent branch identified by index j; it extends from x_{j-1} to x_j and has a diameter d_j (see fig. 2.3B). Two daughter branches arise at x_j. One daughter is identified by index $k1$; it extends from x_j to x_{k1} and has a diameter d_{k1}. The other daughter is identified by index $k2$; it extends from x_j to x_{k2} and has a diameter d_{k2}. Corresponding to each diameter, there is a value of λ defined by eq. 2.13 and a value of G_∞ defined by eqs. 2.30 and 2.31. It has been usual to assume that the resistivities, R_i and R_m, are the same everywhere, but their values could be different and would then need to be specified for each branch. For the first daughter branch ($k1$), the value of its input conductance (at $x = x_j$) can be expressed (based on eq. 2.37) as

$$G_{in_{jk1}} = G_{\infty k1} \frac{\tanh(L_{k1}) + B_{k1}}{1 + B_{k1}\tanh(L_{k1})} \tag{2.38}$$

where

$$L_{k1} = (x_{k1} - x_j)/\lambda_{k1} \quad \text{and} \quad B_{k1} = G_{out_{k1}}/G_{\infty k1} \tag{2.39}$$

Similarly, for the other daughter branch, we have

$$G_{in_{jk2}} = G_{\infty k2} \frac{\tanh(L_{k2}) + B_{k2}}{1 + B_{k2}\tanh(L_{k2})} \tag{2.40}$$

where L_{k2} and B_{k2} are defined in a corresponding manner. Now, continuity at the branch point is accomplished by setting the leakage (*out*) conductance of the parent branch G_{out_j} (at x_j) equal to the sum of the input conductances (eqs. 2.38 and 2.40) of the two daughter branches. If this sum is divided by the reference G_∞ value of the parent branch, we get

$$B_j = \frac{G_{out_j}}{G_{\infty j}} = \left(\frac{G_{\infty k1}}{G_{\infty j}}\right) \frac{\tanh(L_{k1}) + B_{k1}}{1 + B_{k1}\tanh(L_{k1})}$$

$$+ \left(\frac{G_{\infty k2}}{G_{\infty j}}\right) \frac{\tanh(L_{k2}) + B_{k2}}{1 + B_{k2}\tanh(L_{k2})} \tag{2.41}$$

which can then be used to get the input conductance of the parent branch, at $x = x_{j-1}$; this can now be expressed as

$$G_{in_{j-1}} = G_{\infty j} \frac{\tanh(L_j) + B_j}{1 + B_j\tanh(L_j)} \tag{2.42}$$

in analogy with eqs. 2.38–2.40. Thus, we have shown how the (distally directed) input conductance of an arbitrarily chosen branch (index j) can be expressed in terms of lengths, diameters, and resistivities of this branch and its two daughter branches, together with the distal boundary conditions (encapsulated in B_{k1} and B_{k2}) of the two daughter branches.

If the daughter branches are terminal branches with sealed ends, the values of B_{k1} and B_{k2} are set equal to zero; however, if these daughter branches end in branch points from which higher-order branches arise, then B_{k1} and B_{k2} are calculated from these higher-order branches by means of equations analogous to eq. 2.41 above. If the parent branch is in fact the trunk of the dendritic tree, then eq. 2.42 defines the input conductance of that tree; otherwise, one must consider it together with its sibling branch to calculate their combined effect on their parent branch (index $j-2$), and work back through lower branch orders until one has the input conductance at the origin of the trunk of this tree. In effect, we have here explained the iterative method of calculating the input conductance of a dendritic tree composed of cylindrical branches with uniform cable properties (Rall 1959); an equivalent description is provided very explicitly in chapter 3, following eq. 3.14. Note that a similar iterative method can be used to calculate the input conductance at any other point in the tree.

When the values of R_m and R_i are the same for all branches, the ratio of $G_{\infty k1}$ to $G_{\infty j}$ (in eq. 2.41) can be replaced by the 3/2 power of the diameter ratio, d_{k1}/d_j, and similarly for the ratio of $G_{\infty k2}$ to $G_{\infty j}$; however, in the general case, where R_m may be different for different branches, it is important to use eq. 2.41 as written.

2.4.2 Family of Trees Related to an Equivalent Cylinder

Many useful insights have resulted from the fact that an extensively branched dendritic tree can be represented as an equivalent cylinder, if several conditions are satisfied. The branching need not be symmetric, and it is not necessary that all subdivisions of the tree contain the same number of orders of branching. The necessary conditions are (1) the values of R_m and R_i are the same in all branches; (2) all terminal branches end with the same distal boundary condition (usually taken to be the sealed end condition); (3) all terminal branches end at the same electrotonic distance, L, from the trunk origin (i.e., L equals the sum of x/λ values along the path from $x = 0$ to the distal end of every terminal branch; this L is the electrotonic length of the tree and of the equivalent cylinder); 4) at every branch point, the diameters of the two daughter branches need not be equal but they must satisfy the constraint that the sum of their 3/2 power values must equal the 3/2 power of the parent branch diameter, which can be expressed as

$$(d_j)^{3/2} = (d_{k1})^{3/2} + (d_{k2})^{3/2} \tag{2.43}$$

where the subscripts match those used above in fig. 2.3B. These conditions are sufficient if we are concerned only with the disturbances initiated at $x = 0$ or anywhere in the trunk, because then the spread of current and voltage out into the branches will yield the same voltage time course at all branch locations corresponding to the same electrotonic distance from $x = 0$. However, if inputs are delivered to dendritic branch locations, then we have one more condition; (5) proportional inputs would have to be delivered to all corresponding locations such that an equal input voltage time course would be generated at all electrotonically equivalent dendritic locations. Then the voltage time course in the dendritic tree can be mapped onto an equivalent cylinder by means of the electrotonic distance, X, measured from $X = 0$. A method of solution, using the superposition approach, has been devised for the case of input to a single branch of a tree that is otherwise equivalent to a cylinder; the steady-state superposition is described and discussed in Rall and Rinzel (1973), while transient superposition is described and discussed in Rinzel and Rall (1974).

It should be obvious that natural dendritic trees are unlikely to satisfy all of these constraints. Also, it may be noted that these constraints on dendritic branching were not presented as a law of nature; they were used to define a mathematical idealization that provides a valuable reference case. In fact, it has been found that some natural dendritic trees do approximately satisfy the 3/2 power law constraint at individual branch points; for motoneurons of cat spinal cord, the major discrepancy is found to result from the fact that many high-order branches are missing because their potential parent branches terminate at electrotonic distances (from the soma) that are significantly less than for terminal branches of higher order; consequently, the sum of $d^{3/2}$ for successively higher-order branches is found to decrease very significantly. Such dendritic trees are not equivalent to a cylinder; they more nearly approximate a tapered core conductor or several cylinders of different length, placed electrically in parallel with a common soma. However, other neuron types have been reported to exhibit much less of this problem, with the result that they sustain a fairly constant sum of $d^{3/2}$ out to terminations at almost equal electrotonic distance from the soma (Bloomfield et al. 1987; also some cells in hippocampus).

It may be noted that a different theoretical approach to dendritic trees that are equivalent to a cylinder was provided by deriving the PDE for a hypothetical system with continuous taper and branching; by generalizing the concept of electrotonic distance, this approach provided the basis for a transformation of the PDE to a form that becomes equivalent to that for a cylinder, when the taper parameter is set to zero (see Rall 1962a; or Jack et al. 1975). Here, however, we merely demonstrate the effect that constraints 1–4 have on eqs. 2.38–2.42. Suppose that branches $k1$ and $k2$ are terminal branches; then constraints 2 and 3 imply that $B_{k1} = B_{k2} = B_k$ and that $L_{k1} = L_{k2} = L_k$, with the consequence that the two quotient expressions in eq. 2.41 become the same. However, the branch diameters (and the coefficients they imply in eq. 2.41) can be different and must be considered next. Because R_m and R_i are assumed everywhere the same (constraint 1), the several G_∞ values are proportional to the 3/2 power of the several branch diameters; this means that eq. 2.41 can now be expressed

$$B_j = \left(\frac{(d_{k1})^{3/2} + (d_{k2})^{3/2}}{(d_j)^{3/2}} \right) \frac{\tanh(L_k) + B_k}{1 + B_k \tanh(L_k)} \tag{2.44}$$

where the quantity inside the large parentheses becomes reduced to unity when we impose the constraint on branch diameters (eq. 2.43). Then, B_j is exactly equal to what it would be if the parent cylinder (index j), which originally extended from $x = x_{j-1}$ to $x = x_j$ with diameter d_j, were extended (with unchanged diameter) by an electrotonic distance, $L_k = (x_k - x_j)/\lambda_k$, and terminated with a boundary condition corresponding to B_k. For the case of a sealed end boundary condition, we have $B_k = 0$, and then eq. 2.44 becomes simplified to $B_j = \tanh(L_k)$; for this case, eq. 2.42 can be expressed

$$\frac{G_{in_{j-1}}}{G_{\infty_j}} = \frac{\tanh(L_k) + \tanh(L_j)}{1 + \tanh(L_k) \tanh(L_j)} = \tanh(L_j + L_k) \tag{2.45}$$

where the expression at far right follows from a standard identity (included in standard books of mathematical tables). This input conductance ratio is thus the same as that for an equivalent cylinder of electrotonic length, $L_j + L_k$, with its distal end sealed. While this demonstration has been explicit for the input conductance, it carries over to the steady-state solution of eq. 2.25; the same constraints hold also for the PDE and its transient solutions.

2.4.3   Dendritic Surface Area and Input Conductance of Tree

A particularly useful property of dendritic trees that satisfies the constraints for equivalence to a cylinder is that they have the same membrane surface area as that of an unbranched cylinder that has the same diameter as the trunk of the tree and the same electrotonic length, L_D, as the whole dendritic tree (note that $L_D = L_j + L_k$ in the simple example above). This result for membrane area was deduced as a part of the general treatment of the PDE presented in Rall (1962a,b); here, however, we show it for the example above. The surface area of the parent (trunk) branch equals $\pi d_j \ell_j$, where $\ell_j = x_j - x_{j-1}$. The surface areas of the two daughter branches are $\pi d_{k1} \ell_{k1}$ and $\pi d_{k2} \ell_{k2}$, respectively. The diameters and lengths of these daughter branches are usually different, but we do know that these two daughters have the same electrotonic length, $L_k = \ell_{k1}/\lambda_{k1} = \ell_{k2}/\lambda_{k2}$; we also know that $\ell_k = \lambda_j L_k$ represents the length that must be added to the parent trunk to get the equivalent cylinder for the tree (note that this physical length is larger than that of either daughter branch for the usual case where both daughter branches have smaller diameters and λ-values than the trunk). Now, what we need to show is that the surface area, $\pi d_j \ell_k$, added to the trunk is exactly equal to the sum of the areas of the two daughter branches. We note that each λ is proportional to $d^{1/2}$ (because the underlying resistivities are held constant), and that the three ℓ values (for subscripts k, $k1$, and $k2$) are proportional to their corresponding λ values (because the value of L_k is the same for all three cases). Consequently, for each subscript, the value of surface area ($\pi d\ell$) must be proportional to $d^{3/2}$. It follows that the surface areas match when

$$(d_j)^{3/2} = (d_{k1})^{3/2} + (d_{k2})^{3/2}$$

which is exactly the constraint (eq. 2.43) for equivalence to a cylinder. In other words, this constraint ensures that the dendritic surface area remains the same for few or many orders of branching, when constraints 1 and 3 are also satisfied.

Now we can appreciate the usefulness of a relation between the input conductance, G_D, of a dendritic tree, its membrane surface area, A_D, and its electrotonic length, L_D. That relation can be expressed

$$G_D = G_m A_D \frac{\tanh(L_D)}{l_D} \qquad (2.46)$$

which holds exactly for all dendritic trees that satisfy the equivalent cylinder constraints with a sealed end at $X = L_D$ of all terminal branches. This expression follows from eq. 2.32, together with the second version of eq. 2.31, and the fact that $A_D = \pi \ell d = \pi L_D \lambda d$. When we know the value of G_m (either in a simulation or in a favorable experimental situation) eq. 2.46 provides a valuable relation between dendritic surface area and dendritic input conductance. In experimental situations, however, one must beware of complications that may result from soma shunting caused by microelectrode penetration of the membrane; this is considered explicitly below in eq. 2.49.

For very small values of L_D, $\tanh(L_D) = L_D$, making $G_D = G_m A_D$; the physical meaning is that because there is negligible voltage decrement in a very short dendritic tree, the dendritic membrane is essentially isopotential, and this explains why the input conductance is simply the product of the surface area and the membrane conductance per unit area. On the other hand, for very large values of L_D, $\tanh(L_D) = 1$; then (because $A_D/L_D = \pi \lambda d$) this makes $G_D = G_m \pi \lambda d = G_\infty$, as it should because the voltage decrement with distance is essentially the same for very large lengths (greater than four times λ) as for semi-infinite length. For L_D values of 0.5, 1.0, and 1.5, the ratio of $\tanh(L_D)$ to L_D has the values 0.924, 0.762, and 0.603, respectively. These values are less than 1.0 by amounts that are related to the nonisopotentiality of the dendritic membrane potential during a steady-state input conductance measurement.

Although eq. 2.46 is strictly valid only for dendritic trees that are equivalent to a cylinder, the physically intuitive understanding provided in the preceding paragraph suggests that a similar result must hold also for dendritic trees that depart from equivalent-cylinder constraints. It should be possible to explore this for different types of departure from the idealized reference case, and to provide guidelines for approximate results for these different types. Only preliminary work has been done on this so far; for some cases (such as taper, or terminal branches at different electrotonic distances from the trunk) it may prove fruitful to use an effective value, L_{efD}, defined as the inverse hyperbolic tangent of the ratio G_D/G_∞, which can be computed by the iterative method described above. Another way this more general approach can be expressed is as follows:

$$G_D = G_{md} A_D F_{dga} \qquad (2.47)$$

where G_{md} represents dendritic membrane conductivity per unit area, and F_{dga} represents a factor, to be determined for each branching type; of course eq. 2.46 shows that we have an exact expression for F_{dga} in the idealized reference case of trees equivalent to a cylinder.

2.5   Input Conductance of a Neuron

Now we consider a whole neuron composed of several dendritic trees attached to a common soma. When our focus is on the passive membrane properties of the soma and dendrites, we often omit an explicit axon. Some neuron types (such as granule cells of olfactory bulb and amacrine cells of retina) do not have axons; other neuron types (such as motoneurons and pyramidal cells) have axons whose dimensions and passive membrane properties make a relatively very small contribution to the input conductance of the whole neuron. However, under conditions where the nonlinear properties of axonal membrane become important (i.e., for an axon of large diameter), explicit addition of the axon to the model must be evaluated, according to the questions being asked.

Because the input conductances of the several dendritic trees are electrically in parallel with the soma membrane, the input conductance, G_N, of the whole neuron can be expressed

$$G_N = G_S + \sum_{j=1}^{n} G_{Dj} = (\rho + 1)G_S \qquad (2.48)$$

where G_S represents the soma input conductance, and the summation is for the input conductances of n dendritic trees; also, the expression at far right makes use of the parameter ρ that was used (Rall 1959) to represent the dendritic-to-soma conductance ratio, $\sum G_D/G_S$.

The soma input conductance, G_S, must now be made more explicit.

$$G_S = G_{shunt} + G_{ms}A_S = \beta G_{md}A_S \qquad (2.49)$$

Here the shunt conductance caused by microelectrode penetration is included because it can be very large; also, A_S represents the soma surface area, and G_{ms} represents the soma membrane conductance per unit area (excluding the shunt conductance); this could be different from G_{md}, the dendritic membrane conductance per unit area (here assumed constant for all of the dendrites). The expression at far right constitutes a definition of β; this parameter can be thought of as the soma shunting factor, or as the ratio of G_{md} to an apparent G_{ms} (implied by the shunt together with the actual G_{ms}). Note that the value of β could be as large as 1,000 when the shunt conductance is very large; on the other hand, $\beta = 1$ when $G_{ms} = G_{md}$ and the shunt conductance is zero.

It is important to understand that as the value of the soma shunt is increased, both the value of G_S and the value of the parameter $\beta = G_S/G_{md}A_S$ are increased; however, the value of the parameter $\rho = \sum G_D/G_S$ is decreased. It is significant that the product, $\rho\beta$, remains constant; this is because the value of G_S cancels, leaving

$$\rho\beta = \frac{\sum G_D}{G_{md}A_S} = \frac{\sum A_D F_{dga}}{A_S} \qquad (2.50)$$

where the subscript, j, identifying different dendritic trees, has been suppressed only for the sake of less cumbersome expressions, and the expression at far right (making use of eq. 2.47) shows that the value of $\rho\beta$ is determined by membrane surface areas, together with the factor F_{dga}, whose value often lies between 0.75 and 0.9, depending upon the degree of nonisopotentiality of steady-state dendritic membrane potential; if all of the dendritic trees were to have the same effective electrotonic length, the value of F_{dga} would be the same for all of them and this factor could be placed in front of the summation.

Using the results and notations above, we now can provide two useful alternative expressions for the ratio of whole neuron input conductance to dendritic membrane conductivity:

$$G_N/G_{md} = A_S(\beta + \rho\beta) = \beta A_S + \sum_{j=1}^{n} A_{D_j} F_{dga_j} \qquad (2.51)$$

These expressions are important when one wishes to estimate the value of G_{md} from experimental measurements of G_N and the histological surface areas. Clearly, it is important to find good ways of estimating the value of the soma shunting factor, β, and also the values of the factor F_{dga}, for dendritic trees of different types; see comments made with eqs. 2.46 and 2.47.

2.6 Transient Solutions and Properties

2.6.1 Two Classes of Solutions

The PDE (eq. 2.2) has many solutions; the problem is to construct a solution that satisfies not only the PDE but also the boundary conditions and an initial condition. It is helpful to know that there are two rather different basic solutions from which the more complicated solutions are constructed.

One class of solutions comes from the classical method known as the separation of variables. The solution $V(X, T)$ is assumed to be the product of two functions, one of which is a function of X but not of T, while the other is a function of T but not of X. Using this method, one finds a solution that can be expressed

$$V(X,T) = (A\sin(\alpha X) + B\cos(\alpha X))\, e^{-(1+\alpha^2)T} \qquad (2.52)$$

where A and B are arbitrary constants, and α^2 is known as the separation constant. It is easy to verify, by partial differentiation, that this function satisfies the dimensionless cable equation (eq. 2.2). For a cable of finite length with simple boundary conditions, the values of A or B and α, can be determined from the boundary conditions; typically α is found to be restricted to a particular set of values known as eigenvalues, or roots of the characteristic equation (an equation obtained by applying the boundary conditions to the PDE). An example of such a solution is provided below as eq. 2.54.

A different class of solutions can be constructed from what is sometimes called the fundamental solution, or the Green's function, or the instantaneous point source solution, or the response function. This solution can be expressed

$$V(X,T) = C_o(\pi T)^{-1/2} e^{-(T+X^2/4T)} \qquad (2.53)$$

where X can extend from $-\infty$ to $+\infty$; the singularity (instantaneous point charge) is located at $X = 0$ when $T = 0$. If the amount of this charge is Q_o coulombs, then for a semi-infinite length (extending from $X = 0$ to $X = +\infty$), the value of C_o is $Q_o/(\lambda c_m)$ where λc_m represents the membrane capacitance of a λ length of cylinder (in farads), implying that C_o has the dimension of volts. This value for C_o can be confirmed by integrating the charge per unit length, $c_m V(X,T)$, from $X = 0$ to $X = \infty$, and showing that the total charge on the membrane is Q_o when $T = 0$. For the doubly infinite case, the charge spreads in both directions, and the value of C_o is half the above. Although this solution is most natural for infinite lengths, the method of images can be used to construct solutions for finite length (e.g., Jack et al. 1975, pp. 67–71). Also, it is useful to realize that even for finite lengths, eq. 2.53 provides a good approximation for very small values of X and T (i.e., for early times before the spread of charge can be influenced by a distant boundary condition).

2.6.2   Voltage Decay Transient for Cylinder of Finite Length with Sealed Ends

For a finite length, with simple boundary conditions, Fourier first showed how to construct a solution that satisfies an arbitrary initial condition. Several examples of such solutions were presented and discussed for application to experimental neurophysiology by Rall (1969a); a more general separation of variables (for three-dimensional space and time) was also presented and discussed (Rall 1969b).

For a uniform cylinder of finite length, with two sealed-end boundary conditions ($\partial V/\partial X = 0$, at $X = 0$ and at $X = L$), one finds that coefficient A must be set to zero in eq. 2.52, and that the constant α can have infinitely many values, $\alpha_n = n\pi/L$, where n can be zero or any positive integer. Thus we can express a family of solutions in the form of a summation of infinitely many terms:

$$V(X,T) = \sum_{n=0}^{\infty} B_n \cos(n\pi X/L)e^{-[1+(n\pi/L)^2]T} \qquad (2.54)$$

where the coefficients, B_n, are known as Fourier coefficients, which depend on the initial condition, $V(X,0)$, as follows:

$$B_o = (1/L) \int_0^L V(X,0)\, dX \qquad (2.55)$$

and, for positive integer values of n,

$$B_n = (2/L) \int_0^L V(X,0) \cos(n\pi X/L) \, dX \qquad (2.56)$$

A useful alternative expression of this result is the following:

$$V(X,T) = C_o e^{-t/\tau_o} + C_1 e^{-t/\tau_1} + C_2 e^{-t/\tau_2} + \cdots \qquad (2.57)$$

where $C_o = B_o$ and τ_o equals the passive membrane time constant, $\tau_m = r_m c_m$ (because the membrane was assumed uniform and without a short circuit). Also

$$C_n = B_n \cos(n\pi X/L) \qquad (2.58)$$

and the τ_n, called equalizing time constants for $n > 0$, are all smaller than τ_o, as shown by the following expressions:

$$\tau_o/\tau_n = 1 + \alpha_n^2 = 1 + (n\pi/L)^2 \qquad (2.59)$$

Useful physical intuition results from noting the effect of n on the harmonic status of the functions, $\cos(n\pi/L)$, that is associated with each exponential decay in eq. 2.54. Thus, $n = 0$ associates the slowest decay time constant with a uniform voltage (corresponding to the average voltage along the finite length); this uniform component of charge decays only through the resting membrane conductance. In contrast, $n = 1$ associates the first equalizing time constant, τ_1, with decay and rapid equalization of charge between two half-lengths of the cylinder; note that $\cos(\pi/L)$ is positive for values of X from 0 to $L/2$, and negative from $L/2$ to L). Similarly, $n = 2$ associates τ_2 with decay and even more rapid equalization of charge (over shorter lengths involving less core resistance) between the mid-region and both ends of the cylinder; still larger values of n imply higher harmonics with more rapid equalization of charge over still shorter components of cylinder length.

It is important to note that these time constants depend on L, but they are completely independent of the initial condition or the point of observation. This means that the value of L can be calculated from a time constant ratio, using the expression

$$L = \frac{n\pi}{\sqrt{\tau_o/\tau_n - 1}} \qquad (2.60)$$

This useful theoretical result has been applied to experimental data from many neuron types. As explained in Rall (1969a), one can peel the slowest (τ_o) decay of an experimental or simulated passive decay transient (or of the transient response to an applied current step); then, provided that the coefficient C_1 is relatively large, one can obtain an estimate of τ_1, and thus of the ratio τ_o/τ_1, which can then be used (in eq. 2.60 with $n = 1$) to obtain an estimate of L. However, it is important to remember that eq. 2.60 is strictly correct for a uniform cylinder with two sealed ends; when this equation is applied to experimental data from neurons that deviate significantly from equivalence to a cylinder, one should not expect to get a valid estimate of L without evaluating the expected error. See also the comment at the end of section 2.6.4.

The coefficients C_n do depend on the initial condition (which determines B_n by eq. 2.56), and on the point of observation (which is X in eq. 2.58). An idealized initial condition (which serves as a useful reference case) is the case where $V(X, 0)$ is proportional to the spatial delta function, $\delta(X = 0)$. This equals zero for all values of X except $X = 0$, where the delta function has infinite amplitude; but its integral over X from $X = 0$ to $X = L$ has unit value. Such an initial condition is proportional to an instantaneous point charge placed at $X = 0$ when $T = 0$. If the amount of such a charge is Q_o, the Fourier coeffcients can be shown to reduce to

$$B_o = Q_o/(L\lambda c_m), \quad \text{and for } n > 0, \ B_n = 2B_o \qquad (2.61)$$

where the factor $L\lambda c_m$ represents the capacitance of the membrane cylinder, because c_m is the membrane capacitance per unit length of cylinder, and $L\lambda = \ell$ represents the length of the cylinder. It may be noted that when the charge per unit length, $c_m V(X, T)$, is integrated from $X = 0$ to $X = L$, all terms for which $n > 0$ in eq. 2.54 yield zero integrals, and the term for $n = 0$ yields $B_o L = Q_o/(\lambda c_m)$, which equals the voltage expected if the same amount of charge were distributed uniformly along the length of the cylinder.

It is helpful to understand that this value of B_o is the same for any initial distribution of charge, Q_o, along the length of the cylinder, and that the zero order term, $C_o \exp(-t/\tau_o)$ of eq. 2.57, corresponds to the passive decay of this total charge, regardless of its initial distribution. Next, it is important to understand that the values of B_n, for $n > 0$, do depend on the initial distribution. The higher-order decay terms, $C_n \exp(-t/\tau_n)$, result from rapid equalizing current flow (charge redistribution) between regions of higher and lower than average membrane potential; they are governed by the equalizing time constants, τ_n, which are smaller than τ_o; see eq. 2.59.

An instructive special example is provided by the initial condition that is proportional to $\delta(X = L)$, corresponding to an instantaneous point charge located at $X = L$. For this case, $B_n = 2(-1)^n B_o$, meaning that we have alternating signs; the values of B_n are negative for odd integer values of n, while they are positive for even values of n. Using eq. 2.58, we see that at $X = 0$, the value of $\cos(n\pi X/L) = 1$ for all n; thus the C_n have the same alternating signs as B_n (but note that at $X = L$, the C_n would all be positive). With alternating signs, such a sum can produce a smooth transient that resembles a synaptic potential; readers who have never summed such a series may find this an interesting example to compute.

Another instructive example is the initial condition that is proportional to $\delta(X = L/2)$, corresponding to an instantaneous point charge located at the midpoint, $X = L/2$. For this case, $B_n = 0$ for all odd integer values of n (because, in eq. 2.56, $\cos(n\pi X/L)$ becomes $\cos(n\pi/2)$, which is zero when n is odd); also, for even values of n, we have alternating signs, with negative values whenever $n/2$ is odd. In this case, the symmetry leads us to expect the same transient (with alternating signs) at $X = 0$ and at $X = L$; however, at $X = L/2$, the values of C_n (for n even) are all positive.

A different example, which has a rough resemblance to an initial charge distributed over a lumped soma, is to have the initial charge distributed uniformly over a short length, from $X = 0$ to $X = A$, with a zero initial voltage everywhere beyond $X = A$ to $X = L$. Then eqs. 2.55–2.58 imply a coefficient ratio for the decay transient at any location X, that can be expressed

$$\frac{C_n}{C_o} = \frac{2\sin(n\pi A/L)}{n\pi A/L}\cos(n\pi X/L) \qquad (2.62)$$

The maximum value of this ratio is 2, which is obtained only in the limiting case where $A = 0$ and $X = 0$; this means that unless the initial condition is restricted to a point ($A = 0$) and the observation is made at the same point ($X = 0$), this coefficient ratio will be less than 2. For example, if A/L and X/L are both set equal to 0.1, this ratio is 1.87 for $n = 1$, and it is 1.51 for $n = 2$. This result provides a warning that parameter estimates based on the coefficient ratios found in experimental data should take this effect into consideration.

2.6.3   Lumped Soma Coupled to One Equivalent Cylinder

When a lumped soma is coupled to one or more equivalent cylinders, the mathematical solution of the PDE is more complicated. By losing the zero slope boundary condition at $X = 0$, we lose the earlier simple expressions for the eigenvalues α_n, the time constants τ_n, and the coefficients C_n. As explained in Rall (1969a), we now have to specify α_n as the roots of a transcendental equation that can be expressed as

$$\alpha L \cot(\alpha L) = -\rho_\infty L \qquad (2.63)$$

where $\rho_\infty = G_\infty/G_S = \rho \coth(L)$; note that the equivalent cylinder could represent several dendritic trees, provided that they have the same value of L and satisfy the specified constraints. A figure showing how the resulting ratio of τ_o/τ_1 depends on the values of L was provided in Rall (1969a), but is not reproduced here. However, it is useful to know that these results can be approximated by the expression

$$\alpha_n \approx n\pi/L_N \qquad (2.64)$$

where L_N represents an effective L value for the whole neuron (soma + dendrites); this L_N is greater than the L value of the dendritic equivalent cylinder, now labeled L_D. Intuitively this means that the soma membrane (although isopotential) adds something to the apparent electrotonic length of the dendrites. Excluding very small values of ρ, it was found that useful approximations could be expressed

$$L_N/L_D \approx \sqrt{(\rho+1)/\rho} \approx 1 + 0.5/\rho \qquad (2.65)$$

Here we include no details on the effect of soma coupling on the values of the coefficients C_n, or on the related sets of C_n one obtains for an applied current step at $X = 0$; see Rall (1977, pp. 83, 84); see also Durand (1984), Kawato (1984), and Poznanski (1987), who consider the effect of a different soma membrane time constant (as would occur with significant soma shunting).

2.6.4 Soma Coupled to Cylinders of Different Lengths

If there are k dendritic equivalent cylinders having different L_D values, these can be distinguished by an index, j; then the previous transcendental equation (eq. 2.63) becomes generalized to

$$\alpha = -\sum_{j=1}^{k} \rho_{\infty j} \tan(\alpha L_{Dj}) \qquad (2.66)$$

A useful numerical example (Rall 1969a) assumed the values $\rho_{\infty 1} = 3$, with $L_{D1} = 1$ for one dendritic equivalent cylinder, and $\rho_{\infty 2} = 5$, with $L_{D2} = 2$ for the other. Noting that $\alpha_0 = 0$ is a root, we find that

$\alpha_1 \approx 1.10$, $\alpha_2 \approx 1.97$, and $\alpha_3 \approx 2.92$ are also roots of eq. 2.66. For $n > 3$, it was found that $\alpha_n \approx n\pi/3$; what makes this noteworthy is that this agrees with eq. 2.64, for $L_N = 3$, and in this example, $(L_{D1} + L_{D2}) = 3$. Furthermore, in view of the earlier approximation (eq. 2.65) that adds something for the soma, one could try $L_N \approx 3.2$; using this, eq. 2.64 suggests α_n values of 1.96 and 2.94 for n of 2 and 3 respectively; these values are very close to the approximate values of α_2 and α_3 noted above. On reflection, this result is not difficult to understand; if the two ρ_∞ values were equal, the two cylinders would have the same diameter; their combined cylinder length would correspond to $L_D = 3$, and their combined value of $\rho = \rho_\infty(\tanh L_{D1} + \tanh L_{D2})$. Then, a ρ_∞ value of 4 would imply a combined ρ value of about 6.9, and eq. 2.65 would imply $L_N/L_D \approx 1.07$, or a value of about 3.2 for L_N; if ρ_∞ were very large, then one would expect the soma to contribute negligible effective length. This kind of result has been verified with other examples.

It is important to emphasize that the voltage decay corresponding to τ_1 may not be apparent in experimental or simulated data, because the coefficient associated with this time constant may be very small. In particular, when $L_{D1} = L_{D2}$, the eigenvalue $\alpha_1 = \pi/L_N = \pi/(2L_{D1})$ exists, but the corresponding coefficient, C_1, (for observation and input at the soma) is zero; this means that τ_2 but not τ_1 would be observed. If one were to apply eq. 2.60 knowing τ_o and this τ_2, one would get $L = L_N$, but if one did not know that the true τ_1 was absent from the data and then treated τ_2 as though it were τ_1, the application of eq. 2.60 would then yield $L = 0.5L_N = L_{D1} = L_{D2}$. The same result should be expected when the two cylinders differ slightly in their electrotonic lengths, because then the value of C_1, although not zero, is still very small relative to C_0 and C_2. This insight can be extended to the case of a soma coupled to several dendritic cylinders, provided that their electrotonic lengths differ by less than 20% (Segev and Rall 1983).

2.7   Insights Gained from Equivalent Cylinder Computations

Several early computations provided quantitative results that led to qualitative insights that apply also to dendritic trees that deviate from equivalent-cylinder constraints. Many of these early computations were done by hand (using a slide rule and math tables), and can now be done easily with a hand calculator that includes trigonometric and hyperbolic functions. In today's climate of computer work stations, it is important to remember that computer programs can have errors that produce garbage; it is wise to check a few key values by hand calculation. The analytical solutions obtained for equivalent cylinders are especially useful for such calculations.

2.7.1   Steady-State Decrement of Voltage with Distance

The belief that cable theory implies a simple exponential voltage decrement to $1/e$ for a λ distance is correct for a very long (many λ) cable that has uniform properties and is unperturbed (i.e., by any input, leak, short circuit, or voltage clamp). It is also correct for a finite length with one particular boundary condition that can be expressed as $G_L/G_\infty = 1$ at $X = L$; see fig. 2.2 and eq. 2.25. However, as that figure and that equation make clear, such a simple voltage decrement is a very special case. These theoretical results show that the general case of voltage decrement with distance depends upon both the length of uniform cable and the boundary condition at $X = L$. The special case $G_L = 0$ corresponds to the sealed-end boundary condition $dV/dX = 0$ at $X = L$. The special case $G_L = \infty$ corresponds to the voltage clamp $V = 0$ at $X = L$; it is important to remember that this does not correspond to a membrane short circuit; it means that the membrane potential difference is clamped to its resting value; infinite G_L accomplishes this because it is a conductance not to ground but to what is better thought of as an infinite resting membrane capacitance. A true membrane short circuit means that V is clamped to $-E_r$. Also, note that eq. 2.22 holds for clamping $V = V_L$ at $X = L$.

The attenuation factor $V(X = 0)/V(X = L)$ is defined by eq. 2.24, except for cases of voltage clamp that differ from $V = 0$ at $X = L$. For a sealed end at $X = L = 1.0$, this attenuation factor is 1.54, meaning that the steady voltage decrements from 100% to about 65% for this case.

Although this section has referred, so far, only to one cylinder extending from $X = 0$ to $X = L$, it applies also to dendritic trees that are equivalent to a cylinder, provided that the decrement is from the trunk into the branches. For inputs to dendritic branches, similar equivalent-cylinder results apply only when all branches at the same electrotonic distance, X, receive their proportional share of the input, ensuring that $V(X)$ is the same in all of these branches. Thus, if a steady voltage were applied to all of the terminals of such a tree with $L = 1$, and if the trunk were sealed at $X = 0$, the decrement would be from 100% at the terminals to 65% at $X = 0$. The same decrement would also be expected from the dendritic terminals to the soma in an idealized neuron composed of several such trees coupled at $X = 0$ (assume no lumped soma, but a proximal bit of each trunk can be regarded as soma), provided that all dendritic terminals of all trees had the same steady voltage and the same value of L. In this case, the symmetry about $X = 0$ would cause all of these trees to have $dV/dX = 0$ at $X = 0$, meaning that they would all have effectively sealed ends at $X = 0$, even though they were still connected to each other; in fact, this case can be represented by a single equivalent cylinder with voltage applied at $X = L$ and voltage decrement to a sealed end at $X = 0$.

In contrast to all of these cases, one would expect significantly greater attenuation if only one of these trees received input, while the other trees received none. For that case, and also for input to a single branch of one tree, the method described by Rall and Rinzel (1973) can be used to obtain results like those illustrated below in fig. 2.4.

2.7.2   Input Conductance and Input Resistance

The reference values G_∞ and R_∞, for semi-infinite length, are defined by eqs. 2.28–2.31. For example, if $R_m R_i = \pi^2 10^5 \ ohm^2 cm^3$, and if $d = 10 \ \mu m = 10^{-3} \ cm$, then it follows that R_∞ would equal 20 $megohm$, and that G_∞ would equal 50 nS.

For finite length with a sealed end, the input conductance is smaller than the reference value by an amount defined by eq. 2.32; this smaller input conductance corresponds to the less steep initial slopes shown for curves F, H, and J, compared with curve E in fig. 2.2. For L values of 0.5, 1.0, and 2.0, the values of G_{in}/G_∞ are about 0.46, 0.76, and 0.96, respectively, and the values of R_{in}/R_∞ are about 2.2, 1.3, and 1.04, respectively.

For finite length with $G_L/G_\infty = 4$ at $L = 1$ (see curve G of fig. 2.2) we can use eq. 2.37 to find that G_{in}/G_∞ is about 1.18, which is greater than 1.0, as expected from a comparison of initial slopes in fig. 2.2, and as expected from knowing that G_L is greater than for a semi-infinite extension of the reference cylinder. On the other hand, a value less than 1.0 (i.e., about 0.85) is implied when $G_L/G_\infty = 1/4$ at $L = 1$; see curve C of fig. 2.2.

2.7.3   Steady State for Current Injected to One Branch

Here fig. 2.4 illustrates an idealized dendritic neuron consisting of six equal dendritic trees. Current is injected at a single branch terminal, here designated I; this input branch is distinguished from its sibling branch S, and its first and second cousin branches (C-1) and (C-2). The resulting steady voltage distribution in the various branches of the input tree (shown in this figure) was computed from the general solution

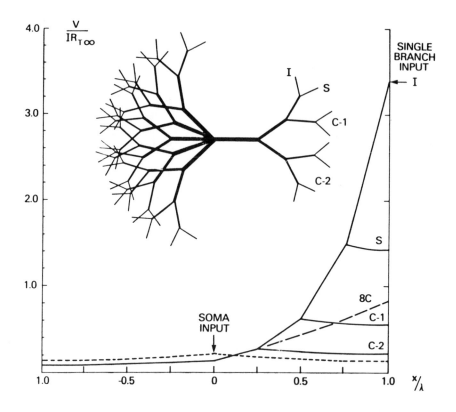

Figure 2.4
Diagram of idealized neuron model composed of six dendritic trees, and plot of steady-state voltage values for three different cases. Solid curve shows voltages computed for current input to a single distal branch terminal, designated I for input branch; in this case, the sibling branch (S), the first cousin branches (C-1), and the second cousin branches (C-2) receive no input; they have sealed ends. Curve with long dashes (labeled 8C) corresponds to the same amount of input current divided equally among all eight terminal branches (cousins) belonging to the same tree. Curve with short dashes correponds to the same amount of total input current applied at the soma. (Modified from Rall and Rinzel 1973, which can be consulted for the mathematical statement and solution of this problem.)

of this problem (Rall and Rinzel 1973), based on superposition methods and considerations of symmetry.

One noteworthy feature of these results is the contrast in voltage decrement in the input branch, compared with its sibling branch. Both branches have the same length and diameter in this idealized tree; the essential difference lies in the boundary conditions. The proximal end of the input branch is open to current flow into its parent branch; this permits a large flow of current along its cytoplasmic core, resulting in a steep voltage decrement along the length of the input branch. In contrast, the sealed terminal of the sibling branch allows zero current to flow out of that end; also, little current flows across the high resistance of the cylindrical branch membrane; with so little current flowing either in or out of this sibling branch, its voltage profile is almost isopotential. A similar contrast holds true also for the very small terminal branches known as dendritic spines. When a spine head receives synaptic input there is significant attenuation along the spine stem, from a large membrane depolarization at the spine head to a smaller depolarization at the spine base and the parent dendrite where the spine stem is attached. For spines with excitable spine head membrane, the large depolarization at the spine head enhances the probability of reaching spike threshold; also, for an excitable spine that does not receive synaptic input, the nearly isopotential spread of depolarization from the parent dendrite through the spine stem out to the spine head increases the probability that such a spine may also reach spike threshold and thus contribute to a chain reaction that may result in the firing of clusters of excitable spines (Rall and Segev 1987).

Another feature of these results is the contrast in input resistance values when the distal input location is compared with a central input location (at the soma). In this figure, the dashed curve shows the lower voltage values obtained when the same amount of current is injected at the soma as that previously injected at the distal branch. In this example, the distal input resistance is sixteen times larger than the somatic input resistance, and still larger factors can result from additional orders of branching; see Rall and Rinzel (1973), where it is also shown that the increased depolarization at a distal location cannot be more effective in its spread to the soma, because steady-state voltage attenuation (from the distal input site to the soma) always exceeds the input resistance ratio. Nevertheless, the large local synaptic depolarization produced at distal dendritic locations is important for graded dendro-dendritic synaptic interactions that depend on the local dendritic depolarization;

it is also important to the attainment of threshold conditions in excitable dendritic spines located on distal dendritic branches.

2.7.4 Synaptic Excitation Distributed over Half of an Equivalent Cylinder

One early transient calculation (Rall 1962a) is summarized by fig. 2.5; this shows voltage (membrane depolarization) transients for the case of an equivalent cylinder that had a synaptic excitatory conductance distributed uniformly over one-half of its length. The excited half could represent either the proximal or the distal half of the dendritic surface area of a dendritic tree. The synaptic intensity, defined as the ratio of synaptic conductance per unit area to the resting membrane conductance per unit area, was set equal to 2; it was turned on at $T = 0$ and left on for the three curves shown in part A of the figure; however, for the three curves in part B, the synaptic conductance was turned off at $T = 0.2$, implying a brief square on-off transient of synaptic conductance that generates a crude synaptic potential (EPSP). In both A and B, the middle curve was calculated at the midpoint ($X = 0.5$) of the cylinder, the upper curve was calculated at one end (the "hot" end belonging to the excited half of the cylinder) and the lower curve was calculated at the other "cold" end of the cylinder.

There are several points to be noted about these results. One is the difference in the shapes of the transients in part B. As noted in the original paper, "the transient at the 'hot' end rises and falls more rapidly. The transient at the 'cold' end begins very slowly, but it continues to rise after the conductance pulse is over; this is due to an equalizing flow of current between the two halves of the dendritic tree." Considering an experimental EPSP to be recorded near the proximal end of a dendritic tree, we note that the upper curve shows the steeper rise to a larger peak, as well as the rapid early decay obtained for proximally located synaptic input, while the lower curve shows the slower rise to a later and more rounded peak (with no rapid early decay) of an EPSP produced by distally located synaptic input. These are the kinds of differences in EPSP shape that were pursued further with compartmental computations (Rall 1964, 1967), leading to shape indices defined as the half-width and the rise time (or time-to-peak) and to the shape index plot, which facilitated the comparison of theory and experiment (Rall et al. 1967) and helped to establish the importance of the dendritic location of a synaptic input; see fig. 2.7 below.

Another point of interest is that the late decay is the same for all three curves; this is an exponential decay with the passive membrane

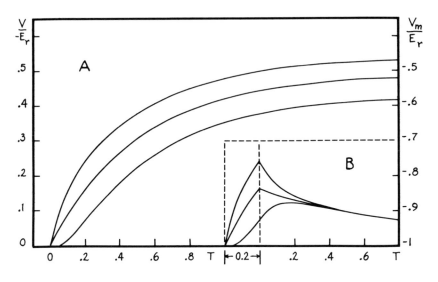

Figure 2.5
Transients of membrane depolarization at three locations in a dendritic tree or its
equivalent cylinder (for $L = 1$), when a uniform synaptic excitatory conductance was
applied to a half-length of the equivalent cylinder. The middle curves in A and in B
correspond to the midpoint ($X = 0.5$); the other curves correspond to the two ends
($X = 0$, or $X = 1.0$); the upper curves in A and in B show the voltage transient at
the "hot" end (i.e., end of the half-cylinder that received synaptic excitatory input),
while the lower curve in A and in B correponds to the "cool" end of the equivalent
cylinder. For A, the synaptic conductance ($G_\epsilon = 2G_r$) came on as a step, when
$T = 0$, and stayed on. For B, the on-step at $T = 0$ was followed by an equal off-step
at $T = 0.2$; thus, the input was a square conductance pulse over half of the membrane
surface. (From Rall 1962a, which can be consulted for the mathematical statement
and solution of this problem.)

time constant. However, the early decay is significantly modified by the rapid equalizing current flow between regions of unequal potential; the equalizing time constants governing this equalizing flow were implied by the eigenvalues (γ_n^2 of Rall 1962a); these time constants were made explicit as τ_n in a later publication (Rall 1969a); see eqs. 2.57–2.59 above, which hold for passive decay to the resting potential. It is important to note that while the synaptic conductance is on, the perturbed membrane (the portion of membrane that receives this input) would have its local membrane conductivity tripled; an isolated patch of this perturbed membrane would have a time constant only 1/3 of that for passive resting membrane; however, the system composed of both regions of this cylinder has eigenvalues and time constants determined by eqs. 44–46 of Rall (1962a). Consequently, the rate of rise of the upper curves in fig. 2.4 is much steeper than the rate of late decay in part B of this figure. These points can be understood better by looking at the equation that was used to represent synaptic excitation and inhibition in this boundary value problem (Rall 1962a); see the next section.

2.7.5 Formal Representation of Synaptic Excitation and Inhibition

The membrane equivalent circuit used for synaptic mediated excitation and inhibition (Rall 1962a, 1964) is shown in fig. 2.6; this is closely related to the models introduced by Fatt and Katz (1953) and by Coombs, Eccles, and Fatt (1955). The membrane capacity per unit area, C_m, is electrically in parallel with three conductance pathways per unit area; G_r represents the resting membrane conductance that lies in series with the resting battery, E_r (e.g., $-70\ mV$, interior relative to exterior); G_ϵ represents the synaptic excitatory conductance that lies in series with its reversal potential, E_ϵ (e.g., zero, interior relative to exterior); G_j represents the synaptic inhibitory conductance that lies in series with its reversal potential, E_j (e.g., $-80\ mV$, interior relative to exterior). Then, following Kirchhoff's current law , the membrane current density across a space-clamped patch of uniform membrane can be expressed

$$
\begin{aligned}
I_m = \quad & C_m(dV_m/dt) + G_r(V_m - E_r) + G_\epsilon(V_m - E_\epsilon) \\
& + G_j(V_m - E_j)
\end{aligned}
\tag{2.67}
$$

For time periods during which the membrane parameters remain unchanged, and $I_m = 0$, this equation can be rearranged to the following form:

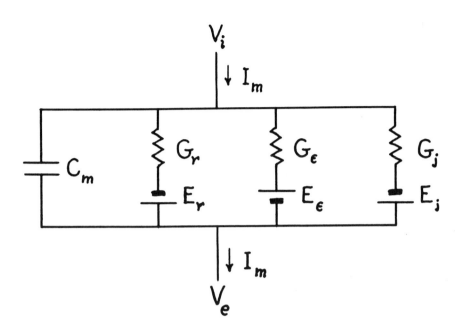

Figure 2.6
Equivalent electric circuit for membrane that can receive synaptic excitation and/or synaptic inhibition, based on Fatt and Katz (1953) and Coombs, Eccles, and Fatt (1955). The membrane current, I_m, per unit area, can divide into four pathways: one is capacitative, and three are conductive pathways in series with associated reversal potentials, shown as batteries. The resting conductance, G_r, per unit area, could be the sum of the resting conductance values for several ion species, and the reversal potential, E_r, could be a weighted sum of several different ionic reversal potentials. Both G_r and E_r are assumed to remain constant (i.e., independent of V and T). For resting conditions, both G_ϵ and G_j are zero. For synaptic excitatory input, the value of G_ϵ is increased from zero; this can be as a step, a square pulse, or a smooth, brief transient (e.g., an alpha function, proportional to $Te^{-\alpha T}$); the reversal potential, E_ϵ, is a constant that is often taken to be zero, relative to a resting potential, E_r, that may be $-70\ mV$, interior relative to exterior. For synaptic inhibitory input, the value of G_j is increased from zero; its reversal potential, E_j, is a constant that is often taken to be something like $7\ mV$ more negative than E_r, or one can set the ratio, $(E_j - E_r)/(E_\epsilon - E_r)$, to some value (e.g., -0.1).

$$\tau dV/dt = -k^2(V - V^*) \qquad\qquad\qquad\qquad\qquad (2.68)$$

where $\tau = R_m C_m = C_m/G_r$ and $V = V_m - E_r$; also V^* is the steady-state value of V (with $I_m = 0$) as shown by eq. 2.70 below, and k^2 is a factor defined by eq. 2.69. Equation 2.68 implies that V decays exponentially to V^* with a time constant equal to τ/k^2, where

$$k^2 = (G_r + G_\epsilon + G_j)/G_r \qquad\qquad\qquad\qquad (2.69)$$

and

$$V^* = \frac{G_\epsilon(E_\epsilon - E_r) + G_j(E_j - E_r)}{G_r + G_\epsilon + G_j} \qquad\qquad\qquad (2.70)$$

For resting conditions, G_ϵ and G_j are both zero; then $k^2 = 1$ and $V^* = 0$, meaning that V decays to zero with the resting time constant, τ. However, when $G_\epsilon = 2G_r$ with zero G_j, then $k^2 = 3$ and $V^* = (2/3)(E_\epsilon - E_r)$, meaning that V would decay to 0.67 (when V is normalized relative to $E_\epsilon - E_r$) with an effective time constant that is 1/3 the resting value; in fig. 2.5A, the asymptote of the upper curve is less than 0.67 because this half cylinder was not space-clamped and there was a spread of current from the "hot" half to the "cold" half, during the time that $G_e = 2G_r$ was kept on over half of the cylinder. If instead $G_\epsilon = G_r$ over all of the cylinder, then $k^2 = 2$ and the normalized value of V^* would be 0.5; this would produce a transient similar to the middle curve of fig. 2.5, but it would not be identical. Why it would not be identical must be related to the fact that the effective value of λ^2 is reduced over the "hot" region while the synaptic conductance is on; this would upset the symmetry about the "midpoint." Further details are omitted here, but it is noted that nonuniform synaptic inhibition was also explored by hand calculations summarized in figs. 8 and 9 of Rall (1962a).

This theoretical paper provided useful analytical results; the hand calculations provided early insights about EPSP shapes for nonuniform synaptic input distributions, and about interactions of excitatory and inhibitory synaptic inputs. These were explored further in subsequent studies (Rall 1964, 1967, 1969a; Jack et al. 1975; Segev and Parnas 1983).

Although a square pulse of synaptic conductance was adequate for some computations, we often prefer to specify a brief smooth time course for the synaptic conductance. The function used for this purpose by Rall (1967) was used also by Jack et al. (1971), and by others; it is a one-parameter function (often referred to as the alpha function) that can be expressed

$$G(T) = \alpha^2 T \exp(-\alpha T) \tag{2.71}$$

where α and T are both dimensionless. This function is zero for $T = 0$, rises smoothly to a peak at a time $T_p = 1/\alpha$, and then falls a little more slowly back to zero. Halfway up, $T \approx 0.23\ T_p$, and halfway down, $T \approx 2.68\ T_p$, implying a half-width of 2.45 T_p. The peak amplitude equals α/e, and the area under this curve equals unity. Plots of this time course for α values of 10, 20, 40, and 100 can be found in Jack and Redman (1971) and Jack et al. (1975).

2.8   Insights Gained from Compartmental Computations

Compartmental modeling of a neuron was introduced in the 1960s. As explained in Rall (1964), this adaptation from compartmental modeling of metabolic systems was facilitated by interaction with the analytical and computational expertise of Drs. Hearon and Berman in the Mathematical Research Branch at NIH. A single compartment could correspond to a single dendritic branch, a group of branches, or just a segment of a trunk or branch element, according to the needs of a given problem. The region of the neuron represented by a single compartment is treated as isopotential; voltage differences between regions are represented as differences between compartments. Mathematically, the PDE of cable theory is replaced by a system of ODEs for which analytical and computational solutions are already available. The major advantage is flexibility: the membrane properties and the amount of synaptic conductance input or current injection can be different in every compartment; dendritic branching need not satisfy equivalent-cylinder constraints. It is possible to compute the consequences of any branching geometry and any spatio-temporal pattern of input that one chooses to specify.

The necessary equations were explained and illustrated in Rall (1964); they are also discussed in chapter 3, while chapter 13 presents efficient numerical methods for their solution. Here we point briefly to basic early results that were obtained using a simple chain of ten equal compartments. Because they were made equal, these compartments provide a lumped representation of an equivalent cylinder. As indicated by the diagram (upper right in fig. 2.7), this ten-compartment model can represent the entire soma-dendritic extent of the neuron; compartment 1 can be regarded as the soma; compartment 2 represents the trunks of all dendritic trees belonging to this neuron; compartments 3 to 10 represent increasing electrotonic distance away from the soma to the dendritic terminals of all these trees. Each compartment represents an equal amount of membrane surface area available for synaptic input. Given this model, the focus in fig. 2.7 is on the effect of input location on EPSP shape, the effect of spatio-temporal input pattern is shown in fig. 2.8, and the effect of location of synaptic inhibition is shown in fig. 2.9.

2.8.1   Effect of Synaptic Input Location on the EPSP Shape at the Soma

The three voltage transients shown at lower right in fig. 2.7 represent three different EPSP shapes computed for the soma compartment in response to brief synaptic excitatory conductance input to a single compartment for three different choices of input location. The EPSP amplitudes have been normalized; the input locations were compartments 1, 4, or 8, as indicated by the numbers inside the open triangles; the input conductance time course (shown as the dotted curve above them) was the same in each case. The reference EPSP (designated by the black triangle) resulted when the same input time course was applied uniformly to all ten compartments. It is apparent that the EPSP obtained with the most proximal input location (1) rises most steeply to the earliest peak; this is a sharp peak because of rapid early decay, which can be understood as due to rapid equalizing spread of depolarizing charge away from the soma to the dendritic compartments. The rapid rise and rapid early decay are responsible for a relatively short half-width (duration at half maximum). In contrast, the EPSP obtained at the soma in response to the distal input location (8) shows a delayed, slow rise to a later, more rounded peak; this can be understood as due to equalizing spread of depolarizing charge toward the soma from the distal dendritic input location. The slow rise and slow early decay are responsible for a relatively long half-width. The difference between these shapes resembles that seen in fig. 2.5B, with essentially the same explanation.

To facilitate comparison of many experimental EPSP shapes with these theoretical EPSP shapes, we devised the shape index plot (Rall et al. 1967) illustrated at left in fig. 2.7. This was particularly useful because we did not know the input locations for the experimental EPSPs. What we and others could do was to compare the shape scatter of an experimental EPSP population with the two theoretical shape index loci shown in fig. 2.7. The solid line through the black triangle is the locus of shapes computed for uniform synaptic input to all ten compartments, when the input time course is changed by choosing different values of the parameter alpha in eq. 2.71. The dashed curve through

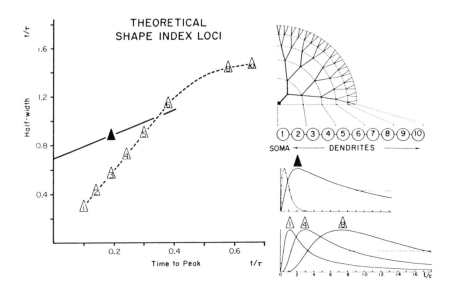

Figure 2.7
EPSP shapes and shape index loci. Diagram (upper right) indicates the mapping
of soma-dendritic membrane into a chain of ten equal compartments, of which 1
represents the soma membrane, and 10 represents all of the most distal dendritic
branches. Four voltage transients (lower right) represent computed EPSPs at the
soma; their shapes differ because they result from different synaptic input locations;
the same brief synaptic excitatory conductance transient (shown as dotted curve with
peak at $t = 0.04\tau$ and a half-width close to 0.1τ) was used for all four cases. The
upper EPSP (black triangle) resulted when the input was equal in all compartments;
the three lower EPSP shapes resulted when the synaptic input was restricted to a
single compartment (open triangles show the number, 1, 4, or 8, that designates the
input compartment for each case). The same EPSP shapes are represented on the
shape index plot (at left), where each abscissa represents the time-to-peak, and each
ordinate represents the half-width (duration at half-maximum). The curve through
the open triangles represents a theoretical locus of EPSP shapes obtained by varying
only the location of the single input compartment; this locus corresponds to one
particular input time course; a shifted locus was found for a faster or slower input;
see (Rall et al. 1967) for examples. The line through the solid triangle represents
a theoretical locus of EPSP shapes obtained by varying only the input time course
(i.e., the parameter α), while the synaptic input remained distributed uniformly over
the soma-dendritic surface. (From Rall et al. 1967; tables of computed values and
other details in Rall 1967.)

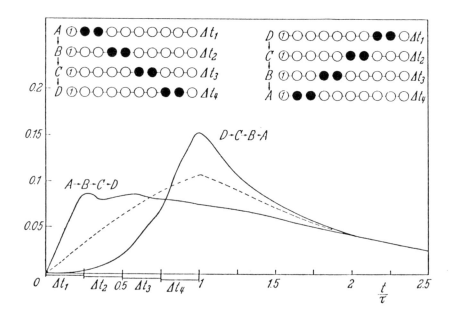

Figure 2.8
Effect of spatio-temporal pattern of synaptic input on the resultant composite EPSP
at the soma, computed with a ten-compartment model. The total amount of synaptic
input was the same in each case; only its spatio-temporal pattern was different. The
diagram at upper left shows the synaptic input sequence, A-B-C-D, meaning proximal
location first, with distal location last; this input produced the soma voltage transient (composite EPSP) labelled A-B-C-D at lower left. The diagram at upper right
shows the opposite synaptic input sequence, D-C-B-A, meaning distal location first,
with proximal location last; this input produced a different soma voltage transient
(composite EPSP), with delayed rise to a larger peak amplitude, labeled D-C-B-A.
In both cases, the input compartments (shown filled) received a synaptic excitatory
conductance pulse ($G_\epsilon = G_r$ for 0.25τ) during one of the four labeled time increments. The same total amount of synaptic input also produced the dashed curve,
when spatio-temporal pattern was eliminated from the synaptic input by spreading
the synaptic conductance uniformly ($G_\epsilon = 0.25G_r$) over compartments 2–9 for the
full duration from $t = 0$ to $t = \tau$. (Modified from Rall 1964).

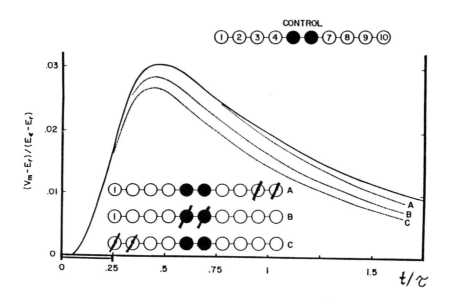

Figure 2.9
Effect of location of inhibition, synaptic, computed with ten-compartment model. The control EPSP at the soma, shown as the solid curve, was produced by a synaptic excitatory conductance in compartments 5 and 6 (shown filled) that was a square pulse from $T = 0$ to $T = 0.25$, with $G_\epsilon = G_r$. Dotted curves show effect of three inhibitory input locations (indicated by diagonal slash in compartmental diagrams); this inhibition was a relatively weak but sustained inhibitory conductance ($G_j = G_r$, with $E_j = E_r$; shunting inhibition). In case A, the inhibitory input location was distal to the control input; this did not reduce the control EPSP amplitude at the soma. In cases B and C the inhibitory input location was either proximal to or the same as the control input; both reduced the EPSP amplitude significantly. Larger reductions of EPSP amplitude would result from larger values of G_j and from hyperpolarized values for E_j. (Modified from Rall 1964).

the open triangles is the locus of shapes computed when the input was restricted to different choices of a single compartment, using the same input time course (i.e., $\alpha = 25$ in eq. 2.71) with each of these locations.

In the original paper by Rall et al. (1967) and in papers by Jack et al. (1971) and others, it was found that the variation in the shapes of EPSPs produced by single Ia afferent fiber input to motoneurons of cat spinal cord is in much better agreement with theoretical loci of the type shown here by the dashed curve with the open triangles. It was concluded that these synapses are distributed over proximal and distal dendritic locations, that unitary EPSP shapes can be accounted for by these locations, and that compound EPSP shapes can be accounted for by two or more input locations. Additional details can be found in the original papers; important experimental confirmation of the correlation of EPSP shape and synaptic location has been provided by the experiments of Redman and Walmsley (1983).

2.8.2   Effect of Spatio-Temporal Pattern of Synaptic Input

The purpose of the computations summarized in fig. 2.8 was to demonstrate that it should be possible to distinguish two synaptic inputs that are equal in amount and differ only in one aspect of their spatio-temporal pattern. This computation used the ten-compartment model, and the synaptic excitatory conductance input sequences, A-B-C-D and D-C-B-A, which were composed of equal square pulses of synaptic conductance; see figure legend and Rall (1964) for details. The resulting composite EPSPs are significantly different, and would be distinguished by a neuron whose spike threshold is 0.12 ± 0.02 in the normalized ordinate scale of this figure; such a difference could be exploited for motion detection, provided that the synapses are appropriately arrayed.

Each of these two spatio-temporal input patterns yields a result that can have functional value. The case A-B-C-D shows how one can obtain a quick rise to a subthreshold plateau; such a plateau provides a bias voltage that would poise the neuron to be ready to fire in response to a relatively small, sharp additional input. The case D-C-B-A shows that greater EPSP amplitude at the soma is attained when the distal input precedes the proximal input.

2.8.3   Effect of Synaptic Inhibitory Input Location

Other computations with the ten-compartment model were used to compare the effects of moderate sustained synaptic inhibitory conductance at three locations; see fig. 2.9 and figure legend. The resulting EPSPs at the soma demonstrate the importance of inhibitory input location relative to the location of the excitatory input. The synaptic inhibition is effective when it has the same location as the synaptic excitation, and also when it is located at the soma (i.e., proximal to the control input location), but it is much less effective when located distal to the control input location. As discussed by Rall (1964), Jack et al. (1975), and Segev and Parnas (1983), the timing is also very important when the synaptic inhibitory conductance is brief.

These computations led to useful insights. Synaptic inhibitory input located at the soma is nonspecific because it is effective against synaptic excitatory depolarization that spreads to the soma from any of several dendritic trees, as well as against excitatory input located at or near the soma. In contrast, synaptic inhibition at dendritic locations is more specific, because it is effective against synaptic excitation located in the same dendritic tree, provided that the inhibitory input location is the same or proximal, but not distal to the excitatory input location (see Rall 1964, 1967; Jack et al. 1975; also Koch et al. 1982, 1983).

2.9   Insights Gained from Other Cable Computations

2.9.1   Transients at Different Locations in a Dendritic Tree for Input to One Branch

The transients of fig. 2.10 were computed for the same neuron model as that of fig. 2.4; the mathematical solution for the transient response to input restricted to one branch terminal (Rinzel and Rall 1974) was based on the same superposition concepts that were used for the steady-state problem. It may be noted that this computation did not require a compartmental model; it did require computational convolution of the input current time course with several response functions. One can see the qualitative effects of electrotonic spread from the input branch toward the soma and into the other trees; the time of peak is increasingly delayed and the peak amplitude is increasingly attenuated. Quantitatively, these peak times and amplitudes, as well as those for the sibling and cousin branch terminals, are available in a table (Rinzel and Rall 1974; also Rall 1977); this table has been used to test a set of comparable compartmental computations (Segev et al. 1985). Discussion of many topics, including the relation between transient charge attenuation and steady-state attentuation, the distribution of charge dissipation over different regions of the model, and the nonlinearities associated with synaptic conductance input, can be found in the original publication.

2.9.2   Computation of Field Potentials in Olfactory Bulb

The diagrams in figs. 2.11 and 2.12 indicate how a compartmental cable model played a role in a theoretical reconstruction of extracellular field potentials generated by synchronous antidromic activation of the mitral cell population in the olfactory bulb (Rall and Shepherd 1968). Computing the intracellular voltage transients required only the compartmental model. To get extracellular potentials, it was necessary to model three-dimensional aspects of the mitral cell population. By assuming a spherical cortical layer with closed radial symmetry (not shown here), one could compute the first set of extracellular potential transients shown in fig. 2.11. Then, by considering the concept of punctured spherical symmetry and by considering the distinction between the primary extracellular current (radial in the cortex) and the secondary extracellular current, which flows out of the cortex to ground and back through the puncture (see Rall and Shepherd 1968, and Klee and Rall 1977, for a detailed explanation and validation of this concept), one could obtain the second set of extracellular potential transients shown in fig. 2.11. These theoretical results agree quite well with the early portion of the experimental records (designated periods I and II in the middle part of fig. 2.12). However, it was important to notice that the field potentials of period III could not have been generated by activity in the mitral cell population, as explained next.

Figure 2.12 shows schematically how the cortical layers of the olfactory bulb are related to four depths at which field potentials were recorded; also, at the right of this figure, the primary extracellular current flow, and its associated field potential polarity, are shown for the mitral cell population (in periods I and II), and for the granule cell population (in period III). The axonless granule cell population extends dendrites over the full depth range shown, hence the long equivalent cylinder. The mitral cell axons (in the granular layer, GRL) have a core resistance per unit length that is much larger than their associated dendritic core resistance (for many dendrites lying electrically in parallel in the EPL); consequently, mitral cell activity generates much less radial current and radial gradient of extracellular potential in the GRL than in the EPL. This statement expresses our explanation of what was actually observed in periods I and II; it also explains our conviction that the large extracelluar potential gradient in the GRL (during period III) cannot have been produced by mitral cell activity. Our interpretation of the field

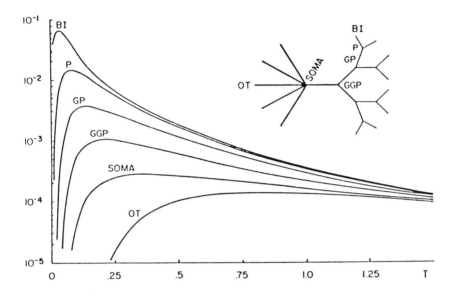

Figure 2.10
Semi-log plot of voltage transients at several locations in an idealized neuron model (inset) in response to injection of a brief current to one branch terminal. BI designates the input branch terminal, while P, GP, and GGP designate the parent, grandparent, and great-grandparent nodes (branch points) along the main line from BI to the soma; OT designates the distal terminals of the other trees. This model had six equal dendritic trees (see fig. 2.4); the input tree had three orders of branching, with each branch length equal to $1/4$ of λ. Thus $L = 1$ for this tree, and also for the five other trees (here indicated by schematic equivalent cylinders). Additional details about this figure and about several related figures, including a table of peak times and amplitudes (for these and other locations), can be found in the original publication (Rinzel and Rall 1974).

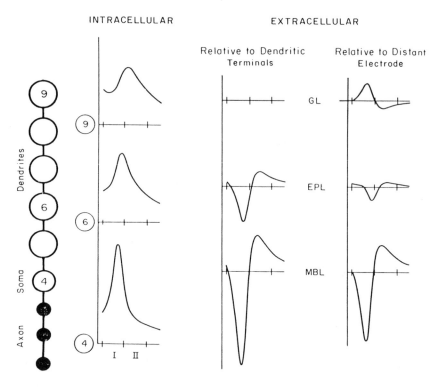

INTRACELLULAR

EXTRACELLULAR

Relative to Dendritic
Terminals

Relative to Distant
Electrode

Figure 2.11
Computed intracellular and extracellular voltage transients in response to synchronous antidromic activation of the mitral cell population in a model of the olfactory bulb. Leftmost diagram shows a compartmental model of a simplified mitral
cell; the three axonal compartments (shown filled) and the soma compartment (4)
had excitable membrane; the five dendritic compartments had passive membrane in
this computation (but they had excitable membrane in other computations). Computed voltage transients are shown only for compartments 4, 6, and 9, assumed to
correspond to three depths (layers) in the olfactory bulb; as shown also in fig. 2.12,
these layers are the mitral body layer (MBL), the external plexiform layer (EPL),
and the glomerular layer (GL). The intracellular voltage transients $V_i(t)$ show the
computed passive electrotonic spread, from an action potential at the soma to the
attenuated passive transients in the dendrites; for each time, t, the values of $V_i(X)$
imply a voltage gradient and a corresponding intracellular core current; this implies
an equal and oppositely directed extracellular current flowing radially in the olfactory bulb. This extracellular current generates radial extracellular voltage gradients
from which one can compute the two sets of extracellular potentials shown. See also
comments in text about reversal of extracellular potential in time periods I and II.
The equations and results are presented and discussed in Rall and Shepherd (1968);
numerous associated insights are discussed there and in Rall (1970), as well as Klee
and Rall (1977).

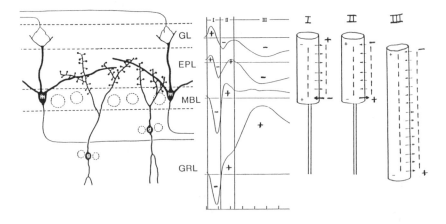

Figure 2.12
Diagram showing depth distribution of extracellular field potentials in time periods I, II, and III, in relation to cortical layers in the olfactory bulb, and in relation to cable models that distinguish the granule cell population from the mitral cell population. Schematic diagram at left shows two mitral cells and two granule cells in relation to four cortical layers: the glomerular layer (GL), the external plexiform layer (EPL), the mitral body layer (MBL), and the granular layer (GRL). The voltage transients (at center) are field potentials recorded at depths corresponding to those four layers, relative to a distant reference electrode. The three equivalent cylinder models at right contrast the current flow and extracellular potential difference generated by the mitral cell population in periods I and II with that generated by the granule cell population during period III, according to our modeling and interpretation the data. This contrast was crucial to our expectation of dendro-dendritic syna interactions between mitral cells and granule cells (Rall et al. 1966; Rall and Shep 1968). (Figure modified from Rall 1970).

potentials during period III (as caused by activity in the granule cell population) then required that membrane depolarization in the granule cells would have to be greatest for their dendrites in the EPL, not for those in the GRL; this suggested massive synaptic excitatory input to the granule cell dendrites in the EPL. The timing of these events, together with the proximity of the two sets of dendrites, led to our conviction that there must be dendro-dendritic synaptic interactions between the mitral cell dendrites and the granule cell dendrites in the EPL.

As explained more fully in the original papers (Rall, Shepherd, Reese, and Brightman 1966; Rall and Shepherd 1968) and also discussed in Rall (1970), our theoretical predictions and the histological results of our collaborators converged on the recognition of reciprocal dendro-dendritic synapses in the EPL. Our functional interpretation of these synapses was as follows: first mitral dendritic depolarization activates mitral-to-granule excitatory synapses, and then the resulting depolarization of the granule cell dendrites in the EPL activates granule-to-mitral inhibitory synapses that suppress the excitability of the mitral cells. It is noteworthy that neither of these synapses needs to be activated by an action potential, that both of these synapses are dendro-dendritic, that one of them is excitatory while the other is inhibitory, and that one cell type is axonless while the other has a conventional axon. These synapses provide a pathway for graded recurrent inhibition that could provide both lateral inhibition and self-inhibition; this lateral inhibition could contribute to olfactory discrimination. Both inhibitions could contribute to local damping of mitral cell excitability and to rhythmic activity of these cell populations. Thus, a remarkable set of new facts and insights resulted from this interaction between theory and experiment.

2.9.3 Voltage Clamp at the Soma of a Dendritic Neuron

Many labs now have the ability to voltage-clamp a neuron soma, but they are confronted with uncertainty about how far the effect extends into the dendrites, for steady conditions, for transient conditions, and for sinusoidal steady states. For any neuron whose specific geometry and membrane properties are known, this problem can be investigated with a compartmental model that incorporates all of the known complications. Nevertheless, a valuable idealized reference case is provided by assuming completely linear passive membrane properties and by assuming the soma to be isopotential, and that the dendrites can be represented by an equivalent cylinder. For this idealized case, analytical results and computed examples have been presented and discussed in a recent pub-

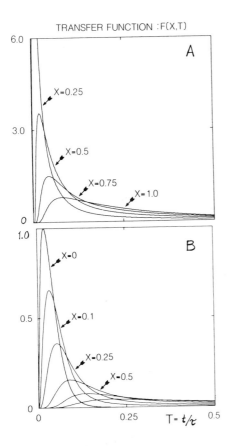

Figure 2.13
Transfer function (in A) and its convolution (in B) for voltage clamping at the soma of a passive soma-dendritic model with $L = 1.5$. Curves have two interpretations: (1) as the voltage transient, $V(X, T)$, at point X, in response to a voltage transient, $V(0, T)$, imposed by the voltage clamp at the soma, and (2) as the current transient, $I(0, T)$, detected by the voltage clamp at $X = 0$, for a synaptic current, $I_i(X, T)$, imposed at point X. In B, the imposed transient is the one labeled $X = 0$. In A, the imposed transient corresponds to a Dirac delta function. Details of equations and interpretations can be found in the original publication (Rall and Segev 1985).

lication (Rall and Segev 1985). Here we illustrate only the computed results shown in fig. 2.13.

If a voltage clamp imposes at the soma ($X = 0$) the voltage time course labeled $X = 0$ in the lower figure (fig. 2.13B), then, by computational convolution of this time course with the transfer functions illustrated in the upper figure (fig. 2.13A), one can predict the voltage time course to be expected at different electrotonic distances away from the soma, as illustrated here for $X = 0.1$, 0.25, 0.5, 0.75, and 1.0 in the lower figure, given a dendritic electrotonic length, $L = 1.5$, together with the idealized assumptions already stated. Similar results can be computed for different examples of imposed voltage time courses at the soma. Also, the voltage decrement with distance, for a voltage step at $X = 0, T = 0$, has been illustrated (fig. 3 of Rall and Segev 1985) for $T = 0.1$, 0.2, 0.5, 1.0, and ∞. These results make it clear that the dendritic membrane is not voltage-clamped, unless the value of L is very small.

Sometimes a voltage clamp at the soma is used to record a current transient that results from synaptic activity. If the synapse is located on the soma, the recorded current equals the synaptic current, except for possible limitations of the instrumentation, and with the qualification that the synaptic current generated by a conductance transient will be slightly different from normal, because of the constant driving potential provided by the voltage clamp compared with a varying driving potential under normal (unclamped) conditions. When the synapse is located on a dendritic branch, one should expect a significant discrepancy between the synaptic current generated at the input site and the current transient detected by the voltage clamp at the soma. As demonstrated and discussed by Rall and Segev (1985), that discrepancy can be defined quantitatively by the same transfer functions and convolutions already illustrated in fig. 2.13. Thus, the curves in the lower figure (for each labeled X value) give the predicted current transient at the somatic voltage clamp in response to synaptic current injected at each labeled value of X, assuming that the injected current time course is given by the curve labeled $X = 0$. These examples illustrate a theoretical basis for better experimental estimation of the synaptic current time course generated at dendritic synaptic locations. Theoretical expressions for sinusoidal steady states can also be found in Rall and Segev (1985).

The address of Wilfrid Rall is Mathematical Research Branch, Building 31, Room 4B-54, National Institutes of Health, Bethesda, Maryland 20892.

CHAPTER 3

Compartmental Models of Complex Neurons

IDAN SEGEV, JAMES W. FLESHMAN, and ROBERT E. BURKE

3.1 Introduction

A complete understanding of information processing at the level of an individual nerve cell requires detailed knowledge of both the anatomical structure and physiological properties of the neuron and its synapses, and a model of the cell that faithfully embodies this information. Several important technical and theoretical advances in the last thirty years have greatly enhanced such an understanding. The electron microscope enables identification of sites, sizes, and, to some extent, types of synapses on dendrites and cell bodies (Gray 1959). Intracellular labeling with horseradish peroxidase (HRP) permits the entire dendritic and axonal domain of nerve cells to be viewed in exquisite detail (Ulfhake and Kellerth 1981; Cullheim, Fleshman, Glenn, and Burke 1987). When combined with ultrastructural studies, this technique provides the most complete knowledge available on the synaptic architecture of neurons (e.g., Conradi, Kellerth, Berthold, and Hammarberg 1979; Kellerth, Berthold, and Conradi 1979; White and Rock 1983).

Recent progress in patch-clamping techniques and in developing voltage- and ion-dependent dyes and antibodies against specific membrane channels is yielding important information on membrane properties that cannot be obtained with conventional microelectrode techniques (e.g., measurement of voltages and channel properties in the membrane of dendrites remote from the cell body; Grinvald 1985; Ross and Werman 1987). Finally, the development of cable theory for dendritic trees by Rall (1959) and its recent extension using compartmental methods and powerful computers have made it possible to construct increasingly realistic models of several types of morphologically and physiologically characterized neurons (e.g., Lux, Schubert, and Kreutzberg 1970; Barrett and Crill 1974; Rall 1981; Brown, Fricke, and Perkel 1981; Koch, Poggio, and Torre 1982; Turner and Schwartzkroin 1984; Segev,

Fleshman, Miller, and Bunow 1985; Shelton 1985; Rall and Segev 1986;
Koch and Poggio 1987; Clements and Redman 1988; Fleshman, Segev,
and Burke 1988).

A nerve cell model is the quantitative embodiment of a set of measurements, guesses, and hypotheses and, as such, it can refine the intuitive
understanding of neuroelectric signal processing. The present chapter
is focused on describing the compartmental approach to modeling nerve
cells. We will briefly summarize the basic features and assumptions of
this class of models and demonstrate how they may be constructed using a widely available circuit simulation program. Examples illustrate
how one can map anatomical and physiological measures onto model
parameters and how such models can be used to constrain estimates of
essential parameters that cannot be measured experimentally.

3.2 Principles of Compartmental Neuron Models

3.2.1 Overview

The one-dimensional cable theory of neurons describes current flow in
a continuous passive dendritic tree using partial differential equations
(with the appropriate boundary conditions; see chapters 2 and 13).
These equations have straightforward analytical solutions for transient
current inputs to an idealized class of dendritic trees that are equivalent
to unbranched cylinders (equivalent cylinder; Rall 1959; Rall and Rinzel
1973; Rinzel and Rall 1974; Jack, Noble, and Tsien 1975). The solutions
are more complicated for passive dendritic trees with a general branching structure, where the voltage trajectory in response to an arbitrary
current injection can be computed recursively (Butz and Cowan 1974;
Horwitz 1981, 1983; Wilson 1984; Koch and Poggio 1985). These algorithms become more complex as well as computationally expensive when
the system is perturbed by *synaptic* currents produced by conductance
changes (Rinzel and Rall 1974; Poggio and Torre 1977; Koch et al. 1982;
Holmes 1986). When the membrane properties are *voltage-dependent*,
as is the case with membranes that show rectification or that support
action potentials, the analytical approach using linear cable theory is no
longer valid. As Rall pointed out early on, these complex cases must
be dealt with using compartmental rather than analytical models (Rall
1964).

In principle, the compartmental approach replaces the continuous differential equations of the analytical model by a set of ordinary differential equations. The assumption is that if the continuously distributed system is divided into sufficiently small segments (or compartments), one makes a negligibly small error by assuming that each compartment is isopotential and spatially uniform in its properties. Nonuniformity in physical properties (e.g., diameter, specific electric properties) and differences in potential occur *between* compartments rather than within them (Rall 1964; Perkel, Mulloney, and Budelli 1981).

A chain of three cylindrical dendritic segments that are sufficiently short to be considered isopotential is shown in fig. 3.1A. Assuming the membrane is passive, these segments may be represented by the equivalent circuit of fig. 3.1B. Focusing on the jth segment, one can see that the "resting" channels of the membrane are represented by a single resistor ($\hat{r}_{m_j}$) in parallel with a capacitive current path ($\hat{c}_{m_j}$) that models the dielectric properties of the lipid bilayer.[1] For convenience, the resting potential is taken to be zero and therefore the battery in series with channels that are open in the resting state is omitted. Adjacent compartments are connected by series resistances (r_j) representing the cytoplasm. It is assumed that the resistance of the extracellular medium is very low relative to r_j. Therefore the extracellular medium is assumed to be everywhere isopotential and is taken as ground. For further discussion of membrane models see Hodgkin and Katz (1949), Fatt and Katz (1953), and Rall (1964).

The advantage of the compartmental approach is that it places no restrictions on the membrane properties of each compartment. Compartments may represent somatic, dendritic, or axonal membrane; they may be passive or excitable and may contain a variety of synaptic inputs. In addition, arbitrarily complex dendritic and axonal branching structures and other morphological irregularities, such as spines, are readily represented in the topology of the compartmental connections. The compartmental approach permits great flexibility in the level of resolution. In this chapter we are concerned with relatively high resolution models, in which each compartment represents a few tens of microns of dendrite. The next chapter treats a single compartmental model with a very complex electrical structure. However, a compartment could also

---

[1] The symbols $\hat{r}_m$, $\hat{c}_m$, $\hat{r}_i$, and $\hat{i}_m$ are used throughout the chapter to represent *per compartment* values, as distinguished from r_m, c_m, r_i, and i_m, which are conventionally taken as *per unit length* values. "Resting" channels are the channels that are open at the resting potential.

A

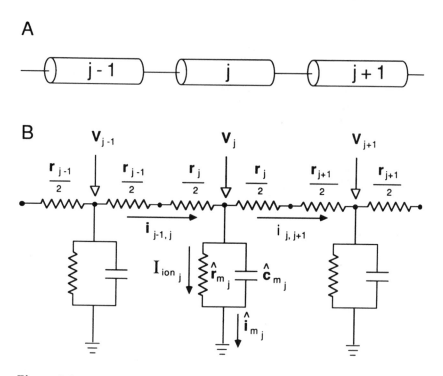

B

Figure 3.1
Equivalent circuit for a compartmental model of a chain of three successive small cylindrical segments of passive dendritic membrane. (A) The constant-diameter jth segment is assumed to be sufficiently short electrically that may be considered as isopotential. (B) The resting-membrane resistance and capacitance of that segment are lumped into one resistor, $\hat{r}_{mj}$ and one capacitor, $\hat{c}_{mj}$. The net current through the membrane is $\hat{i}_{mj}$. The axial resistance of the segment, r_j, is split in half and the membrane $R - C$ elements are placed in between. Membrane potential (V_j) is defined as the displacement from the resting potential. It is assumed that the resistivity of the extracellular medium may be taken as zero, hence the connection of the extracellular side of the membrane $R - C$ to ground. For simplicity, the resting potential is taken as zero, eliminating the need for a battery in series with the membrane resistance. The term $I_{ion,j}$ represents transmembrane ionic current in the jth compartment. Longitudinal resistance between compartment j and $j+1$ (denoted in the text as $r_{j,j+1}$) is the sum of half the longitudinal resistance of segment j and half the longitudinal resistance of segment $j + 1$ (i.e., $r_{j,j+1} = (r_j + r_{j+1})/2$). The corresponding longitudinal current through this resistance is designated as $i_{j,j+1}$.

be designed to represent a complete neuron for use in connectionist network models (e.g., see chapters 9 and 10).

While the compartmental approach has many advantages for neural modeling, it should be regarded as a complement to analytical models derived from Rall's cable theory (chapter 2). Many insights and initial evaluations of key parameters can be obtained by first applying the analytical approach to simplified and idealized approximations of the neuron or neurons under study. Based on these approximations, a subsequent, more detailed compartmental model can be constructed and used to refine the analytical results (see section 3.3 below).

3.2.2   Mathematical Formulation

As mentioned above, the mathematical consequence of compartmental models of neurons is a system of ordinary differential equations (or a corresponding set of difference equations), one for each compartment. Each equation is derived from Kirchhoff's current law, which states that in each compartment, j, the net current through the membrane, $\hat{\imath}_{m_j}$, must equal the longitudinal current that enters that compartment minus the longitudinal current that leaves it (fig. 3.1B). For an unbranched region, where the jth compartment lies between the $j-1$th and the $j+1$th compartments, the membrane current is:

$$\hat{\imath}_{m_j} = i_{j-1,j} - i_{j,j+1} \tag{3.1}$$

where $i_{j-1,j}$ is the longitudinal current that flows from compartment $j-1$ to j and $i_{j,j+1}$ is the current that flows from compartment j to $j+1$ (fig. 3.1B).

The equivalent circuit shows that the membrane current is the sum of capacitative current and the net ionic current (I_{ion}) that flows through the transmembrane resistive pathways ($\hat{r}_m$). For the jth compartment, the membrane current can be expressed as:

$$\hat{\imath}_{m_j} = \hat{c}_{m_j} \frac{dV_j}{dt} + I_{ion_j} \tag{3.2}$$

where V_j is the membrane potential measured with respect to the resting potential. For compartments that are stimulated by an external current source (e.g., an electrode), an additional term (I_{stim}) must be added to the membrane current. The longitudinal current can be described as the voltage gradient between directly connected compartments divided by the axial resistance between these compartments. Thus eq. 3.1 can be rewritten as:

$$\hat{c}_{m_j} \frac{dV_j}{dt} + I_{ion_j} + I_{stim_j} = \frac{V_{j-1} - V_j}{r_{j-1,j}} - \frac{V_j - V_{j+1}}{r_{j,j+1}} \qquad (3.3)$$

or:

$$\hat{c}_{m_j} \frac{dV_j}{dt} + I_{ion_j} + I_{stim_j} = (V_{j-1} - V_j)g_{j-1,j} - (V_j - V_{j+1})g_{j,j+1} \quad (3.4)$$

where $r_{j-1,j}$ (or $1/g_{j-1,j}$) is the axial resistance (conductance) between the $j-1$th and the jth compartments. For the parent compartment at a branch point, current flow into the two daughter branches is represented by adding a second expression that is identical to the right-hand side of eqs. 3.3 and 3.4, with appropriate subscripts to identify the daughter branches (fig. 1 of Parnas and Segev 1979). For the first and last compartments in a chain, only the first term for the longitudinal current appears on the right-hand side of the equations.

The transient solution of eqs. 3.3 and 3.4 (i.e., the values of $V_j(t)$ for $j = 1, \ldots, N$, where N is the number of compartments in the model) depends critically on the description of I_{ion}. This term can embody the properties of the many types of channels in neural membranes and may have a mathematical description that ranges from simple to very complex. The following section divides ion channels into three distinct classes and presents their general formal description together with the corresponding membrane models. More detailed descriptions can be found in chapters 4, 5, and 6.

3.2.3   Membrane Models

The conductive branches in fig. 3.2 summarize the three basic classes of ionic channels that are found in nerve membrane: *passive* or *leak*, *synaptic*, and *active* channels. From a modeling viewpoint, the simplest class of membrane channels is the passive channels. Passive membrane is electrically represented by a constant (time- and voltage-independent) transmembrane conductance (g_{leak}; left branch in equivalent circuit of fig. 3.2) in series with a fixed voltage source (E_{leak}) that designates the reversal potential of the passive channels. The ionic current through this branch obeys Ohm's law and can be expressed simply as:

$$I_{leak} = g_{leak}(V - E_{leak}) \qquad (3.5)$$

Other membrane channels may be controlled by the presence of external or internal chemical agents (e.g., neurotransmitters or second messengers). Synaptic channels change their conductance to a certain ion, or ions, when the appropriate chemical stimulus binds to the receptor

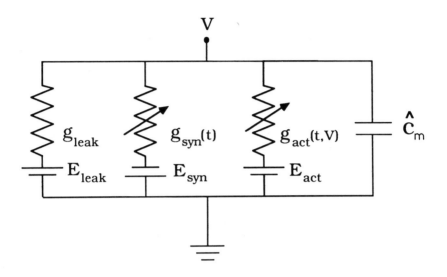

Figure 3.2
Equivalent circuit model of isopotential patch of nerve membrane that consists of the three basic classes of transmembrane channels. The left-most branch represents ohmic leak channels in the patch. It consists of a constant conductance, g_{leak}, in series with a constant battery (E_{leak}) through which the passive ionic current flows. Synaptic (chemically gated) channels are represented by the middle time-varying branch (g_{syn}) which is in series with a battery (E_{syn}), representing the reversal potential of the synaptic processes. Active channels are represented by the rightmost resistive branch. A time- and voltage-dependent resistor (g_{act}) is in series with a battery (E_{act}) whose value is the equilibrium potential of the ionic species involved (Na^+, K^+, Ca^{2+}, etc.).

associated with these channels. Synaptic membrane is most simply modeled as a time-dependent, but voltage-independent, conductive pathway (g_{syn}) in series with a constant voltage source (E_{syn}), which is the reversal potential of the ionic species involved (Rall 1964, 1967).[2] One convenient expression for such a time-varying conductance change is based on the "alpha function" (Rall 1967; Jack et al. 1975) and has the form $g_{syn}(t) = \alpha T e^{-\alpha T}$, where $\alpha = \tau_m/t_{peak}$, $T = t/\tau_m$, τ_m is the membrane time constant (see below), and t_{peak} is the time-to-peak of the conductance transient. The middle conductive branch of fig. 3.2 shows the electrical representation of this class of channels. The synaptic current that flows through this (nonlinear) branch is:

$$I_{syn}(t) = g_{syn}(t)(V(t) - E_{syn}) \tag{3.6}$$

The rightmost conductive branch in fig. 3.2 represents the class of voltage-dependent channels. This branch consists of a voltage source (E_{act}) in series with a *voltage-* and *time-dependent* conductance, $g_{act}(t, V)$, through which the active current flows. The equation describing this current has the same form as the synaptic current in eq. 3.6, with g_{act} and E_{act} replacing g_{syn} and E_{syn}, respectively. Depending on the description of g_{act}, this class of nonlinear channels may produce membrane responses that mimic various sorts of subthreshold membrane rectification or action potentials (Hodgkin and Huxley 1952; Nagumo, Arimoto, and Yoshizawa 1962; FitzHugh 1969; Adams et al. 1986; and chapters 4 and 5 below).

The total membrane current through a patch of membrane that has all three types of ionic channels is the sum of all those currents plus the capacitive current:

$$\hat{i}_m = \hat{c}_m \tfrac{dV}{dt} + g_{leak}(V - E_{leak}) + g_{syn}(V - E_{syn}) \\ + g_{act}(V - E_{act}) \tag{3.7}$$

Combining this equation with eq. 3.4 for the jth compartment (without the stimulus current) and rearranging, the following general form is ob-

---

[2]Some chemical synapses are also voltage-dependent, such as the NMDA receptors (Mayer, Westbrook, and Guthrie 1984; Jahr and Stevens 1987), which are believed to underly the synaptic plasticity (for a discussion of their role in computation see Koch 1987). The assumption that E_{syn} is constant is valid only if the specificity of the channel to the different ions that flow though it is time-independent. For example, a channel that carries both sodium and potassium (i.e., $g_{syn}(t) = g_{Na}(t) + g_K(t)$) can be modeled as a conductive branch with a fixed battery (whose value lies between the Nernst potential values of E_{Na} and E_K) only if the ratio $g_{Na}(t)/g_K(t)$ remains constant throughout the conductance change.

tained for the system of differential equations that are associated with compartmental models:

$$\hat{c}_m \frac{dV_j}{dt} = g_{j-1,j}V_{j-1} - (g_{leak_j} + g_{syn_j} + g_{act_j} + g_{j-1,j} + g_{j,j+1})V_j$$
$$+ g_{j,j+1}V_{j+1} + g_{leak_j}E_{leak_j} + g_{syn_j}E_{syn_j} + g_{act_j}E_{act_j} \quad (3.8)$$

Note that within each of the basic classes of channels there may be several subtypes, for example, active channels that carry Na^+ or K^+ or Ca^{2+} ions, each with its own voltage and time dependencies (see chapter 4 and Hille 1985 for a summary of the properties of different channels).

3.2.4   Methods and Approaches

We have demonstrated that the mathematical consequence of a compartmental approach to nerve cell models is a set, or matrix, of coupled, first-order differential equations of the form given by eq. 3.8. They can also be written as a matrix differential equation of the form

$$\dot{V} = A\vec{V} + \vec{b} \quad (3.9)$$

where $\vec{V}$ is the unknown vector of membrane potentials of the different compartments ($\vec{V} = $ col $(V_1, V_2, \ldots, V_N)$), $\dot{V}$ is the time derivative of V, A is a matrix composed of the coefficients, and $\vec{b}$ is a column vector consisting of the products of batteries and conductances. For constant coefficients, a linear system of equations is obtained and classical numerical methods can be employed to invert matrix A and directly obtain the required transient solution (Hearon 1963; Rall 1964; Perkel et al. 1981). However, when the coefficients are not fixed, as is the case with synaptic perturbation and with active (nonlinear) currents, matrix A and vector b change from instant to instant. For these cases one usually replaces the matrix differential equations with a corresponding matrix of difference equations and employs numerical methods (e.g., linearization, direct elimination, integration, etc.; for more details see Rall 1964; Parnas and Segev 1979; Carnevale and Lebeda 1987). We will not discuss these methods any further and point the interested reader to chapters 4, 7, and 13. We would like to note that a common feature of all matrix representations of multicompartmental neuron models is that they are very sparse, that is, most of the matrix terms are zero. Thus, any numerical approach to the solution should utilize sparse matrix algorithms that only store and operate on nonzero terms. This will increase the efficiency of the computation and allow solution of very large systems of equations.

There are two ways to approach the solution of such systems. One may write a computer program designed to solve a specific set of equations (see, e.g., Perkel et al. 1981; Carnevale and Lebeda 1987) or one may use a more generalized equation-solving or modeling system (e.g., Rall 1964, using the SAAM program by Bergman, Shahn, and Weiss; Shepherd and Brayton 1979, using IBM-ASTAP; Segev et al. 1985, using SPICE; Flach, Carnevale and Sussman-Fort 1987, using SABER). The first approach allows one to tailor the program to the needs of the particular model, which could result in significant savings in computer resources. Furthermore, for certain compartmental models it may be possible to obtain an analytical solution. In these cases the behavior of the system can be understood in terms of the parameters that govern it (e.g., the time constants that determine transient response; see Perkel et al. 1981 for analytical approaches to compartmental models). Examples of compartmental models designed and implemented for specific neuronal systems can be found in Cooley and Dodge (1966); Rall and Shepherd (1968); Moore et al. (1975); Perkel and Mulloney (1978a,b); Segev and Parnas (1979); Koch, Poggio and Torre (1982); Traub and Wong (1983); Shelton (1985); Clements and Redman (1988); see also the following programs: NODUS (De Schutter 1986, 1988); DENDR (MacGregor 1987); AXON-TREE, (Manor and Segev, in preparation).

The use of more general-purpose computer programs in neural modeling will likely be less efficient than custom-designed programs in terms of computer time, but they offer at least three advantages. First, one does not have to write the program oneself. Second, since such programs are not designed with any specific model in mind, one can easily accommodate new data and ask new questions without having to rewrite and debug additional code. Third, a number of modeling packages are available that run on computer systems that range from PCs to engineering workstations, minicomputers, mainframes, and even supercomputers. This makes it easier to share data and models and may allow one to take advantage of computer resources best matched to the complexity of the modeling problem.

Computer programs have long been used to design and test electrical circuits (e.g., NET2, ADVICE, ASTAP, SCEPTRE) and, as first suggested by Shepherd and Brayton (1979), it was natural to investigate their utility in constructing compartmental models of nerve cells. Most circuit simulation programs share the same basic structure. The input data describes the electrical elements (resistors, capacitors, diodes, batteries, etc.) and their interconnections, in pictorial or list form. An analysis subprogram performs one or more of several possible types of analysis (e.g., transient, DC, or AC). This portion of the program translates the circuit description into a system of equations and computes the numerical solution. For neuronal modeling one typically performs a transient analysis, as one does experimentally, in which the time-domain response of the system is computed at discrete time steps, Δt, over a specified interval, $0, \ldots, T$. AC analysis may be used to describe model behavior in the frequency domain (see experimental studies by Smith, Wuerker, and Frank 1967; Nelson and Lux 1970; Fox and Chan 1985; Hateren 1986; and modeling studies by Guthrie and Westbrook 1984, Rall and Segev 1985, and Segev et al. 1985). Finally, an output subprogram provides the results of the analysis in the form of a tabulation or a graph.

One of the most popular programs of this type is called SPICE, originally developed in the Department of Electrical Engineering and Computer Science at the University of California at Berkeley (Vladimirescu, Zhang, Newton, Pederson, and Sangiovani 1981). SPICE is capable of simulating very large systems of linear and nonlinear compartments (numbering perhaps in the thousands) that may be required in order to build fine-grained models of large, highly branched cells with complex membrane properties, such as spinal cord α-motoneurons (Bunow, Segev, and Fleshman 1985; Segev et al. 1985; Fleshman, Segev, and Burke 1988). We will show below that programs like SPICE provide neurobiologists with very powerful and useful tools to construct and investigate the behavior of models that describe the properties of neural systems in considerable detail.

Versions of SPICE are available for a nominal fee for several mini- and mainframe computers, including DEC VAX (VMS and UNIX), CDC Cyber, IBM 370, and Cray (contact the EECS Department at UC Berkeley for details). In addition, there are several SPICE-based programs that incorporate additional circuit design and graphic display capabilities (available commercially for greater-than-nominal fees) for personal computers and workstations, as well as larger machines (e.g., "PC Workbench" and "Analog Workbench" from Analog Design Tools; "I-G Spice" from AB Associates; "IS-Spice" from Intusoft; "P-Spice" from Microsim). In later sections we will outline the principles of the SPICE language and in Appendix 3.A we present a complete example of the use of SPICE to model the network in fig. 3.3C.

3.3   From Morphology to Model

In the remainder of this chapter we illustrate the process of transforming an anatomically reconstructed neuron into a compartmental model.
We start with the problem of measuring and encoding neuron morphology, then move from the structure of neurons to the structure of
a SPICE input file and show how the coded structure of a neuron can
be transformed into electrically lumped *passive* compartments. Rall's cable theory for passive dendrites is used to estimate specific parameters
in neurons for which both anatomical and physiological measurements
are available. Computational examples are presented for excitatory and
inhibitory synaptic input. Finally, building models of active compartments is considered.

3.3.1   Encoding Neuron Morphology

If the research question requires a compartmental model that faithfully
represents the details of neuron morphology, then appropriate morpho-
metric data must be obtained. Typically, this involves staining a single
cell with HRP and reconstructing it from serial sections (e.g., Barret
and Crill 1974; Lux et al. 1970; Kellerth and Ulfhake 1981; Cullheim
et al. 1987). The dimensions of the soma and the lengths and diameters of all the dendritic and axonal branches are then measured. For
purposes of the reconstruction and measurement as well as the subsequent computer simulation, it is useful to have a system of nomenclature
that uniquely defines the location of every segment of the cell topology
(see fig. 3.3 and examples in Rall 1959, Segev et al. 1985). The number of segments necessary to represent an entire neuron depends on the
morphology of the cell and on numerical considerations that will be discussed below. In the case of complicated dendritic trees, such as those
of spinal α-motoneurons (Barrett and Crill 1974; Fleshman et al. 1988)
and cerebellar purkinje cells (Shelton 1985), hundreds or even thousands
of anatomical segments may be needed to represent neuronal morphology accurately. For less extensively branched cells, such as the spine-less
vagus motoneurons, a few dozen segments are sufficient (Nitzan, Yarom,
and Segev, in preparation). There are tradeoffs among the number of
compartments used in a model, the amount of error one can tolerate, and
the amount of computer memory and time required to do the analyses.
This problem is discussed in more detail in Segev et al. (1985).

   It is important to note that the process of making quantitative measurements of neuron morphology necessarily involves at least three types
of errors. First, there are limitations in the staining techniques (incom-

plete filling of the cell with HRP, for instance, or shrinkage of the tissue during fixation). Second, there are inherent limits in any measuring method that discretizes a continuous structure. Third, it is necessary to choose geometrical entities (e.g., spheres, cylinders, cones) to represent the irregularly shaped neuronal segments. Discussion of these points may be found in Rall (1959), Segev et al. (1985), Cullheim et al. (1986), Clements and Redman (1988), and Fleshman et al. (1988). For the present demonstration it is assumed that measurements of cell morphology are trustworthy, that dendritic and axonal segments are adequately represented by short cylinders, and that the soma is reasonably modeled by an isopotential ellipsoid.

Figures 3.3A and 3.3B show an example of the process of decomposing a stained neuronal structure into geometrical subunits. A camera lucida drawing of the two-dimensional projection of a three-dimensional HRP-filled dendrite and soma of a guinea pig vagal motoneuron is shown in fig. 3.3A. Dendritic lengths were corrected for the thickness of the histological sections using the Pythagorean rule; diameters were measured at the midpoint of each segment (see also Cullheim et al. 1987). As shown, dendrite diameters were not necessarily uniform between branch points. Therefore it was necessary to choose a criterion for segmenting the dendrites. In the example illustrated, whenever the diameter of a dendritic segment changed by more than 0.2 μm, it was replaced by two segments (segmentation is shown by crossing lines on dendrite in panel A). Using this sampling rule, 12 segments were needed to represent the relatively simple dendrite of fig. 3.3A and one more was used for the soma. The compartmental representation of this structure by geometrical entities (cylinders and an ellipsoid) is shown in panel B. The corresponding electrical circuit equivalent of this anatomical segmentation is given in panel C. We used a system of nomenclature similar to the one used by Segev et al. (1985) to label the circuit nodes in fig. 3.3C. The first digit in the node number is the branch order (1 to 3 in this case). The second digit is the branch number, which, for binary branching, will vary from 0 to $2^{m-1} - 1$, where m is branch order. Parent branch number k will have daughter branches numbered $2k$ and $2k + 1$. The third digit is the segment number starting at 0 for the most proximal segment. The soma compartment in our convention is assigned node number 1.

3.3.2   Circuit Simulation Using SPICE

A main part of our goal is to embody anatomical data in a format that can be acted on by the SPICE program. This section provides a brief overview of the structure and formalisms of the SPICE input format.

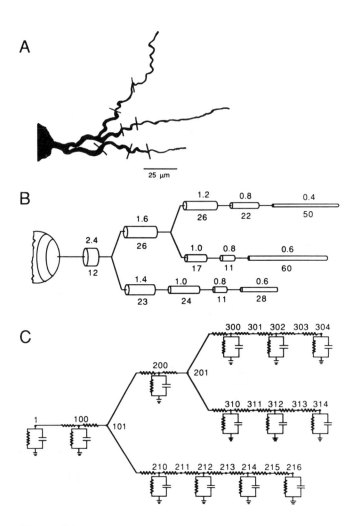

Figure 3.3
Stages in abstraction from an anatomical dendritic tree to an electrical circuit analog.
(A) Two-dimensional projection of part of the soma and one dendrite of a vagus
motoneuron in the guinea pig. Points at which unbranched dendrites were broken
into successive cylindrical segments are indicated by lines. (B) Representation of the
same dendrite as a branched system of cylindrical segments, indicating the length
(below) and diameter (above) of each dendritic segment (in μm). Diameters are not
drawn to the same scale as the lengths, but both are in the correct proportions.
The motoneuron soma (shown partially) had a maximum diameter of 20 μm and
minimum diameter of 15 μm. (C) Circuit analog of B (see fig. 3.1) showing the
pattern of connections at branch points and the numbers assigned to circuit nodes
within (even numbers) and between (odd numbers) successive segments.

The input file is a text file that contains the circuit description (network list) and control statements. The network list describes the type, value, and connections of every electrical element in the circuit, one element per line. Each circuit element must have a unique name, the first letter of which identifies the element type (e.g., R for resistors, C for capacitors, I for independent current sources, etc.). Connections are specified using positive integer node numbers. Node 0 is reserved for ground. Element values may be given in integer or floating point format, or by SPICE mnemonics that indicate powers of 10 (e.g., $P = 10^{-12}$, $N = 10^{-9}$, $U = 10^{-6}$, $M = 10^{-3}$, $MEG = 10^6$). An example is given below of an $R - C$ circuit comprised of a 1 $M\Omega$ resistor and a 1 nF capacitor connected between node 1 and ground which receives a current pulse with an initial value of 0, a pulse value of 1 nA, delay time of 0.5 $msec$, 0 $msec$ rise and fall times, and a duration of 0.2 $msec$:

```
RM   1 0 1MEG
CM   1 0 1NF
IP   0 1 PULSE 0 1NA 0.5MS 0 0 0.2MS
```

Note that the "F" in NF and the "S" in MS above are for the convenience of the user and have no meaning to SPICE. Control statements start with a period in the first column, for example:

```
.TRAN 50US 5MS
.PRINT TRAN V(1)
```

The first statement directs SPICE to perform a transient analysis computing the results at time increments no longer than 50 μsec for a total analysis period of 5 $msec$ (101 time points). The second statement specifies that SPICE is to print the value of the voltage at node 1 at each time point. A SPICE input file must start with a title line and end with a .END line. Those additions to the five lines above would constitute a valid input file.

A limitation in the generic SPICE program is that it provides only predefined elements and functions. There is no direct way to define arbitrary functions. This limitation makes SPICE numerically robust with good convergence properties, but the program is somewhat cumbersome when simulating membrane nonlinearities with specific voltage and time dependencies. There are at least two possible "work-arounds" for the absence of user-defined functions. One can either approximate the desired function using polynomials or piecewise linear functions, which may be defined in SPICE, or one can design an electrical circuit whose output is the desired function (just as one would use an analog computer to solve

differential equations). We have used the latter approach to produce an
"alpha-shaped" conductance transient that represents chemical synaptic
input (Segev et al. 1985). A similar approach was also used to represent
the Hodgkin-Huxley equations in SPICE format (Bunow et al. 1985).
The synapse circuit is described below.

We would like to produce an alpha function of the form

$$V(t) = Ate^{-t/t_{peak}} \qquad\qquad (3.10)$$

where t_{peak} is the time-to-peak of the function and A has units of V/sec.
This equation is the solution of the differential equation

$$\frac{dV}{dt} = -\frac{1}{t_{peak}}V + Ae^{-t/t_{peak}}; \quad V(0) = 0 \qquad\qquad (3.11)$$

One can "rewrite" this equation using electrical elements as follows:

```
C1dV/dt     =     -V/R1     +    I1(EXP(-t/T1))
Capacitive        Resistive       Exponential
 current           current         current
```

Matching the parameters of eq. 3.10 with the corresponding SPICE pseu-
docode above requires that t_{peak} = R1C1 = T1 and A = I1/C1. The
SPICE input file that implements this circuit equation is:

```
R1 5000        0  0.2MEG
C1 5000        0  1NF
I1   0      5000  EXP 0 1 0.6MS 0 0 0.2MS
```

The EXP function creates an exponential waveform, just as the PULSE
function used above specifies a rectangular waveform. In the example,
the output current has an initial value of 0. After a delay of 0.6 $msec$
the current instantaneously rises to 1 A (zero rise-time) and immediately
(zero duration) begins to decay with an exponential time course (fall-
time constant = 0.2 $msec$). This exponentially decaying current causes
a rapid rise in voltage across C1, reaching its peak 0.2 $msec$ after onset,
followed by a slower decay. The time course of this potential will represent the so-called alpha-shaped conductance transient, $g_{syn}(t)$ in the
synapse circuit below (see also eq. 3.6). From eq. 3.10, the peak value of
this potential is $V(t_{peak}) = At_{peak}e^{-1} = (I1/C1)T1/e = 7.36 \times 10^4 \ V$.

The next step is to use this voltage source to produce a synaptic
current, $I_{syn}(t)$. As described in eq. 3.6, the synaptic current is the
product of $g_{syn}(t)$ and the synaptic driving potential. The arithmetic in
eq. 3.6 may be accomplished in SPICE using a "G" element, a voltage-
dependent current source, with two pairs of controlling nodes: (1) the

alpha function, and (2) the synaptic driving potential. In the examples above, the alpha function appears between nodes 5000 and 0. The driving potential is the difference between the synaptic reversal potential, represented by a battery connected at node 6000, and the membrane potential at the synaptic site, which is node 1 in this example. The necessary elements are shown in SPICE format below:

```
VSYN  6000    0   DC 100MV
GSYN    1 6000   POLY(2) 5000 0  1 6000  0 0 0 0 0.068P
```

In the GSYN element, POLY(2) indicates a polynomial in two variables. The variables are the voltages at the controlling nodes, V(5000,0) and V(1,6000). The coefficients of the polynomial term are given by the last five numbers of the GSYN element line. The only non-zero coefficient, $p_4 = 0.068 \times 10^{-12}$, is for the product of the two controlling nodes.

The product of p_4 and the alpha function voltage between node 5000 and zero is the conductance, $g_{syn}(t)$, in units of Siemens. Thus the peak conductance is $0.068 \times 10^{-12} \times 7.36 \times 10^4 = 5 \ nS$, which is the nominal conductance change produced at the single boutons in the cat group Ia–motoneuron synapse, according to Finkel and Redman (1983). This quantity times the driving potential, given by $V(1, 6000)$, is the synaptic current, given exactly in the form of eq. 3.6. Now it is very easy to add more "synapses" identical to the one above at different points in the circuit. Let us say, for example, that we wish to add one synapse at node 2 and two synapses at node 3. Only two additional lines need be added to the input file:

```
GSYN2    2 6000   POLY(2) 5000 0  2 6000  0 0 0 0 0.068P
GSYN3    3 6000   POLY(2) 5000 0  3 6000  0 0 0 0 0.136P
```

The approach described above may be used to create different classes of synapses, for example synapses with differing reversal potentials to represent excitatory and inhibitory synapses or differing in time course or peak conductance. Each synapse type requires an additional group of five SPICE lines: three to produce the desired alpha function and two for the battery and G element. These synapses can be connected to different nodes in the circuit by writing additional G elements, which differ only in name, since element names must be unique, and in their points of attachment to the circuit representing the postsynaptic cell.

3.3.3   Translating Physiological and Anatomical Measurements into a SPICE Input File

Figures 3.1–3.3 show schematically how neuronal structures are transformed and represented as compartmental models, but the electrical elements in these figures have no values specified. How do we assign realistic values to the different resistive and capacitive elements in the model? Obviously, the behavior of the model depends critically on the electrical characterization of its elements.

For the purposes of the following exercise, we assume that the cell is in a resting state, that the membrane conductance is passive, and that the specific electrical properties of the membrane and cytoplasm are identical everywhere in the cell. If one knows the value of the specific membrane resistance (R_m in Ωcm^2) and membrane capacity (C_m in $\mu F/cm^2$), and the specific cytoplasmic resistivity (R_i in Ωcm), it is possible to calculate the value of the (lumped) membrane resistance ($\hat{r}_m$ in Ω) and capacitance ($\hat{c}_m$ in F) and the cytoplasmic resistance ($\hat{r}_i$ in Ω) for each segment in the model. From the relations given by Rall (1977):

$$\hat{r}_m = \frac{R_m}{A}$$

$$\hat{c}_m = C_m \times A \qquad\qquad\qquad (3.12)$$

$$\hat{r}_i = \frac{4R_i}{\pi d^2} \times \ell$$

where A is the membrane area of the segment ($\pi d\ell$ for a cylindrical segment with diameter d and length ℓ and πd_S^2 for a spherical soma with diameter d_S). For example, the area of the soma in fig. 3.3 is 1060 μm^2. Assuming values of $C_m = 1$ $\mu F/cm^2$ and $R_m = 5000$ Ωcm^2, the soma $\hat{r}_m$ is 471.7 $M\Omega$ and the soma $\hat{c}_m$ is 10.6 pF. For the same specific membrane properties, assuming $R_i = 70$ Ωcm, the values for the terminal segment at node 216 in fig. 3.3C ($d = 0.6$ μm and $\ell = 28$ μm) are $\hat{r}_m = 9473.52$ $M\Omega$, $\hat{c}_m = 0.53$ pF, and $\hat{r}_i = 34.66$ $M\Omega$ (see SPICE input file representation for this compartment in Appendix 3.A).

To minimize lumping errors, the electrical length of a compartment, ℓ/λ, should not be too long. Based on comparison of SPICE computations to corresponding analytical results, Segev et al. (1985) suggested, as a rule of thumb, that if the anatomical segmentation resulted in compartments greater than 0.2 λ, they should be subdivided into shorter compartments, with appropriate changes in element values and node numbers.

How can we obtain estimates of the specific values R_m, C_m, and R_i? Linear cable theory permits some relevant information to be extracted from experimental recordings of membrane voltage during current stimulation. The simplest measure one can obtain is the steady-state input resistance (R_N) measured from the cell body. This is done by injecting a current pulse (usually in the hyperpolarizing direction) that is long relative to the membrane time constant (see below), and sufficiently small so as not to evoke nonlinear membrane responses. The resultant voltage change can be measured directly or from the change in the amplitude of a superimposed antidromic spike. In either case, the ratio of the voltage change to the current injected is a measure of R_N (Frank and Fuortes 1956). It is also possible to measure the membrane time constant ($\tau_m = R_m C_m$) by analyzing the transient voltage decay following a current pulse using the peeling method as suggested by Rall (1969), and discussed in section 2.6.2. This method is based on the general solution of the cable equation, which shows that, in any passive system (with no voltage clamp, short circuit, or injury), the voltage decay following a long current pulse can be expressed as the sum of an infinite series of decaying exponentials:

$$V(t) = C_0 e^{-t/\tau_0} + C_1 e^{-t/\tau_1} + C_2 e^{t/\tau_2} + \cdots \qquad (3.13)$$

where $\tau_0 > \tau_1 > \tau_2 > \ldots$ and $\tau_0 = \tau_m$. The coefficients, C_0, C_1, etc., depend on the initial distribution of membrane potential and on the point of observation, but not on time (Rall 1969, and see chapter 2). Thus, given an experimental membrane voltage transient of the form described in eq. 3.13, it is possible to recover the longest time constant, τ_m, from the "tail" of the decay curve using a semilogarithmic plot of the voltage. Under favorable conditions (good signal-to-noise ratio; linear membrane response) it is also possible to separate one or two additional "equalizing" time constants (τ_1 and τ_2) by successive "peeling" of linear portions of the transient. The ratio of time constants can be used to estimate overall electrotonic length (see Rall 1969 for details; see Burke and Ten Bruggencate 1971, and Fleshman et al. 1988, for application of the technique to cat spinal α-motoneurons).

With these measurements of R_N and τ_m, and under the assumption that C_m is approximately 1 $\mu F/cm^2$ (Cole 1968) and that R_m is uniform over the cell surface, it is possible to estimate R_m and R_i for any particular morphology. R_m may be calculated from the experimentally measured membrane time constant, noting that $R_m = \tau_m/C_m$. With this R_m value one can then calculate the value of R_i that matches the experimental R_N value using the algorithm derived by Rall (1959).

Briefly, this algorithm permits one to compute the input conductance
(G_{in}) at the proximal (somatic) side of a cylindrical dendritic segment
if one knows or assumes the output conductance at the distal end of
the segment (G_{out}), the length (ℓ) and diameter (d) of the segment, and
values for R_m and R_i:[3]

$$G_{in} = G_\infty \frac{(G_{out}/G_\infty) + \tanh(\ell/\lambda)}{1 + (G_{out}/G_\infty)\tanh(\ell/\lambda)} \tag{3.14}$$

where G_∞ is the input conductance of a semi-infinite cylinder of diameter
d ($G_\infty = \pi/2(R_m R_i)^{-1/2}d^{3/2}$) and λ is the space (or length) constant
of that cylinder ($\lambda = ((d/4)(R_m/R_i))^{1/2}$).

The calculation begins at the dendritic terminal segments and proceeds proximally to the soma in an iterative manner as follows:

1. Assume a set of boundary conditions at the terminal segments.
   We will assume sealed end boundary conditions, implying that
   $G_{out} = 0$.

2. Calculate the input conductance at the proximal end of terminal
   segment j from eq. 3.14. For the sealed-end case, $G_{in_j} = G_{\infty_j} \times$
   $\tanh(\ell_j/\lambda_j)$.

3. If there is no branch point at the proximally adjacent segment,
   $j - 1$, then $G_{out_{j-1}}$ is equal to G_{in_j}. $G_{in_{j-1}}$ is calculated from
   eq. 3.14, using appropriate values of ℓ and d, and therefore G_∞
   and λ.

4. If there is a branch point, G_{out} for the parent branch is the sum
   of the G_{in} of the two (distal) daughter branches. Using this value
   of G_{out}, G_{in} of the parent branch is calculated as above.

5. These processes are repeated for all branches of the ith dendritic
   tree until one reaches the soma, at which point one has calculated
   the input conductance of the entire tree, G_{in_i}. The input conductance of the whole neuron, G_N, is then simply:

---

[3] The algorithm for computing R_N is applicable for any passive structure. The
specific electrical characteristics need not be the same in all segments (Rall 1959; see
also Fleshman et al. 1988). A similar algorithm can be used to calculate the input
resistance at any point in the tree, as well as the transfer resistance between any two
points (see Miller and Bloomfield 1983; Schierwagen 1986). The algorithm is also
applicable to the frequency (Laplace) domain, enabling one to calculate the input
and transfer impedance in a complex passive tree for any specified input frequency
(Lux 1967; Rall and Rinzel 1973; Barret and Crill 1974; Glasser, Miller, Xuong, and
Selverston 1977; Koch and Poggio 1985; Rall and Segev 1985).

$$G_N = G_S + \sum_{i=1}^{K} G_{in_i} \tag{3.15}$$

where K is the number of dendritic trees (including the axon), G_S is soma conductance ($1/\hat{r}_m$ of soma),[4] and $G_N = 1/R_N$. For a given R_m value, there is only one value of R_i that will match the computed R_N with the experimentally measured value.

If the experimental data are adequate, it is possible to use the higher-order time constants and their coefficients to estimate two other important parameters that help define the electrotonic structure of a neuron: electrotonic length and the dendritic to somatic conductance ratio. These parameters can help to refine the initial estimates of the specific electrical properties. In addition, the size and shape of experimentally recorded synaptic potentials can also be useful in validating these estimates. Discussion of these possibilities is beyond the scope of this chapter, but may be found in Rall (1967), Rall, Burke, Smith, Nelson, and Frank (1967), Rall (1969), Jack and Redman (1971), Jack et al. (1975), Brown et al. (1981), Rall (1982), Durant, Carlen, Gurevich, Ho, and Kunov (1983), Redman and Walmsley (1983), Bloomfield, Hamos, and Sherman (1987), Crunelli, Kelly, Leresheche, and Pirchio (1987), and Fleshman et al. (1988).

3.3.4 Simulation of Synaptic Input

The preceding sections have illustrated how data gathered using intracellular recording, stimulating, and staining techniques can be used to construct a computer model of a dendritic neuron with passive membrane properties. Figure 3.3A shows a reconstruction of the cell body and one of seven dendrites of a vagal motoneuron. Using the methods and assumptions described above, the specific membrane parameters determined as above for this cell were: $R_m = 5000 \ \Omega cm^2$ (with $C_m = 1 \ \mu F/cm^2$) and $R_i = 70 \ \Omega cm$ (Nitzan, Yarom, and Segev, in preparation). Using these values, and with a measured soma area of $1060 \ \mu m^2$ and the dendritic dimensions given in fig. 3.3B, a SPICE file for this dendrite was constructed and is listed in Appendix 3.A.

In addition to the 13 passive compartments comprising the dendrite and soma, the listing includes five excitatory synaptic inputs distributed

---

[4]It is possible to include in this formulation the effect of a known soma shunt conductance (G_{shunt}) that is caused by microelectrode penetration. In this case $G_S = (A_{soma}/R_m) + G_{shunt}$, where A_{soma} is the area of the soma membrane (see chapter 2, eqs. 2.49–2.51).

distally in the dendritic tree and two inhibitory inputs at or near the soma. The excitatory inputs are activated simultaneously (at $t = 0.5$ $msec$). They are brief ($t_{peak} = 0.2$ $msec$; $\alpha = 25$) and reach a peak conductance of 2 nS, with a reversal potential of 100 mV. The two inhibitory inputs are activated at $t = 0$. These inputs have a slower time course ($t_{peak} = 1$ $msec$; $\alpha = 5$), with a peak conductance change of 40 nS and a reversal potential equal to the resting membrane potential (0 mV; shunting or silent inhibition).

Using SPICE 2G.6 running on the VAX11/750 under VMS with a floating point accelerator, the circuit above took 58 sec of CPU time using the Trapezoidal algorithm and 120 sec using the Gear integration method, with less than 1% difference in the computed results. For some nonlinear models (see below) the Gear method proved more accurate. The same circuit was simulated using an OliveHi M24 (IBM XT-type) personal computer with a math coprocessor and two commercial versions of SPICE. IS-SPICE required 230 sec using the trapezoidal method; P-SPICE required 90 sec using the same integration algorithm. Solution by the Gear method (see Chapter 13) took 780 sec for the IS-SPICE program. That option is not available in P-SPICE.

Figure 3.4 shows the computed synaptic potentials. The continuous curves show the potentials measured at two dendritic locations (see inset) and the soma in response to activation of the five excitatory synapses described above. The dashed lines reflect the addition of the two proximal inhibitory inputs. The relatively small attenuation in EPSP peak amplitude from node 304 to the soma (node 1) indicates that this system is electrically compact. It should be noted that the conductance load that would be contributed by the other six dendrites in the complete cell is missing in this simulation. When inhibitory inputs near the soma are activated, the peak depolarization at the soma is significantly reduced while the peak amplitude of the EPSPs at the distal sites are almost unaffected. However, due to the effect of this strong inhibitory conductance on the soma time constant, the time course of the EPSP is markedly shortened at all locations. For more discussion of the effects of dendritic location on the behavior of synaptic potentials, see Rall (1967), Rall and Rinzel (1973), Rinzel and Rall (1974), and Segev et al. (1985).

3.3.5   Electrically Excitable Compartments in SPICE

In a previous study we showed how SPICE can be used to model Hodgkin and Huxley-like (1952) kinetics for the Na^+ and K^+ currents (Bunow et al. 1985). To achieve this goal we "wrote down" the four differential equations describing the Hodgkin and Huxley model using SPICE

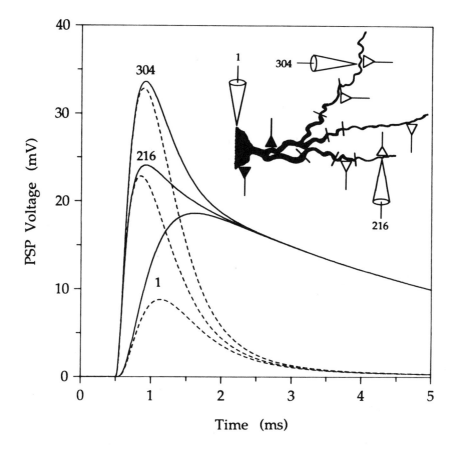

Figure 3.4
The effect of synaptic inputs on the cell model in fig. 3.3. Five excitatory synaptic inputs were activated simultaneously along distal segments of the tree (open triangles in inset). The resulting EPSPs (continuous lines) were measured at three locations: nodes 304, 216, and 1 (soma), as shown by "electrodes" in the inset. The dashed lines are the PSPs at the same points when two proximal inhibitory inputs (filled triangles in inset) were activated in addition to the five excitatory inputs. Passive parameters for the cell were: $R_m = 5000 \ \Omega cm^2$, $C_m = 1 \ \mu F/cm^2$, and $R_i = 70 \ \Omega cm$. Parameters for the excitatory inputs were: $g_{peak} = 2 \ nS$, $t_{peak} = 0.2 \ msec$ ($\alpha = 25$), $E_{syn} = 100 \ mV$; activated simultaneously at $t = 0.5 \ msec$. Inhibitory inputs: $g_{peak} = 40 \ nS$, $t_{peak} = 1 \ msec$ ($\alpha = 5$), $E_{syn} = 0 \ mV$ (rest), both activated simultaneously at $t = 0 \ msec$. The corresponding SPICE file for this simulation is listed in Appendix 3.A.

elements, just as we did for the alpha function to simulate synaptic inputs. Simulating the Hodgkin and Huxley model in this way is rather cumbersome, requiring about 60 lines of code per Hodgkin and Huxley compartment. Here we do not intend to repeat this model, but rather to demonstrate a different approach to simulating nonlinear membrane properties, specifically those characterized by excitation thresholds, using simplified polynomial models. These models have proven to be very useful in the analysis of excitation threshold and propagation in excitable cells (chs. 9–12 of Jack et al. 1975, and chapter 5 below).

For present purposes we chose a membrane model characterized by an instantaneous N-shaped current-voltage relation. In the example shown in fig. 3.5A we used a cubic equation for $I_{act}(V)$ of the form

$$I_{act}(V) = g_{rest}(V + aV^2 + bV^3) \tag{3.16}$$

where $g_{rest} = 2.12\ nS$ ($471.1\ M\Omega$) is the resting conductance of the soma compartment in the SPICE model above (dashed line in fig. 3.5A); $a = -57\ V^{-1}$ and $b = 357\ V^{-2}$. As discussed by Jack et al. (1975) and Rinzel and Ermentrout in chapter 5, this kind of current-voltage relation qualitatively describes a Hodgkin and Huxley-like membrane when the fast Na^+ activation (m) process occurs instantaneously, while the slower K^+ activation (n) process and the Na^+ inactivation (h) process are held constant at their resting values. The function in eq. 3.16 crosses the V axis at three points: 0, 20, and 140 mV, corresponding to the resting potential, the threshold for excitation with uniform polarization, and the peak of the "action potential," respectively.

SPICE provides a class of nonlinear voltage-dependent current sources (G elements) that may be used to describe a nonlinear conductance characterized by the current-voltage relation in eq. 3.16. As with the synapse, this is done by making the controlling nodes identical to the output nodes, this time using a one-dimensional polynomial function,

```
GCUBIC 1 2 POLY(1) 1 2  0 2.123N -121N 757N
```

which produces a current between nodes 1 and 2 (in A) that depends on the voltage (in V) between these same controlling nodes, as required in eq. 3.16:

$$
\begin{aligned}
I(1,2) &= 2.123 \times 10^{-9} V(1,2) - 121 \times 10^{-9} V(1,2)^2 \\
&\quad + 757 \times 10^{-9} V(1,2)^3
\end{aligned} \tag{3.17}
$$

Figure 3.5B shows the response of an isolated patch of this membrane to excitatory synaptic inputs of different strengths ($g_{peak} = 1.5$,

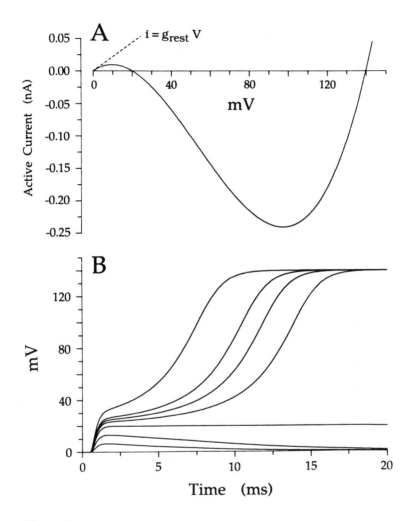

Figure 3.5
Threshold phenomena in a SPICE model of a membrane patch with a cubic N-shaped current-voltage relation. (A) $I - V$ curve described by eq. 3.16. The dashed line is the resting slope conductance, g_{rest}, which is 2.12 nS (471.1 $M\Omega$). (B) Response to seven different intensities of excitatory synaptic input. The three lower traces are for inputs below and very near threshold (20 mV); the four upper traces show synaptic inputs above threshold, all of which produce an all-or-none "action potential" with an amplitude of 140 mV. Parameters for the synapse are, from bottom to top: $g_{peak} =$ 1.5, 3, 4.5, 5.25, 5.6, 6, and 7.5 nS, with $t_{peak} = 0.2$ $msec$ and $E_{syn} = 100$ mV, activated at $t = 0.5$ $msec$.

3, 4.5, 5.25, 5.6, 6, and 7.5 nS, curves from bottom to top, respectively).
The SPICE input file for the smallest synaptic conductance (1.5 nS) is
given below. Here the RSOMA element in the the previous SPICE example is replaced by GCUBIC, so that this patch of membrane has the
same resting properties as the soma compartment in the passive example
above.

```
CUBIC I-V CURVE TO SIMULATE THRESHOLD RESPONSE
*
*I_act = g_rest*(V -57*V^2 + 357*V^3)
*gives V_th = 20 mV; V_peak = 140 mV
*
GCUBIC 1 0 POLY(1)   1 0   0 2.123N -121N 757N
CMSOMA 1 0 10.6PF
RGRD   1 0 1T
*
*alpha function (with t_peak = 0.2 ms) and an excitatory synaptic
*battery
*
RALPHA 5001 0 0.2MEG
CALPHA 5001 0 1NF
IALPHA 0 5001 EXP 0 1 0.5MS 0 0 0.2MS
VSYN 1000 0 DC 100MV
*
*excitatory synaptic input with g_peak = 1.5 nS
*
GSYN 1 1000 POLY(2) 1 1000   5001 0   0 0 0 0 0.02PF
.TRAN  50US   20MS
.PRINT TRAN  V(1)
.OPTIONS LIMPTS=600
.END
```

Note the very large resistance (RGRD = 10^6 $M\Omega$) that is connected
from node 1 to ground. This is necessary because SPICE does not consider that the GCUBIC element is connected to ground during the error-
checking that occurs at the beginning of a SPICE run. Since SPICE
requires that all nodes have a DC path to ground, the RGRD resistor is
necessary to avoid aborting the job. If the resistor is sufficiently large
the behavior of the circuit is not affected.

The simple model presented above displays several important features of excitable membrane. It can be seen that a weak synaptic input
(fig. 3.5B, lowest trace) produces an EPSP that is well below the voltage
threshold for excitation of 20 mV. This response decays passively to the
resting potential with a single time constant, $\tau_m = C_m/g_{rest}$. Slightly in-

creasing the synaptic conductance (second trace from bottom) produces an EPSP with an amplitude (about 12 mV) that is already within the negative slope of the $I - V$ curve, producing a "local response" that is revealed by a broadening of the EPSP. A still larger synaptic input approaches 20 mV (third trace from bottom), where the unstable point of threshold is reached and a prolonged, very slowly decaying EPSP is produced. Larger inputs produce an all-or-none regenerative "action potential" with an amplitude of 140 mV. Further increases in the synaptic strength result in a spike with a faster rise-time but a constant amplitude.

The same approach can be used to model other types of membrane nonlinearities, such as outward rectification or inward rectification with no excitation threshold. It is also possible to use higher-order polynomials with the G elements and to introduce time-dependence for modeling more complicated cases of excitation threshold, such as those of Goldstein and Rall (1974), Bunow et al. (1985), and chapter 5 below).

3.4   Discussion

The computer-based compartmental model is a powerful method for simulating the morphological and electrical properties of nerve cells, especially when the experimental question requires a fine-grained model that embodies a great deal of anatomical or physiological detail. General-purpose network simulation programs such as SPICE make it relatively straightforward to simulate complicated nerve cells that may require a large number, perhaps thousands, of compartments. Compartmental models are very flexible; they do not place constraints on the morphology of the modeled cell, its electrical properties, or the way synaptic inputs are distributed. Despite the advantages of compartmental models, it should be remembered that idealized cable models remain essential for the estimation of key parameters upon which the compartmental models are based. With these parameters, a detailed exploration of the compartmental model can be performed and the model can be further refined by comparison with experimental data (e.g., Fleshman et al. 1988).

A serious problem in attempts to develop realistic models of experimental systems is the uniqueness, or lack thereof, of the parameters that define the model. In compartmental models, a value must be computed for $\hat{r}_m$, $\hat{r}_i$, and $\hat{c}_m$ in every compartment. Appropriate experimental constraints and reasonable assumptions are necessary to reduce the degrees of freedom in making the choices on which these computations depend (see Rall 1988 for discussion of these points). A common assumption is that the specific electrical properties of the membrane and cytoplasm (R_m, C_m, and R_i) are uniform throughout the cell. Similarly, it is often assumed that dendrites terminate with sealed end boundary conditions and that the extracellular resistivity is uniform and effectively zero. Given a set of constraints and assumptions, it is possible to assign particular parameters to every compartment that result in a satisfactory match between experimentally determined morphological and electrical properties (see figs. 3.4 and 3.5). Relaxing one or more of these constraints (e.g., assuming that R_m may be spatially nonuniform) may cause problems of nonuniqueness (i.e., there may be many different models that match the empirical measurements equally well; Fleshman et al. 1988; Clements and Redman 1989). In such cases additional experimental data, such as measurements of higher-order time constants or the size and shape of synaptic potentials, may allow one to reduce the number of possible models.

The approach to the construction of compartmental models of nerve cells presented in this paper may be summarized as follows. First, obtain a set of experimental data that characterize the cell of interest morphologically and physiologically. Second, construct a cable model of the passive (resting) state of the cell. This requires choosing a set of assumptions and several key parameters that result in a model best accommodating the experimental data (morphological measurements, R_N, τ_m, etc.). Third, use these key parameters and constraints to build a detailed compartmental model of the cell. This initial model can be refined by incorporating additional data or relaxing one or more of the original constraints, then determining the effects of these changes on the performance of the model. For example, one may wish to incorporate nonlinear membrane properties in some compartments (Bunow et al. 1985). Finally, when the model is judged to be sufficiently well behaved and in accord with known experimental data, it can be used predictively to examine model behavior under input conditions specific to experimental questions of interest. A common outcome of modeling exercises is the redirection of experimental work toward questions that will improve the model and, therefore, one's understanding of the underlying system.

3.4.1 Applications of SPICE-Based Models

This section presents a few examples of the kinds of questions for which SPICE models have proven useful. Consider the problem of threshold conditions for evoking an orthodromic action potential in cat spinal α-motoneurons following group Ia input (Bunow et al. 1985). In fully reconstructed motoneurons in which membrane properties and the spatiotemporal distribution of Ia synaptic inputs were taken into account, it was shown that a very high density of excitable sodium channels is needed in the soma and initial segment to overcome the passive conductance load imposed by the large surface area of motoneuron dendrites. Predictions were made of the number of excitable channels necessary to generate an action potential.

Another question studied by Bunow et al. was the extent to which an orthodromic action potential generated in the initial segment and soma attenuates as it spreads passively into the dendrites. The model suggested that the effect of such an action potential on ambient membrane potential in the dendrites is negligible. This result is relevant to models of learning and memory at the cellular level that are based on Hebb's hypothesis (1949), in which plastic changes are held to occur in the synapses between cells, dependent on the synchronization of firing of the pre- and post-synaptic cells. The question raised by the modeling results is how would a Hebbian dendritic synapse "know" that action potentials were generated in the soma? Is there a chemical signal that spreads from the soma back to the synapses? Does the signaling mechanism require dendritic spikes, or are there other possible mechanisms for such plastic changes (see Gamble and Koch 1987)?

A third application of SPICE models is found in the study of Rall and Segev (1987), who explored the functional implications of excitable channels in dendrites. For this study, compartmental models of complex dendritic trees covered with dendritic spines were constructed. Dendritic spines were represented by two compartments, one for the spine head membrane and one for the spine stem. Excitable channels (with Hodgkin and Huxley-like kinetics) could be distributed at different regions of the cell model, including the spine head compartments. The study demonstrates that the large number of spines and synaptic contacts per neuron can provide a rich repertoire of logical operations implemented by excitable spine clusters.

Finally, an example using SPICE to analyze the synaptic architecture that may underlie directional selectivity in electrophysiologically characterized ganglion cells of the rabbit retina is given in Plate 1. The spatial distribution of voltage along the dendritic tree at four different times is coded in different colors. The figure demonstrates how different spatiotemporal patterns of activity of excitatory and inhibitory synapses (in this case shunting inhibition) may be responsible for the directional selectivity of the cell (see O'Donnell et al. 1985).

3.4.2   SPICE and Other Programs for Nerve Cell Modeling

There are several reasons to recommend SPICE as a tool for nerve cell modeling: (1) SPICE is available for many different computer systems, from PCs to large mainframe computers. (2) There is no intrinsic limit on the size of the neuron model. We have simulated cat spinal α-motoneurons with as many as 5,000 passive compartments on a relatively small VAX. However, there are machine-specific limits on model size. (3) The SPICE input list is easily modified, for example by adding synapses or an excitable soma and axon to an existing model. (4) In our work to date, the program has proven very robust for transient analysis. (5) A subcircuit facility in SPICE permits hierarchical modeling. This feature enables the user to group elements together into a model (a single dendritic spine, a patch of excitable membrane, or a whole cell), which can then be invoked as a unit to construct more complex systems.

Despite these advantages, SPICE has two major limitations: (1) arbitrary mathematical expressions cannot be defined directly. As we demonstrated above, one is forced to use electrical components and their defining equations for this purpose, a procedure that complicates the modeling of arbitrary functions (e.g., Hodgkin and Huxley-type descriptions of time- and voltage-dependent conductances, ion concentrations that change as a function of cell activity, etc.) (2) The SPICE program uses a uniform temporal spacing of sampling points for transient analysis. While it automatically adjusts the internal integration step to maintain accuracy, the maximum step size is always less than the user-specified sampling interval. This restriction improves the robustness of the program, but it can greatly increase the computer time required for problems in which closely spaced intervals are needed over only a fraction of the analysis period, for example to resolve rapidly changing currents and voltages, such as the rising phase of an action potential.

Recently, a new general-purpose simulator called SABER was recommended to us (Flack et al. 1987; Shepherd, Carnevale, and Woolf, 1988).[5] Unlike SPICE, this commercially available program can incorporate arbitrary functions and thus can handle ion fluxes, voltage-dependent conductances, and other important features of nerve cells in a more straightforward manner. SABER also supports a number of plotting and graphic

---

[5] For more information regarding the use of SABER in neuronal simulations contact Dr. Ted Carnevale at the Department of Neurology, State University of New York, HSC T12 Room 20, Stony Brook, New York, 11794. His electronic mail address is ted@sbcs.sunysb.edu. SABER is the product of Analogy, Incorporated, P.O.Box 1669, Beaverton, Oregon 97075.

routines. However, at this moment, we do not have enough information to provide a critical evaluation of the program.

Another interesting simulator is called NODUS, designed by E. De Schutter (Department of Neurology, University of Antwerp, Belgium) for Macintosh computers (De Schutter, 1986, 1988). It uses the graphics features of that machine to aid in constructing compartmental models and for on-line display of currents and voltages. One can simulate passive as well as Hodgkin-Huxley-like conductances with NODUS and analyze the behavior of the model in the time domain.

It is likely that more simulation programs will be developed to answer the specific needs of neurobiologists who are interested in the compartmental approach to modeling individual nerve cells and neural networks. As these programs proliferate and become more powerful and easier to use, compartmental models of electrochemical processes at the cellular level will likely become increasingly important tools for neurobiologists. Judicious and creative use of these tools can help to deepen our understanding of the role of channels, membranes, synapses, and cell structure in neural information processing and brain function as a whole.

Idan Segev's address is Department of Neurobiology, Institute of Life Sciences, Hebrew University, Jerusalem, Israel; his BITNET address is idan@hujivms.bitnet. James Fleshman's address is Systems Research Center, University of Maryland, College Park, Maryland 20742; his ARPAnet address is jim@eneevax.umd.edu. Dr. Fleshman's contribution to this chapter was supported by FDA order number 306464 and by a grant from the Whitaker Foundation. Robert Burke's address is Laboratory of Neural Control, National Institute of Neurological and Communicative Disorders and Stroke, National Institutes of Health, Bethesda, Maryland 20892. His BITNET address is rrb@nihcu.bitnet.

The authors dedicate this chapter to the memory of Marcos Solodkin, a friend and colleague who was just beginning his modeling studies and who died very much too young.

Appendix 3.A: Example Listing

A complete SPICE input file describing the cell shown in fig. 3.3 is listed below, with five excitatory and two inhibitory synapses. Lines beginning with asterisks serve to introduce comments in a SPICE file and may be used to group related lines of code.

```
MODEL FOR DENDRITE IN FIGURE 3.3, WITH 5 EXCIT. + 2 INHIB. INPUTS
*
*R_m = 5000; C_m = 1; excit. synapses at 302,304,314,214,216;
*inhib. synapses at 1,100
*
RMSOMA          1            0            471.70MEG
CMSOMA          1            0             10.60PF
*
RI1             1          100              1.34MEG
RI2           100          101              1.34MEG
RM100         100            0           6631.46MEG
CM100         100            0              0.75PF
*
RI3           101          200              4.53MEG
RI4           200          201              4.53MEG
RM200         200            0           3825.84MEG
CM003         200            0              1.31PF
*
RI5           201          300              8.05MEG
RI6           300          301              8.05MEG
RM300         300            0           5101.12MEG
CM300         300            0              0.98PF
*
RI7           301          302             15.32MEG
RI8           302          303             15.32MEG
RM302         302            0           9042.90MEG
CM302         302            0              0.55PF
*
RI9           303          304            139.26MEG
RM304         304            0           7957.75MEG
CM30          304            0              0.63PF
*
RI10          201          310              7.57MEG
RI11          310          311              7.57MEG
RM310         310            0           9362.06MEG
CM310         310            0              0.53PF
*
```

```
RI12        311         312         7.66MEG
RI13        312         313         7.66MEG
RM312       312          0       18085.80MEG
CM312       312          0          0.28PF
*
RI14        313         314        74.27MEG
RM314       314          0        4420.97MEG
CM314       314          0          1.13PF
*
RI15        101         210         5.23MEG
RI16        210         211         5.23MEG
RM210       210          0        4942.70MEG
CM210       210          0          1.01PF
*
RI17        211         212        10.69MEG
RI18        212         213        10.69MEG
RM212       212          0        6631.46MEG
CM212       212          0          0.75PF
*
RI19        213         214         7.66MEG
RI20        214         215         7.66MEG
RM214       214          0       18085.80MEG
CM214       214          0          0.28PF
*
RI21        215         216        34.66MEG
RM216       216          0        9473.52MEG
CM216       216          0          0.53PF
*
*
*EXCITATORY SYNAPSES.
*
*Generation of ''alpha function'' voltage source,
*starts at t = 0.5 ms, with t_peak = 0.2 ms.
*
RALPHA 5001    0 0.2MEG
CALPHA 5001    0 1.0NF
IALPHA     0 5001 EXP 0 1 0.5MS 0 0 0.2MS
*
*Excitatory battery.
*
VEX 1000 0 DC 100MV
*
*Nonlinear voltage-dependent current sources (5 excitatory
*synaptic inputs), each synapse with g_peak of 2 nS.
```

```
*
GSYNE1 214 1000 POLY(2) 214 1000 5001 0 0 0 0 0 0.0272P
GSYNE2 216 1000 POLY(2) 216 1000 5001 0 0 0 0 0 0.0272P
GSYNE3 302 1000 POLY(2) 302 1000 5001 0 0 0 0 0 0.0272P
GSYNE4 304 1000 POLY(2) 304 1000 5001 0 0 0 0 0 0.0272P
GSYNE5 314 1000 POLY(2) 314 1000 5001 0 0 0 0 0 0.0272P
*
*INHIBITORY SYNAPSES.
*
*Generation of "alpha function" voltage source,
*starts at t = 0 ms, with t_peak at 1 ms.
*
RALPHAI 6001 0 0.2MEG
CALPHAI 6001 0 5.0NF
IALPHAI     0 6001 EXP 0 2 0 0 0 1MS
*
*Inhibitory battery.
*
VIN 2000 0 DC 0MV
*
*Nonlinear voltage-dependent current sources (2 inhibitory
*synaptic inputs), each synapse with g_peak of 40nS.
*
GSYNI1   100 2000 POLY(2)   100 2000 6001 0 0 0 0 0 0.136P
GSYNI2     1 2000 POLY(2)     1 2000 6001 0 0 0 0 0 0.136P
*
.TRAN   10US   5MS
.PRINT TRAN   V(1) V(304) V(216)
.OPTIONS LIMPTS=501   ABSTOL=0.01P TRTOL 10 METHOD=GEAR RELTOL=0.1M
CHGTOL=1F
.END
```

The .OPTIONS card sets user-selectable parameters that override default parameters. For example, LIMPTS changes the default number of points that can be printed to 501, since the analysis, as defined in the .TRAN card, contains 501 points (default is 201); ABSTOL sets the absolute error tolerance for the current (default $= 1\ pA$); METHOD $=$ GEAR specifies the Gear integration method, which, although slower, is more accurate than the default Trapezoidal algorithm for many cases that are relevant to neural modeling. For more on the .OPTIONS and on other SPICE capabilities the reader is urged to consult the SPICE manual.

CHAPTER 4

Multiple Channels and Calcium Dynamics

WALTER M. YAMADA, CHRISTOF KOCH, and PAUL R. ADAMS

4.1 Introduction

The cornerstone of modern neurobiology is the analysis by Hodgkin and
Huxley (1952) of the initiation and propagation of the action potential in the squid giant axon. Their description accounted for two ionic
currents, the fast sodium current, I_{Na}, and a delayed potassium current, I_K. Almost without exception, impulse conduction along axons
can be successfully analyzed in terms of one or both of these currents
(see Waxman and Ritchie 1985, Parnas and Segev 1979, and Joyner,
Westerfield, and Moore 1986, for examples of experimental and theoretical studies investigating action potential propagation in invertebrate
and vertebrate axons with various branching patterns). When modeling
active structures other than the squid axon, researchers have usually
adopted Hodgkin and Huxley's system of coupled four-dimensional nonlinear differential equations since models more applicable to vertebrate
neurons have not been fully developed. However, while the Hodgkin-
Huxley formulation has been singularly important to biophysics, their
equations do not describe a number of important phenomena such as
adaptation to long-lasting stimuli or the dependency of some conductances on various ionic concentrations. Moreover, the transmission of
electrical signals within and between neurons involves more than the
mere circulation of stereotyped impulses. Impulses must be set up by
subthreshold processes and the shape of impulses is variable. These differences reflect the roles of voltage-dependent ion currents additional to
those described by Hodgkin and Huxley.

In recent years a plethora of ionic membrane currents have been described (Hille 1984). They differ in principal carrier, voltage- and time-
dependence, dependence on internal calcium, and susceptibility to modulation by synaptic input and second messengers. Our understanding
of these currents, and to a lesser extent the role they play in impulse
formation, has accelerated rapidly in recent years as a result of various
technical innovations such as single-cell isolation and patch clamping.

However, in order to understand more completely the functional role of these currents in determining membrane responses we must develop empirical equations that approximate the behavior of the currents under physiological conditions and compare numerical simulations of these equations with the physiological preparation.

This chapter will focus on modeling the electrical properties of one particular neuron type whose various macroscopic currents have been described in detail, the bullfrog sympathetic ganglion "B" type cells. These are the largest cells in the ganglion, having a mean diameter of $35\mu m$ (Honma 1970; for a scanning electron micrograph study of the bullfrog sympathetic ganglion see Baluk 1986). They receive inputs from rapidly conducting presynaptic axons, the terminals of which engulf the soma and axon hillock. There are several reasons why these cells have proven to be unusually favorable objects for these studies. They are indubitably neuronal. They can be studied in their fully mature form at various levels of simplification: within the intact ganglion, in explant cultures, or after complete dissociation. They can be studied using a variety of different techniques: two-electrode voltage clamp, single electrode voltage clamp, who cell and single channel patch recording, and intracellular injection. They present few space-clamp problems because dendrites are absent and all synapses are formed on or near the cell body. Thus, the soma of these cells can be modeled accurately by a single spherical compartment. Finally, the voltage-dependent conductances of these cells are targets for various types of unusual "modulating" slow synaptic actions that now seem to be far more prevalent in the nervous system than originally suspected (Weight and Votava 1970; Adams and Brown 1982; Kuffler and Sejnowski 1983; Siegelbaum and Tsien 1983; Cole and Nicoll 1984). Thus the bullfrog sympathetic ganglion cells provide an ideal environment for studying cellular adaptation, slow synaptic transmission, and other such phenomena crucial for understanding information processing operations that occur on time scales from milliseconds to many minutes.

Our aim in this chapter is to provide the reader with a complete model for this typical vertebrate cell, a cell that is geometrically rather simple but electrically quite complex, and to describe the numerical algorithms relevant to this work.

Apart from the work discussed here, at least two other detailed models describing the electrical properties of excitable structures exist: Connor and Stevens's (1971) early analysis of a mollusc neuron in terms of three currents, and the model by DiFrancesco and Noble (1985) describing the Purkinje fiber cell system of the heart. The model described in this chapter is in the same spirit as Connor and Stevens's system in that both models attempt to describe the electrical properties of a membrane in terms of underlying ionic membrane currents.[1] DiFrancesco and Noble's model had a different purpose; they explored the effects of ionic pumps on the shape and frequency of rhythmic potential changes in cardiac fibers. The approach in all cases is, however, essentially identical. The experimentalist attempts to dissect out or hold constant as many of the features of the system under study as possible and to describe the remaining features with empirical equations of sufficient detail to determine what role these features may assume to affect the behavior of the system as a whole. Simulations then are not restricted to the merely educational purpose of displaying a system that has already been described in detail, but rather enable the modeler to test his understanding of the integrative aspects of the system under study by allowing the subsystems observed in isolation (e.g., channels recorded under patch clamp or currents measured in isolation by pharmacologically blocking other currents) to interact with the other components of the system. Furthermore, features of the system that are experimentally inaccessible or not easily controlled (e.g., the activation state of a given current) can easily be visualized with the aid of the computer.

We will begin with a rather detailed description of the various inward and outward currents using the rate constant formalism perpetrated so successfully by Hodgkin and Huxley. Section 4.5 deals with the synaptic input and section 4.6 treats calcium diffusion and buffering, a topic of ever-increasing importance. We will then discuss how these ingredients can be incorporated into a single system, solved numerically, and will show pertinent results.

4.2   Modeling Ionic Current Flow

In this section we describe briefly the general methodology used to describe ionic currents. We will do this by example of one current found in the bullfrog, the fast sodium current. For a more detailed discussion see Hille (1984). We begin by assuming that all ionic current flow occurs through channels or pores and that the instantaneous voltage-current relation is linear. The ionic current, $I(t)$, is then related to the voltage across the membrane, V, by Ohm's law:

$$I(t) = g(t, V) \cdot (V - E) \qquad (4.1)$$

---

[1] Very recently, the techniques described in this chapter have been applied to the study of somatic response of hippocampal pyramidal neurons; Borg-Graham (1988).

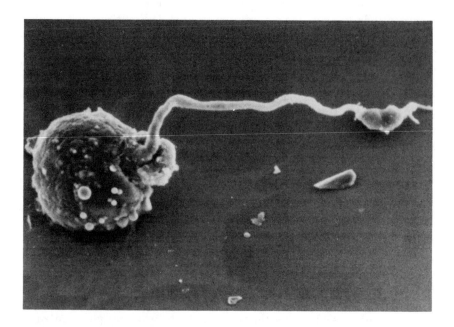

Figure 4.1
Electron micrograph of an isolated bullfrog sympathetic ganglion "B" type cell
(x1600). The complete absence of dendritic processes, a single nonbranching axon
and the spherical shape of the soma, make this cell an excellent preparation for electrophysiological study. The diameter of the cell body is $\approx 30~\mu m$. Courtesy of Barry
Burbach and Paul Adams.

where E is the Nernst potential for the ionic current under study and $g(t, V)$ is the conductance associated with the channel. In general, this conductance depends on time and on the membrane potential but may also depend on various chemical mediators such as intracellular calcium. The use of Ohm's law is best justified by the results of past simulations using Ohm's law that have successfully predicted membrane voltage responses, most notably Hodgkin and Huxley's original 1952 study. However, the relationship between instantaneous current and voltage of most membranes is not a linear relation but shows some degree of rectification. Rectification is the membrane property that causes ionic current flowing in one direction to be preferred over the other and is due to extracellular and intracellular ionic activity differences. A complete discussion of this phenomenon is beyond the scope of this chapter. From a modeling perspective, however, one must be aware that under certain circumstances, such as the large and fast changes in calcium concentration seen in dendritic spines (Gamble and Koch 1987; Qian and Sejnowski 1986), nonlinear models such as the one by Goldman (1943) and Hodgkin and Katz (1949) may become imperative (for a discussion of rectification see Jack, Noble, and Tsien 1975; Hille 1984; Tuckwell 1988).

We assume that all ionic movement across the membrane is via channels that are permeable to a single ionic species and have two states, open or closed. The total conductance associated with any particular population of channels can then be expressed as the maximal conductance of the particular membrane patch under investigation, $\overline{g}$ (given by the conductance of a single channel in the open state times the channel density), times the fraction of all channels that are open. This fraction is determined by hypothetical activation and inactivation variables m and h raised to some integral power. In general, we have

$$g(t, V) = \overline{g} \cdot m(t, V)^i \cdot h(t, V)^j \tag{4.2}$$

where i and j are positive integers. The dynamics of the variables m and h obey first-order kinetics of the form

$$\frac{d\, m(t, V)}{dt} = \frac{m_\infty(V) - m(t, V)}{\tau_m(V)} \tag{4.3}$$

where the steady-state value of m, m_∞, and the time constant, τ_m, are defined functions of voltage. In the original Hodgkin and Huxley study, m_∞ and τ_m were expressed in terms of rate constants, α_m and β_m, that

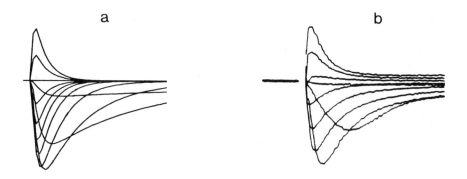

Figure 4.2
I_{Na} elicited by clamping the somatic potential to a fixed potential. The model (a) is compared with experimental data (b) taken from dissociated bullfrog cells with external Mn^{2+} used to block calcium currents (Jones 1987). Both traces are 5 $msec$ long. The trajectories illustrate the sodium current elicited by voltage steps from -80 mV to -30, -20, -10, 0, +10, +20, +30, +40, +50, +60, and +70 mV. Inactivation leads to the complete reduction of I_{Na} after several $msecs$ at most voltage values. I_{Na} becomes an outward current (positive current values) if the voltage is stepped beyond the Nernst potential for sodium (50 mV).

can be thought of as the forward and backward rates governing the transition of the channel between hypothetical "open" and "closed" states. The rates themselves depend on the potential across the membrane in a well-specified manner. For some currents, such as I_C and I_{AHP}, the rate constants depend as well (or solely) on the concentration of intracellular calcium. These rate constants, which ultimately specify the behavior of the current, must be measured experimentally on the basis of extensive voltage-clamp experiments in conjunction with the application of pharmacological agents to block other currents. Such data are shown in fig. 4.2 for the case of the somatic   fast sodium current recorded in dissociated cells. The axonal contribution of I_{Na} to the total current recorded at the soma is minimal in this preparation because the axon is dissociated from the cell body. It is from this data that one derives appropriate numerical values for the activation and inactivation variables. In other words, the description of an individual current measured under voltage-clamp conditions and in isolation provides the input data for our model. The appropriate activation and inactivation variables as a function of voltage are shown in fig. 4.3. Note that the steady-state variable (m_∞ in this case) for an activation variable is a monotonic *increasing*

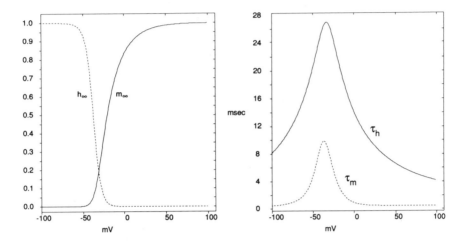

Figure 4.3
The time constants as well as the steady-state values of the activation and inactivation variables for the fast sodium current I_{Na} as a function of voltage. This current is very similar to data published for the node of Ranvier (Frankenhæuser and Huxley 1964), except that the curves for m_∞ and h_∞ are both shifted toward more depolarized values. The detailed equations are given in Appendix 4.A.

function of voltage while inactivation variables are monotonic *decreasing* functions of voltage. With the single exception of I_{Ca} inactivation, we will use this rate formalism to describe all currents present in the bullfrog sympathetic ganglion (a complete set of all equations can be found in Appendix 4.A).

The Hodgkin and Huxley research program has been enormously important for the development of biophysics, linking the level of membrane potential in a quantitative and deterministic manner to the underlying level of macroscopic membrane conductances and rate constants. However, though Hodgkin and Huxley offered a conceptual interpretation of these variables in terms of "gating particles" vacillating between open and closed states, their model is a phenomenological one based on empirical equations describing currents resulting from the   activity of membrane elements that at that time were still the object of much controversy. The advent of the patch clamp recording technique (Sakmann and Neher 1983) has revealed ionic channels to be all-or-nothing pores that behave very much in a probabilistic manner. Several researchers have successfully addressed the issue of how action potentials ca be constructed from the time- and voltage-dependent kinetics of stochastic single-channel currents (in particular, Clay and DeFelice 1983). In this interpretation, the macroscopic rate constant, $n(t)$, is equivalent to the open channel probability. If the channel is closed, the probability that a channel gate will remain closed for a time, T, is $e^{-\alpha T}$, and if it is open the probability that the channel will remain open is $e^{-\beta T}$. If several hundred channels are simulated in this manner, consistency between the macroscopic and the microscopic domain can be demonstrated. However, for our purposes, this deterministic phenomenological description is quite sufficient.

4.3   Inward Currents

The ganglion cell bodies exhibit two rapidly activating inward currents, I_{Na} and I_{Ca}, which closely resemble those already described in a variety of axonal, glandular, or invertebrate preparations. Closer examination of I_{Na} reveals that it is the summation of several distinct sodium conductances, each of which can be distinguished by its sensitivity to various pharmacological agents (tetrodotoxin, cadmium) and by different activation thresholds and kinetics (Jones 1987; for an overview see Barchi 1987). We restrict our model to the largest component of the sodium ionic current, I_{Na}. Peak sodium conductance, G_{Na}, increases sigmoidally with depolarization with an effective threshold near $-20\ mV$. Both activation and inactivation seem to be shifted to more positive values than in the frog node of Ranvier (Frankenhaeuser and Huxley 1964). In intact cells, the threshold for initiating action potentials is more negative than the threshold in isolated cells, possibly due in part to this shift in activation and inactivation voltage dependence (Jones 1987). I_{Na} is described as

$$I_{Na} = \overline{g}_{Na} m_{Na}^2 h_{Na} \cdot (V - E_{Na}) \tag{4.4}$$

Both intra- and extracellular changes in sodium ion concentration are very small, justifying our assumption of a constant Nernst reversal potential, (E_{Na}).

The calcium current is smaller and slower than I_{Na}, contributing little to the electric charge entering the cell during an action potential. However, since I_{Ca} inactivates very slowly, it dominates the inward current during long depolarizations (Adams, Brown, and Constanti 1982b). Of the three types of calcium currents described by Nowycky and colleagues

(1983), it most closely resembles the L form. Inactivation is primarily current rather than voltage-dependent and thus reflects channel block as a result of internal calcium accumulation in the space just below the cell membrane (Eckert and Chad 1984). Removal of inactivation (and thus presumably of internal calcium) takes several seconds following closure of the calcium channels. The voltage-dependent inactivation present in other calcium currents (Carbone and Lux 1984) is present to a much lesser extent in bullfrog sympathetic ganglion cells. The threshold for activation of I_{Ca} is about $-32\ mV$. Hyperpolarization to $-80\ mV$ does not reveal any rapidly inactivating low threshold calcium current, unlike the situation in many other cells (Jahnsen and Llinas 1984; Carbone and Lux 1984). I_{Ca} is described as

$$I_{Ca} = \overline{g}_{Ca} m_{Ca} h_{Ca} \cdot (V - E_{Ca}) \tag{4.5}$$

Activation is modeled as in eq. 4.3, and the equilibrium potential for calcium, E_{Ca}, is described in section 4.6. Inactivation is dependent on the concentration of intracellular calcium below the membrane by a mechanism that has yet to characterized. Therefore, we used the simplest Michaelis-Menten equation to describe calcium current inactivation.

$$h_{Ca} = \frac{K}{K + [Ca^{2+}]_n} \tag{4.6}$$

where the halfway inactivation concentration, K, is a constant and the concentration of free calcium in the shell just below the membrane, $[Ca^{2+}]_n$, is described in section 4.6.

4.4 Outward Currents

The remaining five ionic currents are potassium currents. A number of experimental limitations preclude detailed descriptions of these currents. They are much more difficult to separate than the inward currents because there exist no completely selective blockers. Two of these currents, I_C and I_{AHP}, are activated as a result of calcium influx. Though much progress is being made in developing kinetic schemes for both I_C and I_{AHP}, the exact time course of the calcium concentration changes within the cell during clamp steps or action potentials is uncertain, and so it is not yet possible to develop a detailed kinetic description for these currents (Moczydlowski and Latorre 1983; Gurney et al. 1987). The remaining currents, I_M, I_K, and I_A, are controlled by membrane voltage alone, although varying external calcium may affect the size and kinetics of I_K (Lancaster and Pennefather 1986). Understanding the interplay of these currents is best solved via modeling.

The potassium currents fall into three functional groups. First, the large and fast currents, which can in principle rapidly change membrane potential, I_K and I_C. I_K closely resembles the delayed rectifier current of squid axon and amphibian node of Ranvier (Frankenhaeuser 1963), showing a sigmoidal onset, very slow inactivation, and sensitivity to millimolar external tetraethylammonium (TEA). However, unlike the node of Ranvier, I_K has little responsibility for the rapid repolarizarion of the cell to near resting potentials after depolarization during the spike. This role is served by I_C, which develops its maximum value within 3 $msec$ during pulses that cause large calcium entry (e.g., to 0 mV). Repolarization to resting potential quickly shuts off this conductance. This simple picture of I_C is consistent with the role of this current in repolarizing the cell rapidly toward E_K and turning off immediately in readiness for another spike. I_K and I_C are described by the following equations:

$$I_K = \bar{g}_K m_K^2 h_K \cdot (V - E_K) \qquad\qquad (4.7)$$

and

$$I_C = \bar{g}_C m_C \cdot (V - E_K) \qquad\qquad (4.8)$$

where the activation variable for I_C, m_C, depends on both voltage and intracellular calcium concentration. We have chosen a particularly simple calcium dependency (Appendix 4.A), in which binding to a single calcium channel suffices to effect the transition from a closed to an open channel configuration. Although this is a gross oversimplification (see for instance Moczydlowski and Latorre 1983, for more realistic, albeit more complex, transition schemes), it approximates the calcium dependency of I_C well enough for our purposes. Since the ratio of intracellular to extracellular potassium varies significantly during spiking activity in these cells, the Nernst potential for potassium, E_K, has to reflect this change and thus is continuously reevaluated throughout the simulation (see section 4.6).

If I_C was the only calcium-dependent current activated by a single spike, the spike afterhyperpolarization (AHP) would promptly return to rest with a time constant equal to the membrane time constant. However, healthy cells show a much slower decaying component of AHP, which reflects another calcium-dependent potassium conductance

(Pennefather et al. 1985a). It has been shown that this conductance is quite distinct from the fast calcium-dependent calcium conductance: it is small, is maximally activated by pulses of 1–2 $msec$ duration, deactivates very slowly following brief depolarizations, is not voltage-dependent, and is partially blocked by the bee venom toxin apamin.

I_{AHP} thus falls into the second functional group, that of small currents that can show prolonged activity at potentials between threshold and rest. The other member of this group is I_M, a small, slow, non-inactivating potassium current that is almost completely inhibited by muscarinic receptor stimulation. Both I_M and I_{AHP} can best be thought of as subtracting from small suprathreshold applied current stimuli and can thus prevent spike firing. Both currents therefore contribute and control spike frequency adaptation but in different ways. The AHP and M currents are modeled using the following equations:

$$I_{AHP} = \overline{g}_{AHP} m_{AHP}^2 \cdot (V - E_K) \tag{4.9}$$

where m_{AHP} is dependent solely on the internal calcium concentration, and

$$I_M = \overline{g}_M m_M \cdot (V - E_K) \tag{4.10}$$

The third type of outward current requires hyperpolarization for its activation. This is I_A, which in molluscan cells is largely responsible for generating good proportionality between firing rate and stimulus current even at very low firing frequencies (Connor and Stevens 1971; see also chapter 6). This current is present in bullfrog cells and can strongly affect responses to hyperpolarizing current injections, but does not appear to have a major physiological role, since hyperpolarizing synaptic input is absent in bullfrog "B" type sympathetic neurons. I_A is modeled using the following equation:

$$I_A = \overline{g}_A m_A h_A \cdot (V - E_K) \tag{4.11}$$

Finally, the passive voltage-independent leak current is described by

$$I_{leak} = g_{leak} \cdot (V - E_{leak}) \tag{4.12}$$

where both g_{leak} and E_{leak} are constants that partially reflect impalement damage.

4.5 Synaptic Input

Type "B" ganglion cells receive synaptic input from one (sometimes several) preganglionic axons arising from motoneurons in the spinal cord. Since bullfrog sympathetic ganglion cells possess no dendrites, all of the typical 40 synaptic boutons made by the axon at the axon hillock and over the cell body (Sargent 1983) are located close to the recording electrode. These synapses release acetylcholine (ACh). Axonal stimulation of "B" type cells in the bullfrog sympathetic ganglion results in a fast EPSP, caused by ACh binding to nicotinic receptors, and a much slower EPSP, associated with a muscarinic receptor. The fast EPSP, usually triggering an action potential, reaches a peak in 1–2 $msec$ and decays in about 15 $msec$. It is generated by a brief inward current, lasting about 20 $msec$ (Adams et al. 1986). We modeled this "conventional" synaptic input by a time-varying conductance, $g_{syn}(t)$, associated with a synaptic reversal potential, $E_{syn} = -10mV$:

$$I_{syn} \;=\; g_{syn}(t) \cdot (V - E_{syn}) \qquad\qquad\qquad (4.13)$$

The time course of the synaptic induced conductance change is given by a standard alpha function (Jack et al. 1975),

$$g_{syn}(t) \;=\; const \cdot t \cdot e^{-t/t_{peak}} \qquad\qquad\qquad (4.14)$$

which reaches its maximum value, $const \cdot t_{peak} \cdot e^{-1}$, at $t = t_{peak}$. For $t_{peak} = 2.5\ msec$, the resulting time course of the inward current agrees well with experimental records (Kuba and Nishi 1979).

The second synaptic event begins rising 50–100 $msec$ after the end of the fast EPSP, reaches a peak after 1–2 sec, and lasts about 1 min. The underlying inward current has a similarly slow time course. This small EPSP (several mV) is accompanied by a dramatic change in the response of the cell to long depolarizing test pulses. While normally the cells respond to extended superthreshold current steps with only one or several action potentials, during the slow EPSP the cell responds much more vigorously to extended current stimuli. In other words, the cell has lost most of its adaptation to action potential firing. The underlying mechanism is the almost complete blockage (90%) of I_M current (indeed, the M in I_M stands for muscarine, the application of which leads to inhibition of this current) and the partial block (less than 30%) of I_{AHP}. We can reproduce this loss of adaptation by partially blocking these two currents (see Plate 2). In hippocampal neurons the role of I_{AHP} in controlling repetitive firing appears to be more striking than that of

I_M. We did not explicitly model the time course of the slow EPSP (see, however, fig. 4.9).

4.6 Calcium Diffusion and Buffering

Any detailed description of neuronal excitability must take into account the behavior of certain ionic species inside and outside the cell, most notably calcium and potassium. The dynamics of free, intracellular calcium are of particular interest, because the level of calcium controls activation of certain potassium conductances as well as being crucial for the initiation of phenomena believed to underly synaptic plasticity (for reviews see Kandel 1981; Alkon 1984; Smith 1987).

The most complex and sensitive aspects of this model are those involving the simulation of free intracellular calcium. Four processes that affect intracellular calcium concentration are modeled: the entry of calcium into the cell via I_{Ca}, the diffusion of calcium throughout the cell, the action of intracellular calcium binding proteins (buffers), and the efflux or uptake of calcium via the action of membrane-bound pumps. This list neglects the uptake and release of free intracellular calcium (which can be both voltage and/or calcium-dependent) from intracellular organelles, in particular mitochondria and the endoplasmic reticulum (Fifkova, Markham, and Delay 1983; for a review see McBurney and Neering 1987). However, since their relative contributions to the regulation of $[Ca^{2+}]$ is far from clear, we have neglected these processes in our model.

4.6.1 Calcium Current

The voltage-dependent calcium current discussed above, I_{Ca}, is the only direct liaison in our model between the membrane voltage and intracellular calcium. The change in intracellular calcium concentration due to the influx of calcium ions (carrying $2e$ charge per ion) is given by

$$\frac{\partial [Ca^{2+}]_n}{\partial t} = \frac{-I_{Ca}}{2FV_n} \tag{4.15}$$

where F is Faraday's constant ($9.649 \cdot 10^{13}\ Coulomb/mM$), $[Ca^{2+}]_n$ is the calcium concentration in the shell just below the membrane, and V_n is the volume of this shell. The value of the reversal potential for calcium is then determined by the Nernst equation:

$$E_{Ca} = 12.5 log \frac{[Ca^{2+}]_o}{[Ca^{2+}]_n} \qquad (4.16)$$

where $[Ca^{2+}]_o$ is the constant extracellular calcium concentration $(4\,mM)$.

4.6.2 Calcium Diffusion

Given the absence of dendrites and the near-spherical nature of the cell body, we solve the diffusion equation in spherical coordinates (for an introduction to the mathematics of diffusion see Crank 1975). We then neglect tangential components of diffusion, thus reducing the three-dimensional diffusion equation to a one-dimensional equation. If $[Ca^{2+}]$ is the free calcium concentration and r is the distance from the center of the sphere, the diffusion equation can be written as

$$\frac{\partial r[Ca^{2+}]}{\partial t} = D \frac{\partial^2 r[Ca^{2+}]}{\partial r^2}, \qquad (4.17)$$

(Crank 1975), where $D = 6 \cdot 10^{-6}\ cm^2 sec^{-1}$ is the diffusion constant of calcium in aqueous solution (Hodgkin and Keynes 1957). Solving this equation requires discretization in both space and time. Because we are primarily interested in the action of calcium on the voltage trajectory of the cell, it is crucial to model the space just below the cellular membrane as accurately as possible, since it is here that the binding of intracellular calcium to calcium-dependent potassium channels occurs. Our model assumes a relatively large, well-mixed central core compartment with a radius given by r_{core} (typically 19 μm), surrounded by a number of equally spaced shells (of thickness Δr; typically we use 10 shells with $\Delta r = 0.1\ \mu m$). The last shell corresponds to the intracellular space just below the cell's membrane (see fig. 4.4). This model bears some resemblance to an onion, with a large number of thin shells and a large core.

We could use a simple, explicit forward Euler integration scheme that is stable and bound to converge for small enough Δx and Δt. However, in order to be able to use much larger values of Δt, we use a mixed explicit-implicit scheme for solving eq. 4.17, first proposed by Crank and Nicolson (1947; for a more thorough discussion see Chapter 13). Here the derivative of the function to be evaluate at t is replaced by half of the sum of the derivative at time t and the derivative at $t + \Delta t$. Equation 4.17 then transforms into

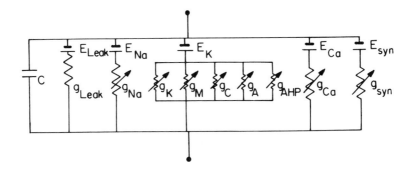

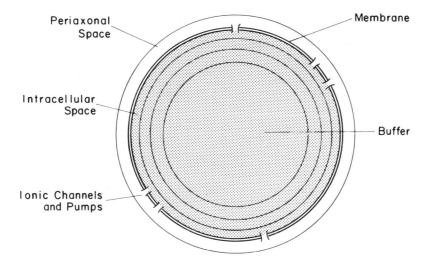

Figure 4.4
Basic structure of the model. The drawing at the top shows the equivalent electrical circuit of our model bullfrog sympathetic type "B" ganglion cell. The membrane conductances $g_{Na}, g_{Ca}, g_K, g_M, g_C, g_A, g_{AHP}$, and g_{syn} all depend on time. The first six conductances also depend on the membrane potential, and g_C and g_{AHP} depend on the calcium concentration $[Ca^{2+}]$ in the shell just below the membrane. The schematic at the bottom illustrates the underlying assumption for modeling the extracellular accumulation of potassium ions as well as the intracellular diffusion of calcium ions. Nondiffusible buffer is distributed inside the cell. Not drawn to scale.

$$\frac{r_i}{\Delta t}([Ca^{2+}]_{i,t+\Delta t} \quad - \quad [Ca^{2+}]_{i,t}) = \tag{4.18}$$

$$\begin{aligned}
\frac{D}{2\Delta r^2} \quad (\quad & (r_i + \Delta r)([Ca^{2+}]_{i+1,t+\Delta t} + [Ca^{2+}]_{i+1,t}) \\
- \quad & 2r_i([Ca^{2+}]_{i,t+\Delta t} + [Ca^{2+}]_{i,t}) \\
+ \quad & (r_i - \Delta r)([Ca^{2+}]_{i-1,t+\Delta t} + [Ca^{2+}]_{i-1,t}) \quad)
\end{aligned}$$

where r_i is the radial distance between the center of the sphere and the midpoint of shell number i, $r_i = r_{core} + i\Delta r$. The central core corresponds to compartment $i = 0$ and the shell just below the membrane to $i = n$. The local truncation error of this scheme is quadratic in both Δr and Δt, while the straightforward, explicit Euler scheme is quadratic in Δr but only linear in Δt (Smith 1985).

To solve this partial differential equation, we need proper initial as well as boundary conditions. As initial conditions, we assume that intracellular free calcium is distributed homogeneously across the cell with $[Ca^{2+}]_{initial} = 50 \ nM$. The boundary condition for the nth shell just below the membrane can be obtained by visualizing an imaginary $n+1$th shell beyond the nth shell and then setting $[Ca^{2+}]_{n+1} = [Ca^{2+}]_n$. The boundary condition at the central core ($i = 0$) is somewhat tricky because the geometry is nonhomogeneous. One way to obtain this condition is to assume another imaginary shell at $i = -1$ inside the central core, setting $[Ca^{2+}]_0 = [Ca^{2+}]_{-1}$, and recalling that the flux across the central sphere will be a factor of three greater than through any given shell. A different approach reverts back to Fick's first law underlying the diffusion equation (Crank 1975) for the innermost compartment. Both methods yield the same result for the limit as $\Delta r / r_{core} \to 0$.

4.6.3 Calcium Buffers

We now have to consider the change in calcium due to its binding to various calcium buffers, such as the ubiquitous protein calmodulin, with four separate calcium binding sites, paravalbumin, calbindin, calcineurin, and others (McBurney and Neering 1987). However, since we are only interested in the free calcium and not in the behavior of the buffer, our model assumes that calcium binds to a single binding site on the buffer. Adapting the model to multiple binding sites is straightforward (Gamble and Koch 1987). We assume this buffer to be so large in terms of its molecular weight that diffusion of buffer molecules can be neglected over the time scale of interest to us. The forward (f) and backward (b) rates of the binding reaction are $10^8 Molar^{-1} sec^{-1}$ and $100 sec^{-1}$ respectively ($K_D = b/f = 1\mu Molar$). Furthermore, we assume that the total concentration of the buffer, that is free buffer, $[B]_i$, plus calcium bound to the buffer, $[CaB]_i$, is equal to $[B]_{i,Total}$, with $[B]_{i,Total} = 30\mu Molar$ in the shell just below the membrane ($i = n$) and $3\mu Molar$ everywhere else. These numbers are similar to those estimated for calcium buffering in the squid axon (Simon and Llinas 1985) and for calmodulin (Klee and Haiech 1980). We then have a second-order reaction (first-order in calcium) of the form

$$B + Ca^{2+} \; \underset{b}{\overset{f}{\rightleftharpoons}} \; CaB \tag{4.19}$$

It then follows that

$$\frac{\partial [Ca^{2+}]}{\partial t} = \frac{\partial [B]}{\partial t} = b[Ca \cdot B] - f[Ca^{2+}][B] \tag{4.20}$$

as well as

$$[B] + [Ca \cdot B] = [B]_{Total} \tag{4.21}$$

Because we are using a second-order numerical method to solve the diffusion equation, we are forced to use an equally accurate method to solve the buffering equation, since any less accurate method, such as first-order Euler, will result in us losing any gain due to the more accurate second-order scheme. Applying the Crank and Nicolson (1947) scheme, we replace the differential in eq. 4.20 by the difference equation

$$\begin{aligned}
\frac{[Ca^{2+}]_{i,t+\Delta t} - [Ca^{2+}]_{i,t}}{\Delta t} = & \; b \cdot [B]_{i,Total} - \frac{b}{2}([B]_{i,t+\Delta t} + [B]_{i,t}) \\
& - \frac{f}{2}([B]_{i,t+\Delta t}[Ca^{2+}]_{i,t+\Delta t} + [B]_{i,t}[Ca^{2+}]_{i,t})
\end{aligned} \tag{4.22}$$

Equation 4.22 is quadratic, that is, it contains terms in both buffer and calcium concentration. This nonlinearity is rather difficult to solve in a straightforward manner but can be circumvented by exploiting a slightly different mixed explicit-implicit integration scheme.

$$\begin{aligned}
\frac{[Ca^{2+}]_{i,t+\Delta t} - [Ca^{2+}]_{i,t}}{\Delta t} = & \; b \cdot [B]_{i,Total} - \frac{b}{2}([B]_{i,t+\Delta t} + [B]_{i,t}) \\
& - \frac{f}{2}([B]_{i,t+\Delta t}[Ca^{2+}]_{i,t} + [B]_{i,t}[Ca^{2+}]_{i,t+\Delta t})
\end{aligned} \tag{4.23}$$

Using a Taylor expansion around i, t one can show that eqs. 4.22 and 4.23 both have a local truncation error of the order of $(\Delta t)^2$, commensurate with the order of the numerical scheme we use to estimate the contribution of diffusion toward calcium dynamics. The equation for updating the buffer concentration $[B]$ is analogous to eq. 4.23:

$$\frac{[B]_{i,t+\Delta t} - [B]_{i,t}}{\Delta t} = b \cdot [B]_{i,Total} - \frac{b}{2}([B]_{i,t+\Delta t} + [B]_{i,t}) \qquad (4.24)$$

$$- \frac{f}{2}([B]_{i,t+\Delta t}[Ca^{2+}]_{i,t} + [B]_{i,t}[Ca^{2+}]_{i,t+\Delta t})$$

We thus have $2n$ linear equations for the entire sphere. As initial conditions for $[B]$, we compute the stationary value of eq. 4.24 for $[Ca^{2+}]_{initial} = 50 \ nM$.

4.6.4 Calcium Pumps

Although the calcium-buffering system discussed above reduces the amount of free intracellular calcium, the remaining calcium ions must ultimately be removed from the cell if calcium homeostasis is to be maintained. Two major transport systems have been identified (DiPolo and Beauge 1983; McBurney and Neering 1987): a sodium-dependent Ca^{2+} efflux, in which the energy required for the extrusion of calcium ions is derived from the inward movement of Na^+ ions down their electrochemical gradient, and a calcium-extrusion system that works independent of Na^+ and requires ATP as an energy source. The former extrusion system is a high-capacity but low-affinity system (half activated at 1–10 μM) while the ATP-driven pathway is active at much lower values of $[Ca^{2+}]$ ($K_m = 0.2 \ \mu M$) but has a smaller capacity. We neglect the Na^+-Ca^{2+} exchange system in our model and describe the ATP-driven pump by a first-order equation, with a voltage-dependent time constant so as to mimic the voltage trajectory of recovery from inactivation.

$$\frac{d[Ca^{2+}]}{dt} = \frac{[Ca^{2+}]_{equil} - [Ca^{2+}]_n}{\tau_{pump}(V)} \qquad (4.25)$$

where $[Ca^{2+}]_{equil}$ is the equilibrium concentration of the pump (50 nM), $[Ca^{2+}]_n$ the concentration of calcium in the nth shell just below the membrane, and $\tau_{pump}(V) = 17.7e^{(V/35)} \ msec$ is the pump's time constant. The appropriate difference equation is

$$\frac{[Ca^{2+}]_{n,t+\Delta t} - [Ca^{2+}]_{n,t}}{\Delta t} = \frac{[Ca^{2+}]_{equil}}{\tau_{pump}(V)} - \frac{[Ca^{2+}]_{n,t+\Delta t} + [Ca^{2+}]_{n,t}}{2\tau_{pump}(V)} \quad (4.26)$$

Note that these membrane-bound pump proteins have to move Ca^{2+} against an extremely large calcium gradient (5 orders of magnitude).

4.7   Potassium Accumulation

A number of phenomena, such as the magnitude of the repolarization phase of a spike, cannot be properly understood without simulating the reduction of the potassium battery, E_K, due to extracellular accumulation of potassium. Potassium accumulation is handled by assuming the existence of a well-mixed shell (pericellular space) surrounding the neuron that corresponds to the anatomical space between the nerve cell membrane and the glial sheath (Frankenhaeuser and Hodgkin 1956). The dynamics of extracellular potassium $[K^+]_o$ is governed by the influx of potassium from inside the cell via the five potassium currents (I_K $_{total}$) and the efflux of potassium by glial cell uptake as well as outward diffusion into the surrounding tissue. Faraday's law is used to convert the current due to the K^+ ions into concentration change. The shell is assumed to lose its potassium load with a time constant $\tau_{K-diff} = 7$ $msec$ and to be about 70 nm thick, these values being based on electrophysiological and anatomical estimates (Taxi 1976; Lancaster and Pennefather 1986).

$$\frac{d[K^+]_o}{dt} = \frac{I_{K\ total}}{V_{peri}F} - \frac{([K^+]_o - [K^+]_{rest})}{\tau_{K-diff}} \quad (4.27)$$

where F is Faraday's constant ($9.649 \cdot 10^{13}$ $Coulomb/mM$), V_{peri} is the pericellular volume, and $[K^+]_{rest}$ is the resting extracellular potassium concentration (2.5 mM). The value of the potassium-reversal battery is given by the Nernst equation:

$$E_K = 25 \cdot log\frac{[K^+]_o}{[K^+]_i} \quad (4.28)$$

where $[K^+]_i$ is the intracellular potassium concentration, which is held constant at 140 mM throughout the simulation, since the relative size of the concentration change is too small to be significant. Only the small volume of the periaxonal space coupled with the much lower extracellular concentration (4 mM) requires us to take extracellular potassium accumulation into account.

4.8   Integration

We are now faced with the formidable task of integrating all seven conductances, described by 11 different rate constants, with the passive properties of the cell as well as the varying concentrations of calcium, calcium buffer, and potassium. Conceptually, the system can be dissected into two different subsystems: the seven membrane-bound ionic conductances (as well as potassium accumulation) mainly governed by voltage, V, and the calcium system throughout the cell, which includes calcium diffusion, buffering, and extrusion. The calcium subsystem is linked to the voltage subsystem via the calcium current I_{Ca}, while linkage in the reverse direction is effected via the calcium-dependent currents I_{Ca}, I_C, and I_{AHP} and, to a much lesser extent, via the calcium battery, E_{Ca}. Solving this system requires the simultaneous solution of a set of highly nonlinear ordinary and partial differential equations in fifteen dimensions! To our knowledge, nobody has attempted this task.

We simplify this problem by updating the two subsystems in series, that is, explicitly, rather than using an implicit simultaneous update. Specifically, when advancing the voltage by one time step to $V(t + \Delta t)$, we use the value of the calcium concentration at t. Subsequent to this step, we compute the new distribution of calcium throughout the cell at $t + \Delta t$ as an explicit function of $V(t + \Delta t)$. The rationale for this approximation is the fact that the concentration of calcium and buffer changes on a slower time scale than the membrane conductances. Over the range of Δt value we use (10–100 μsec), which appears to be a good approximation. We will now discuss the two algorithms we use to update both subsystems.

4.8.1   Voltage Update

We use the simplest possible second-order predictor-corrector scheme to solve both for the membrane potential and for the rate constants. Voltage is predicted using an explicit first-order Euler scheme,

$$V(t + \Delta t) = V(t) + \Delta t \frac{d\,V(t)}{dt} \tag{4.29}$$

and corrected using a second-order mixed explicit-implicit integration method,

$$V(t + \Delta t) = V(t) + \frac{\Delta t}{2}\left(\frac{d\,V(t + \Delta t)}{dt} + \frac{d\,V(t)}{dt}\right) \tag{4.30}$$

These two voltage values are compared against each other. If they fall within a predetermined convergence criterion (here $7 \cdot 10^{-5}$ mV), the new voltage value is accepted. Otherwise the new value is used to recompute a better approximation of voltage until the convergence criterion is satisfied. Within the range of Δt chosen, the algorithm converges after at most two such iterations. The rate constants are updated in a similar fashion using this mixed second-order method. The three calcium-dependent rate constants (inactivation of I_{Ca} and activation of both I_C and I_{AHP}) use the calcium concentration in the shell, $[Ca^{2+}]_n$, at time t. All the details are described by Cooley and Dodge (1966), who used the same scheme to numerically integrate the Hodgkin and Huxley equations in an unmyelinated axon. The potassium concentration, $[K^+]_o$, and battery, E_K, are updated using a straightforward first-order Euler scheme.

4.8.2   Calcium Update

The calcium update routine must simultaneously solve for calcium diffusion, buffering, pumping, and the influx of calcium current. This can simply be achieved by combining eqs. 4.15, 4.18, 4.23, and 4.26 into a single set of $2n$ simultaneous equations. The last four equations are based on the mixed explicit-implicit Crank and Nicolson method. Thus, in principle, we must also evaluate the calcium influx due to the calcium current in a similar fashion, i.e., in the form of $d[Ca^{2+}]_n/dt = (I_{Ca}(t + \Delta t) + I_{Ca}(t))/(4FV_n)$. However, to our knowledge, no technique is currently available to solve efficiently this implicit nonlinear equation, and, as stated above, we decouple the voltage and calcium systems by the use of eq. 4.15. For the outermost shell, n, we have

$$
\frac{r_n}{\Delta t}([Ca^{2+}]_{n,t+\Delta t} \quad - \quad [Ca^{2+}]_{n,t}) = \tag{4.31}
$$

$$
\frac{D(r_n - \Delta r)}{2\Delta r^2} \quad (\quad [Ca^{2+}]_{n-1,t+\Delta t} + [Ca^{2+}]_{n-1,t}
$$

$$
- \quad ([Ca^{2+}]_{n,t+\Delta t} + [Ca^{2+}]_{n,t}))
$$

$$
+ \quad \frac{I_{Ca}}{2FV_n}
$$

$$
+ \quad b[B]_{total} - \frac{b}{2}([B]_{n,t+\Delta t} + [B]_{n,t})
$$

$$
- \quad \frac{f}{2}([B]_{n,t+\Delta t}[Ca^{2+}]_{n,t} + [B]_{n,t}[Ca^{2+}]_{n,t+\Delta t})
$$

$$+ \quad \frac{[Ca^{2+}]_{equil}}{\tau_{pump}(V)} - \frac{[Ca^{2+}]_{n,t+\Delta t} + [Ca^{2+}]_{n,t}}{2\tau_{pump}(V)}$$

The equation describing calcium concentration changes for the shells between the core and the membrane is

$$\frac{r_i}{\Delta t}([Ca^{2+}]_{i,t+\Delta t} \quad - \quad [Ca^{2+}]_{i,t}) = \qquad\qquad (4.32)$$

$$\frac{D}{2\Delta r^2} \quad (\quad (r_i + \Delta r)([Ca^{2+}]_{i+1,t+\Delta t} + [Ca^{2+}]_{i+1,t})$$

$$- \quad 2r_i([Ca^{2+}]_{i,t+\Delta t} + [Ca^{2+}]_{i,t})$$

$$+ \quad (r_i - \Delta r)([Ca^{2+}]_{i-1,t+\Delta t} + [Ca^{2+}]_{i-1,t}) \,)$$

$$+ \quad b[B]_{total} - \frac{b}{2}([B]_{i,t+\Delta t} + [B]_{i,t})$$

$$- \quad \frac{f}{2}([B]_{i,t+\Delta t}[Ca^{2+}]_{i,t} + [B]_{i,t}[Ca^{2+}]_{i,t+\Delta t})$$

The equation describing the calcium concentration change within the core is

$$\frac{r_{core}}{\Delta t}([Ca^{2+}]_{0,t+\Delta t} \quad - \quad [Ca^{2+}]_{0,t}) = \qquad\qquad (4.33)$$

$$\frac{3D}{2\Delta r_{core}^2} \quad (\quad (r_{core} + \Delta r)([Ca^{2+}]_{1,t+\Delta t} + [Ca^{2+}]_{1,t}$$

$$- \quad ([Ca^{2+}]_{0,t+\Delta t} + [Ca^{2+}]_{0,t}) \,)$$

$$+ \quad b[B]_{total} - \frac{b}{2}([B]_{0,t+\Delta t} + [B]_{0,t})$$

$$- \quad \frac{f}{2}([B]_{0,t+\Delta t}[Ca^{2+}]_{0,t} + [B]_{0,t}[Ca^{2+}]_{0,t+\Delta t})$$

The equation describing buffer concentration change from step to step is identical for each of the n shell:

$$\frac{[B]_{i,t+\Delta t} - [B]_{i,t}}{\Delta t} \quad = \quad b \cdot [B]_{i,Total} \qquad\qquad (4.34)$$

$$- \quad \frac{b}{2}([B]_{i,t+\Delta t} + [B]_{i,t})$$

$$- \quad \frac{f}{2}([B]_{i,t+\Delta t}[Ca^{2+}]_{i,t} + [B]_{i,t}[Ca^{2+}]_{i,t+\Delta t})$$

With the appropriate boundary conditions for $i = n$ and $i = 0$, we finally arrive at a set of $2n + 2$ linear equations in $2n + 2$ unknowns with constant coefficients. The simplest technique to solve this system is to substitute $[B]_{i,t+\Delta t}$ (evaluated from eq. 4.34 as a function of $[B]_{i,t}$, $[Ca^{2+}]_{i,t+\Delta t}$, and $[Ca^{2+}]_{i,t}$) into eqs. 4.31–4.33, and to invert the resulting tri-diagonal $n + 1$ by $n + 1$ matrix to arrive at the new value of $[Ca^{2+}]_i$ at time Δt. Efficient recursive algorithms are available for this purpose (e.g., Cooley and Dodge 1966; Press, Flannery, Teukolsky, and Vetterlig 1988).

4.8.3   Variable Time Step

Until now we have assumed that the time step Δt used to integrate the differential equations is fixed. However, during any particular simulation run, the dynamics of the system may first change very fast but later settle down to a more quiescent course. A typical example of this occurs during the application of long-lasting current stimuli. If the stimulus is above threshold, an action potential occurs, requiring a small value of Δt, due to the rapid change in the membrane currents, in particular I_{Na}, I_{Ca}, and I_C, and the large and rapid influx of calcium. A healthy cell will now show spike frequency adaptation (see Plate 2) and will fail to respond to the stimulus with any additional spikes. Since little change occurs during the adapted state, a large value of Δt can be used, substantially reducing the number of iterations required. We thus include a variable time step routine outside the main update loop (described above), which, given a time step Δt, advances the entire system (voltage and calcium) from time t to time $t + 2\Delta t$. Briefly, we advance the system in two steps from t to $t + \Delta t + \Delta t$, by computing the intermediate state at time $t + \Delta t$. Voltage and the value of calcium in the shell below the membrane are then compared against the same variables computed when advancing the system in a single step (using as the step size $2\Delta t$) from t to $t + 2\Delta t$. If the difference is below a given fixed lower threshold, the time step is increased and the system continues at time $t + 2\Delta t$. If the difference is above a given upper threshold, the time step is reduced and the system is reset to its state at time t. If the difference falls between the two thresholds, the system continues with its present value of Δt.

The speedup due to this simple procedure can be substantial, in the case of a simple Hodgkin and Huxley-like piece of squid membrane between one and two orders of magnitude. The increase in speed for partial differential equations is less noticeable, since the system has to be evaluated at every node every step. Moreover, in the case of the bullfrog

soma with an added axon (Yamada, Koch, and Adams 1988), action
potentials propagate from the cell body out into the axon. Thus, the
system cannot take advantage of the relatively slow rate of change at
the soma following the action potential, since compartments along the
axon will be subject to large changes in potential and will thus require
a small value of Δt.

To summarize, we decouple the system into two components, updating
each one of the subsystems independently using a mixed explicit-implicit
integration scheme with a local truncation error of the order of $(\Delta t)^2$ in
time and $(\Delta r)^2$ in space. Superimposed onto these two algorithms is a
routine determining the optimal value of Δt.

4.9   Results

Although the model contains numerous assumptions, it remains realistic in that it accurately predicts the observed voltage-clamp responses
of bullfrog sympathetic "B" cells (Koch and Adams 1984). This agreement is not surprising since the model is largely derived from experimental voltage clamp data (of the type shown in fig. 4.2). It is now
of great interest to see how successfully the model predicts independent current-clamp data under various conditions. Two particular sets
of conditions are examined here: (1) single spikes elicited by large but
very short current pulses, and (2) spike trains elicited by long-lasting
but rather small current pulses. In each case we examined the effects
of various pharmacological manipulations for which we have experimental data (for instance, the block of I_{Ca} via cadmium or the block of
I_{AHP} via curare or apamin). The basic response of the standard model
(fully described in Appendix 4.A) is shown in the panoramas of figs. 4.5
and 4.6. The   computed action potential, the individual ionic currents, the Nernst reversal potential for Ca^{2+} and K^+ and intracellular
calcium all are displayed here. The somatic action potential in this
vertebrate cell shares a number of similarities with the axonal action
potential of the squid (an invertebrate). Threshold, afterhyperpolarization, and repolarization back to the resting potential are all evident
in fig. 4.5a. One noticeable difference to the shape of a Hodgkin and
Huxley action potential is the second, long-lasting phase of the afterhyperpolarization, mediated by the calcium-activated voltage-independent
potassium conductance I_{AHP}. Moreover, the peak of the fast, transient calcium-dependent potassium current, I_C, is about 10 times larger
than the peak of the delayed rectifier current, I_K, and thus is largely

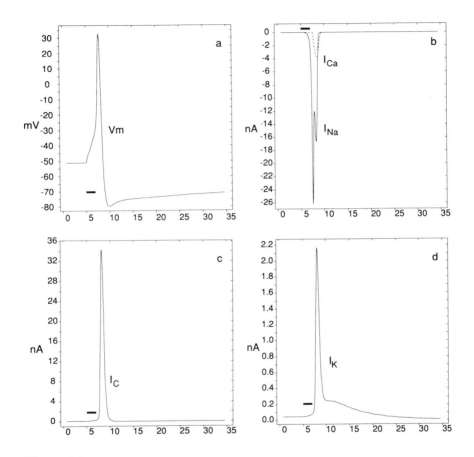

Figure 4.5
The response of the quiescent system (at $-51.26 \, mV$ for our standard parameters) to a brief 2 $msec$ current pulse of 1.75 nA amplitude applied at 5 $msec$ (indicated in this and the following figure by a black bar). This panorama depicts the fast components of the cell's response. The voltage trajectory is shown in (a). Notice the fast and slow components of the afterhyperpolarization following the action potential. (b) illustrates the two inward currents, I_{Na} and I_{Ca}. Only 9% of the incoming charge is carried by the Ca^{2+} ions. (c) shows the delayed rectified potassium current I_K and (d) the fast, calcium-dependent potassium current I_C. Since I_C is much larger than I_K, it is primarily responsible for recharging the cell's membrane potential back to rest.

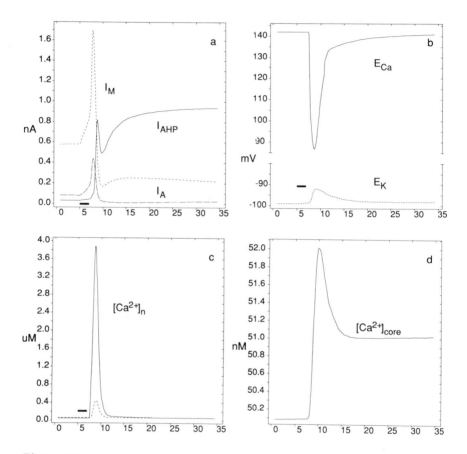

Figure 4.6
The response of the system following the same stimulus as in fig. 4.5. The three
small potassium currents I_A, I_M, and I_{AHP} are plotted in (a). I_{AHP} and, to a lesser
extent I_M, are responsible for the slow phase of the AHP following action potentials
(fig. 4.5a). The change in the Nernst potential for Ca^{2+} and K^+ is illustrated in (b).
The rapid and slow components of increase in E_{Ca} reflect free intracellular calcium
dynamics in the thin ($\Delta r = 0.1\ \mu m$) shell just below the membrane, $[Ca^{2+}]_n$, shown
in (c). Activation of I_{Ca} leads to a rapid influx of Ca^{2+}, which quickly becomes
bound to the buffer. The slow decay results from calcium loss via the pump as
well as diffusion toward the core of the cell. $[Ca^{2+}]$ for the tenth shell below the
membrane is also illustrated in this diagram. The calcium concentration in the core
($19\ \mu m$) is shown in the final diagram.

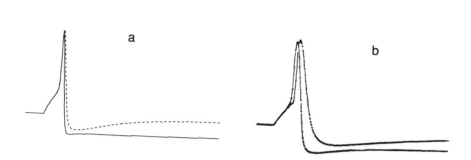

Figure 4.7
Effect of blocking calcium entry on simulated and observed action potentials. (a) shows the superimposed computed action potentials with normal (116 nS) and 5% of the normal value (5.8 nS) of the maximal calcium conductance, $\bar{g}_{Ca}$, during manual clamp to -60 mV. (b) Experimental data recorded before and after application of cadmium to block I_{Ca} show a very similar time course. The peak depolarization is 98 mV. Both traces are 50 $msec$ long.

responsible for repolarizing the potential following the excursion of the membrane potential to 0 mV and beyond. Thus, the I_K of the squid giant axon is replaced by I_C in the bullfrog sympathetic ganglion.

The role of calcium influx, and thus of I_{Ca}, in shaping the action potential is demonstrated in fig. 4.7. Here the standard computed action potential elicited by a brief current pulse is superimposed onto the action potential elicited after reducing the membrane calcium conductance to 5% of its normal value. The rate of repolarization is reduced; the peak afterhyperpolarization occurs later, is smaller, and decays much more rapidly under these circumstances than in control conditions (since I_{AHP} is not being activated). Despite I_C being almost zero under these conditions, this has only a rather small effect on the rapid spike repolarization. This is because even minor spike broadening, due to slower repolarization, can recruit substantial increases in I_K. The same phenomenon is seen in a real cell (fig. 4.7b) exposed to the calcium current blocker cadmium.

Plate 2 illustrates the predicted effects on action potential firing adaptation during various pharmacological manipulations. The upper left panel shows the control, highly adapting response in the absence of any synaptic or pharmacological blockers. Although a suprathreshold input (1.25 nA) is present for 300 $msec$, only a single spike is triggered. After block of I_M, adaptation is reduced but still obvious. Block of I_{AHP} by itself does not suppress adaptation but reveals the afterdepolarization following the spike. Simultaneous block of both I_M and I_{AHP} eliminates almost all of the adaptation, and the model responds as long as a suprathreshold stimulus is present. The synergistic role of these two currents in procuring efficient adaptation is also seen experimentally (Pennefather et al. 1985b). This prominent spike frequency adaptation is characteristic of bullfrog sympathetic ganglion cells and indeed of a large class of vertebrate neurons in the CNS (McCormick et al. 1985; Connor and Kriegstein 1986). As pointed out in section 4.5, both currents are reduced under natural conditions by the release of acetylcholine from presynaptic terminals and their subsequent binding to muscarinc receptors on the sympathetic ganglion cell.

We have modeled nicotinic synaptic transmission in these cells by incorporating a time-dependent conductance change into our model (fig. 4.8). An action potential can be initiated if the peak synaptic conductance change is 28 nS or larger. During a train of synaptic inputs, only the first synaptic input triggers an action potential in normal, adapted cells, since this action potential recruits sufficient I_M and I_{AHP} to induce adaptation. Following blockage of both of these currents, each synaptic input can elicit an action potential. Figure 4.9 shows the corresponding relationship between the frequency of the action potentials generated (f) and the injected current (I) for these four different conditions. To a first approximation, when blocking I_{AHP} the current threshold for eliciting action potentials remains constant (at about 0.63 nA) while the slope increases by a factor of 2 (from 2.4 spikes per nA to 4.7 spikes per nA). Blocking only I_M leaves the slope relatively unchanged while reducing the current threshold to 5% of its original value, i.e., to 0.03 nA. Blocking both conductances both lowers the threshold and increases the slope, leading to the dramatic removal of spike adaptation observed experimentally.

4.10   Discussion

The function of the large, transient ionic currents, $I_{Na}, I_{Ca}, I_C,$ and I_K in the daily chores of our ganglion cell are obvious: the sodium current generates and carries the action potential, while the remaining three large currents ultimately subserve the patterning of the action potential discharge. In this view, the principal role of the calcium current, I_{Ca}, is to activate the calcium-dependent potassium currents—leading to a fast repolarization and spike frequency adaptation. Moreover, I_{Ca} provides the crucial link—via influx of calcium ions—between electrical activity

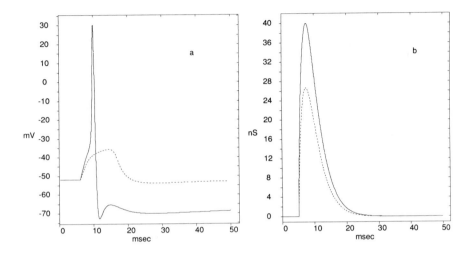

Figure 4.8
Modeling synaptic input. (a) illustrates the calculated ganglion cell response to a
conductance increase having the same time course as the fast nicotinic excitatory
postsynapatic current (EPSC) observed experimentally (Kuba and Nishi 1979). The
two superimposed voltage records were obtained with two different-sized conductance
changes (g_{peak} = 40 and 27 nS). (b) Postsynaptic current following the supra-
and the subthreshold synaptic input, clamped at -52 mV. Notice that the overall
amplitude of both cases does not differ dramatically.

spikes

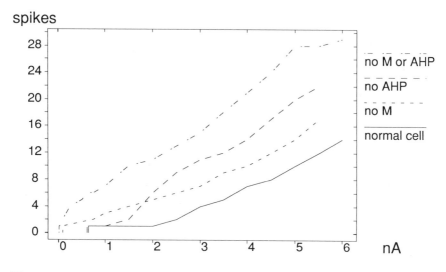

Figure 4.9
Firing frequency versus injected current. The number of calculated spikes following
200 *msec* current steps of variable amplitude in the adapted cell, after the complete
simulated block of either I_{AHP} or of I_M, and after the simultaneous block of both
I_{AHP} and I_M. Blocking I_{AHP} does not appreciably change the current firing threshold but increases the slope of the f-I curve, while blockage of I_M reduces the spiking
threshold.

and the initiation of metabolic events. In contrast, the role of I_{Ca} in
depolarizing the cell body during the action potential is small. Over-
simplifying, one may view the role of the small but persistent currents,
I_M and I_{AHP}, as controlling the transmission of information through
the cells by increasing the excitability of the cell (I_{AHP}) or reducing the
spiking threshold (I_M). Since these currents can be blocked via synaptically released substances, they could be the neuronal substratum for
such neuronal operations as sensory adaptation or routing messages selectively from a single neuron to different postsynaptic targets (Koch
and Poggio 1987).

   The seven currents discussed here are of relevance far beyond the
bullfrog, since very similar currents have been characterized in a host of
other preparations, ranging from mollusc neurons to human neocortical
neurons (for a review see Adams and Galvan 1986). In fact CA1 and CA3
pyramidal cells express all seven currents found in bullfrog cells as well as

a sustained sodium current (Wong, Prince, and Basbaum 1979), a slow, non-inactivating calcium current (Johnston, Hablitz, and Wilson 1980) and a small mixed sodium and potassium current, I_Q, that is activated when the cell is hyperpolarized. The importance of individual currents may vary, though, from cell type to cell type. For example, blocking I_{AHP} in hippocampal pyramidal cells leads to a much more dramatic reduction in spike frequency adaptation than in bullfrog sympathetic cells (Halliwell and Adams 1982; Cole and Nicoll 1984; Madison and Nicoll 1984; Lancaster and Adams 1986). However, the description of these currents in terms of activation and inactivation variables appears to remain relatively invariant across species and cell types.

In the last three decades, we have come to understand the electrical behavior and the integrative function of both nonmyelinated and myelinated axons, the cell body with its numerous currents and passive dendrites in the presence of massive synaptic inputs (see the previous and the following chapters). The daunting challenge facing us now is to extend this understanding to include the possibly highly nonlinear electrical properties of dendrites and synapses. The principal difficulty in this endevor is the fact that most neurons in the central nervous system possess a highly elaborate dendritic tree. Thus, events in the dendritic tree are electrically distant from the recording point, usually in the cell body. This lack of space clamp makes any quantitative evaluation of voltage-dependent currents exceedingly difficult (Rall and Segev 1985). It seems to us that only the judicious application of novel experimental techniques combined with computer simulations such as described in this book will enable us to understand the entire neuron as a computational entity.

The address of Walter Yamada and Christof Koch is Division of Biology, 216-76, California Institute of Technology, Pasadena, California 91125. Paul Adam's address is Howard Hughes Medical Institute, Department of Neurology and Behavior, State University of New York at Stony Brook, Stony Brook, New York 11794. Electronic mail should be addressed to koch@hamlet.caltech.edu or koch@caltech.bitnet.

Appendix 4.A: Modeling Bullfrog Sympathetic Ganglion Cells

PRINCIPAL EQUATION

The principal equation describing the change in intracellular potential at the soma (given in absolute terms by $V(t)$) is

$$C_N \frac{d}{dt}V + I_{Input} + I_{Na} + I_{Ca} + I_K + I_M + I_A + I_C$$

$$+I_{AHP} + I_{leak} + I_{syn} = 0$$

In the following pages, we will describe in detail the kinetics and voltage and calcium dependencies of these currents. Most currents will be described in terms of Hodgkin-Huxley like rate constants with first-order kinetics (all rate constants are normalized to 22° Celsius).

All variables have the following units:

Voltage	mV
Current	nA
Time	$msec$
Concentration	$mmoles\ per\ liter\ (mMolar)$
Conductance	μS
Resistance	$M\Omega$
Capacitance	nF
Volume	l

FAST SODIUM CURRENT

$$I_{Na} = \overline{g}_{Na} m^2 h(V - E_{Na})$$

The rate constants are given by Frankenhaeuser and Huxley (1964), relative to the resting potential, which we set to $-60\ mV$. The activation and inactivation variables, m and h, are further shifted to more positive potentials by $5\ mV$ and $15\ mV$ respectively. The kinetics of both m and h are slowed down by a factor of 2. Although some evidence for a secondary inactivation exists, it did not lead to any observable effect in our model. $\overline{g}_{Na} = 2\ \mu S$. This implies a density of about

$40\ mScm^{-2}$. $E_{Na} = 50\ mV$. The midpoint for m_∞ is $-20.7\ mV$, for m_∞^2 is $-10.8\ mV$, and for h_∞ is $-37.6\ mV$.

Activation variable:

$$\frac{dm}{dt} = \frac{m_\infty - m}{\tau_m}$$

$$\tau_m = \frac{2}{\alpha_m + \beta_m}$$

$$m_\infty = \frac{\alpha_m}{\alpha_m + \beta_m}$$

The forward and backward rate constants are given by

$$\alpha_m = \frac{0.36(V + 33)}{1.0 - e^{-(V+33)/3}} \quad \text{and} \quad \beta_m = \frac{-0.4(V + 42)}{1.0 - e^{+(V+42)/20}}$$

Inactivation variable:

$$\frac{dh}{dt} = \frac{h_\infty - h}{\tau_h}$$

$$\tau_h = \frac{2}{\alpha_h + \beta_h}$$

$$h_\infty = \frac{\alpha_h}{\alpha_h + \beta_h}$$

The forward and backward rate constants are given by

$$\alpha_h = \frac{-0.1(V + 55)}{1 - e^{(V+55)/6}} \quad \text{and} \quad \beta_h = \frac{4.5}{1 + e^{-V/10}}$$

FAST CALCIUM CURRENT

$I_{Ca} = \bar{g}_{Ca} mh(V - E_{Ca})$; where $\bar{g}_{Ca} = 0.116\ \mu S$

We felt it necessary to include a threshold for activation of this current at $-32\ mV$. In other words, $m_\infty = 0$ if $V < -32\ mV$. Inactivation does not depend on potential but on $[Ca^{2+}]_i$. The reversal potential E_{Ca} is variable (natural log assumed) with $E_{Ca} = 12.5 log\frac{[Ca^{2+}]_o}{[Ca^{2+}]_i}$, where $[Ca^{2+}]_o$ is the fixed extracellular concentration of Ca^{2+} is equal

to 4 mM, and $[Ca^{2+}]_i$ is the concentration of Ca^{2+} in the shell just below the membrane (see section 4.6). Initially, we have $E_{Ca} = 141.2\ mV$.
The midpoint for m_∞ is 3 mV and for h_∞ is 0.01 mM.

Activation variable:

$$\frac{dm}{dt} = \frac{m_\infty - m}{\tau_m}$$

$$\tau_m = \frac{7.8}{e^{+(V+6)/16} + e^{-(V+6)/16}}$$

$$m_\infty = \frac{1}{1 + e^{-(V-3)/8}}$$

Inactivation variable:

$$h = \frac{K}{K + [Ca^{2+}]_i};\ where\ K = 0.01\ mM$$

TRANSIENT, OUTWARD POTASSIUM CURRENT

$$I_A = \bar{g}_A mh(V - E_K);\ where\ \bar{g}_A = 0.120\mu S$$

$E_K = 25.0 log\frac{[K^+]_o}{[K^+]_i}$, where $[K^+]_o$ is the variable extracellular and $[K^+]_i$
is the constant intracellular potassium concentration, equal to 140 mM.
The midpoint for m_∞ is $-42\ mV$ and for h_∞ is $-110\ mM$.

Activation variable:

$$\frac{dm}{dt} = \frac{m_\infty - m}{\tau_m}$$

$$\tau_m = 1.38$$

$$m_\infty = \frac{1}{1 + e^{-(V+42)/13}}$$

Inactivation variable:

$$\frac{dh}{dt} = \frac{h_\infty - h}{\tau_h}$$

$$\tau_h = 50\ \ if\ \ V < -80mV\ \ else\ \ 150$$

$$h_\infty = \frac{1}{1 + e^{+(V+110/18)}}$$

Two of our currents, I_A and I_K have time constants that are modeled using either constant value or step functions. These parameters were modeled in this fashion because experimental data in these cases was sketchy; constant value functions lay within the variance of the data.

NON-INACTIVATING MUSCARINIC POTASSIUM CURRENT

$$I_M = \bar{g}_M m(V - E_K); \text{ where } \bar{g}_M = 0.084\mu S$$

The midpoint for m_∞ is $-35 \ mV$.

Activation variable:

$$\frac{dm}{dt} = \frac{m_\infty - m}{\tau_m}$$

$$\tau_m = \frac{1000}{3.3\left(e^{+(V+35)/40} + e^{-(V+35)/20}\right)}$$

$$m_\infty = \frac{1}{1 + e^{-(V+35)/10}}$$

DELAYED, RECTIFYING POTASSIUM CURRENT

$$I_K = \bar{g}_K m^2 h(V - E_K); \text{ where } \bar{g}_K = 1.17\mu S$$

$E_K = 25log\frac{[K^+]_o}{[K^+]_i}$. The midpoint for m_∞ is $-12.1 \ mV$, for m_∞^2 is $-1.6 \ mV$, and for h_∞ is $-25 \ mV$.

Activation variable:

$$\frac{dm}{dt} = \frac{m_\infty - m}{\tau_m}$$

$$\tau_m = \frac{1.0}{\alpha_m(V) + \beta_m(V)}$$

$$m_\infty = \frac{\alpha_m(V - 20)}{\alpha_m(V - 20) + \beta_m(V - 20)}$$

The forward and backward rate constants are given by

$$\alpha_m(V) = \frac{-0.0047(V + 12)}{e^{-(V+12)/12} - 1} \quad \text{and} \quad \beta_m(V) = e^{-(V+147)/30}$$

Inactivation variable:

$$\frac{dh}{dt} = \frac{h_\infty - h}{\tau_h}$$

$$\tau_h = 6000 \text{ if } V < -25 \ mV, \text{ else } 50.0$$

$$h_\infty = \frac{1}{1 + e^{+(V+25)/4}}$$

NON-INACTIVATING CALCIUM-DEPENDENT POTASSIUM CURRENT

$I_C = \bar{g}_C m(V - E_K)$; where $\bar{g}_C = 1.2\mu S$

Calcium-dependent activation variable:

$$\frac{dm}{dt} = \frac{m_\infty - x}{\tau_x}$$

$$\tau_m = \frac{1}{f(V, Ca) + b(V)}$$

$$m_\infty = \frac{f(V, Ca)}{f(V, Ca) + b(V)}$$

The forward and backward rate constants are given by

$$f(V, Ca) = 250[Ca^{2+}]_i e^{+V/24} \quad \text{and} \quad b(V) = 0.1e^{-V/24}$$

VOLTAGE-INDEPENDENT CALCIUM-DEPENDENT POTASSIUM CURRENT

$I_{AHP} = \bar{g}_{AHP} m^2(V - E_K)$; where $\bar{g}_{AHP} = 0.054\mu S$

The midpoint for m_∞ is 44.7 nM and for m_∞^2 is 69.5 nM.

Calcium-dependent activation variable:

$$\frac{dm}{dt} = \frac{m_\infty - m}{\tau_m}$$

$$\tau_m = \frac{1000}{f(Ca) + b}$$

$$m_\infty = \frac{f(Ca)}{f(Ca) + b}$$

The forward and backward rate constants are given by

$$f(Ca) = 1.25 \cdot 10^8 [Ca^{2+}]_n^2 \quad \text{and} \quad b = 2.5$$

PASSIVE COMPONENTS

$$I_{leak} = \overline{g}_{leak}(V - E_{leak}); \text{ where } \overline{g}_{leak} = 0.02 \mu S \ (50 M\Omega)$$

$E_{leak} = -10mV$. The experimentally measured total membrane cell capacity is $C_N = 0.150nF$. The input resistance of our standard cell can be measured by injecting very small de- or hyperpolarizing currents into the soma and measuring the resulting stationary de- or hyperpolarization. In our case, $0.05 \ nA$ of injected current changes the membrane potential by approximately $0.554 \ mV$, corresponding to an input resiance of $\approx 11.1 M\Omega$. The passive values used correspond to an unusual high specific capacity of $\approx 3.0 \mu F cm^{-2}$ (see Yamada, Koch and Adams, 1988) and a specific membrane leak resistance of $\approx 2500 \Omega cm^2$.

FAST, NICOTINIC SYNAPTIC INPUT

$$I_{syn} = g_{syn}(t)(V - E_{syn})$$

with $g_{syn}(t) = const \cdot te^{-t/t_{peak}}$. In order to match experimental data, we assumed $E_{syn} = -10 \ mV$ and $t_{peak} = 2.5 \ msec$ (Kuba and Nishi 1979). The peak conductance change, g_{peak}, achieved at $t = t_{peak}$, varied between 20 and 350 nS. For our standard cell, the minimal peak conductance change necessary to elicit an action potential, $g_{peak} = const \cdot t_{peak} \cdot e^{-1}$, is 26.75 nS.

CHAPTER 5

Analysis of Neural Excitability and Oscillations

JOHN RINZEL and G. BARD ERMENTROUT

5.1 Introduction

Qualitative features of the dynamics of excitable/oscillatory processes are shared by broad classes of neuronal models. These features are expressed in models for single-cell behavior as well as for ensemble activity, and they include excitability and threshold behavior, beating and bursting oscillations, bistability and hysteresis, etc. Our goal here is to illustrate, by exploiting a specific model of excitable membrane, some of the concepts and techniques that can be used to understand, predict, and interpret biophysically these dynamic phenomena. The mathematical methods include numerical integration of the model equations, graphical/geometric representation of the dynamics (phase plane analysis), and analytic formulas for characterizing thresholds and stability conditions. The concepts are from the qualitative theory of nonlinear differential equations and nonlinear oscillations, and from bifurcation theory. In this brief chapter, we will not consider the spatio-temporal aspects of distributed systems, so the methods apply directly only to a membrane patch, to a spatially uniform cell, or to a network with each cell type perfectly synchronized.

One may be familiar with models that exhibit one or two of the different dynamic behaviors, e.g., generation of individual or repetitive action potentials. However, one should realize that a given model, even a seemingly simple one, may display a great variety of response characteristics when a broad range of parameters is considered. This means that a given cell or ensemble may behave in many different modes, e.g., as a generator of single pulses, as a bursting pacemaker, as a bistable "plateauing" cell, or as a beating oscillator, depending upon the physiological conditions (neuromodulator or ionic concentrations) or stimulus presentations (applied currents or synaptic inputs). The nonlinear nature of the models provides the substrate for this broad repertoire; in contrast, linear models may be characterized by exponential and/or oscillatory time courses over their entire parameter ranges. It is important when studying a nonlinear model that stimulus-response properties be considered over ranges of the biophysical parameters.

Here we show that a simple but biophysically reasonable, two-current excitable membrane model is sufficiently robust to exhibit such behavioral richness, as parameters are systematically varied. By adjusting channel densities, activation dynamics, and stimulus intensities, we find that the cell can exhibit quite different threshold characteristics for spike generation (finite or infinite latency, with or without intermediate amplitude responses) and for onset of repetitive firing (finite or zero minimum frequency). The cell shows various types of bistable behavior: two different rest states in one case, and, in another case, a rest state with a coexistent oscillatory response around a depolarized level. The latter situation can provide a mechanism for bursting when an additional slower process (e.g., slow channel kinetics, or a channel affected by slow ion accumulation) responds differently at the two potential levels. Finally, we show that, when the cell is self-oscillatory, phase-resetting behavior for a single brief perturbing stimulus can often be used to predict phase-locking responses to periodic stimulation. These dynamic properties are generic and can, of course, be observed in more complicated, many channel, models. However, by choosing a reasonable but tractable model for illustration we are able to uncover the basic mathematical mechanisms of these behaviors.

The underlying qualitative structure for these behaviors will be revealed here with graphical phase plane analysis, complemented by a few analytic formulas. The concepts we will cover include steady states, trajectories, limit cycles, stability, domains of attraction, and bifurcation of solutions. Phase plane characteristics and system dynamics will be interpreted biophysically in terms of activation curves, current-voltage relations, etc. A user-friendly program, PHSPLAN (developed by G. B. Ermentrout) for IBM-compatible PCs, was used interactively, in the same spirit as an experimental "setup," to generate, explore, and visualize most of the behaviors described here; its numerical procedures are summarized in Appendix 5.B. The concepts apply to higher order systems, and in many cases appropriate projections of phase space, motivated by differences in time scales for certain variables, can lead to similar insights.

5.2   Models for Excitable Cells and Networks

Most models for excitable membrane retain the general Hodgkin and Huxley (1952) format, and can be written in the form:

$$C \frac{dV}{dt} + I_{ion}(V, W_1, ..., W_n) = I(t) \tag{5.1}$$

$$\frac{dW_i}{dt} = \phi \frac{[W_{i,\infty}(V) - W_i]}{\tau_i(V)} \tag{5.2}$$

where V denotes membrane potential (say, deviation from a reference, or "rest" level), C is membrane capacity, and I_{ion} is the sum of V- and t-dependent currents through the various ionic channel types; $I(t)$ is the applied current. The variables $W_i(t)$ are used to describe the fraction of channels of a given type that are in various conducting states (e.g., open or closed or ...) at time t. The first-order kinetics for W_i typically involve V-dependence in the equilbrium function $W_{i,\infty}$ and in the time constant τ_i; ϕ is a temperature-like, time scale factor that may depend on i. If the current, I_j, for channel type j can be suitably modeled as Ohmic, then it might be expressed as

$$I_j = \overline{G}_j \, \sigma_j(V, W_1, ..., W_n) \, (V - V_j) \tag{5.3}$$

where $\overline{G}_j$ is the total conductance with all j-type channels open (product of single channel conductance with the total number of j channels), σ_j is the fraction of j channels that are open (it may depend on several of the variables W_i), and V_j is the reversal potential (usually Nernstian) for this ion species. For some channel types the current-voltage relation may be more appropriately represented by the Goldman-Hodgkin-Katz expression, or by a barrier-kinetics scheme (Hille 1984). In the classical Hodgkin and Huxley model (1952) for squid giant axon, there are three variables W_i, denoted as m, h, and n, to describe the fractions, m^3h and n^4, of open Na^+ channels and K^+ channels, respectively.

For some purposes, it is important that the current balance equation (eq. 5.1) contain terms to account for ionic pump currents. These currents, as well as some channel conductances and ionic reversal potentials, may depend upon time-varying second messengers or ionic concentrations, e.g., in diffusionally restricted intracellular and/or extracellular volumes. For such considerations, additional variables and transport/kinetic balance equations would be included in the model, and these will carry along their own time scales. Indeed, some models that include the dynamics of intracellular free calcium ions introduce time constants that are orders of magnitude longer than channel kinetics and thereby set the time scale for phenomena like bursting oscillations (e.g., as in Chay and Keizer 1983). We also note that the form of eq. 5.2 is not unique; in a phenomenological model of Rall (see Goldstein and Rall 1974), the corresponding equations are nonlinear in the W_i.

Some models for excitability contain many variables and represent numerous channel types, especially if one seeks to account for rather detailed aspects of spike shape and dependence upon many different pharmacological agents. On the other hand, if qualitative or semi-quantitative characteristics of spike generation and input-output relations are adequate, say in network simulations, then a reduced two- or three-variable model may suffice. Such reductions can sometimes be obtained when time scale differences allow certain approximations such as relatively fast variables being instantaneously relaxed to pseudo steady-state values; e.g., if τ_j is small relative to other time constants, then one might set $W_j = W_{j,\infty}(V)$ in eq. 5.2. Likewise, functionally related variables with similar time scales might be lumped together. In this spirit, FitzHugh (1960) considered reductions of the Hodgkin and Huxley model (see also Rinzel 1985) and then introduced (FitzHugh 1961) an idealized, analytically tractable, two-variable model (also see Nagumo, Arimoto, and Yoshizawa 1962) that is widely studied as a qualitative prototype for excitable systems in many biological/chemical contexts. A recent FitzHugh-Nagumo/Hodgkin-Huxley hybrid was formulated and studied by Morris and Lecar (1981) in the context of electrical activity of the barnacle muscle fiber. The model incorporates a voltage-gated Ca^{2+} channel and a voltage-gated, delayed-rectifier K^+ channel; neither current inactivates. The calcium current here plays a role in spike generation analogous to that of the sodium current in the Hodgkin and Huxley model. A simple version of this model is represented by the equations:

$$\frac{dv}{dt} = -i_{ion}(v, w) + i \tag{5.4}$$

$$\frac{dw}{dt} = \phi \frac{[w_\infty(v) - w]}{\tau_w(v)} \tag{5.5}$$

where

$$i_{ion}(v, w) = \overline{g}_{Ca}\, m_\infty(v)\, (v - 1) + \overline{g}_K\, w\, (v - v_K) + \overline{g}_L\, (v - v_L) \tag{5.6}$$

Here quantities are in dimensionless form and written in lower case. In eqs. 5.4–5.6, w is the fraction of K^+ channels open, and the Ca^{2+}

channels respond to voltage so rapidly that we assume instantaneous activation. The nondimensionalization is done so that all dependent variables and many parameters are of order one, thus allowing easier comparison of terms in the equations, and this also helps to identify equivalent groups of parameters (e.g., FitzHugh 1969). The procedure is as follows. First, by dividing eq. 5.1 by V_{Ca} we can scale all voltages relative to V_{Ca} (thus, in eq. 5.6, $v_{Ca} = 1$). Similarly, dividing by a reference $\overline{G}_{Ca}$, with value $\overline{G}_{ref}$, the $\overline{G}$ of eq. 5.3 were scaled. These scalings mean that in eq. 5.4, i is $I/(V_{Ca}\,\overline{G}_{ref})$. Dimensionless t has been introduced as physical t divided by the reference τ, equal to $C/\overline{G}_{ref}$. In eq. 5.5, τ_w has been scaled so its maximum is now one, and ϕ equals τ divided by the pre-scaled maximum ($= 1/\overline{\lambda}_W$ in Morris and Lecar 1981). The voltage-dependent functions, m_∞, w_∞, and τ_w, and the reference parameter sets are given in Appendix 5.A. We note that the value of $\overline{G}_{ref}$ is somewhat arbitrary. If it is closer to the resting value of conductance for Ca^{2+} then τ will be closer to the resting membrane time constant and ϕ would generally be quite small, indicating that the K^+ conductance system is slower. All the computations and figures in this chapter are based on eqs. 5.4–5.6.

Even network models in certain approximations can reduce to a few variables. One example is the Wilson-Cowan model (Wilson and Cowan 1972), while another is discussed in chapter 8 below:

$$\mu_e \frac{d\mathcal{E}}{dt} = -\mathcal{E} + S(\alpha_{ee}\,\mathcal{E} - \alpha_{ie}\,\mathcal{I} - \theta_e) \qquad (5.7)$$

$$\mu_i \frac{d\mathcal{I}}{dt} = -\mathcal{I} + S(\alpha_{ei}\,\mathcal{E} - \alpha_{ii}\,\mathcal{I} - \theta_i). \qquad (5.8)$$

Here, $\mathcal{E}$ and $\mathcal{I}$ represent the respective firing rates of a population of excitatory and inhibitory interneurons. The parameters μ_e, μ_i are the membrane time constants; θ_e, θ_i are the firing thresholds; $\alpha_{ee}, ...$ are the "synaptic weights"; and $S(\cdot)$ is a nonlinear saturating function similar in form to $m_\infty(V)$.

5.3 Understanding Dynamics via Phase Plane Analysis

While an experimenter typically can measure membrane potential, it is usually impossible to monitor other dynamic variables (e.g., conductances) during nonclamped activity. For a theoretical model, we must compute explicitly the time courses of all dependent variables. Thus we

have predictive power and, in principle, more information from which
we can obtain additional insight by comparing the time courses and by
identifying the contributions and temporal relationships of the different
dynamic variables. A valuable way to view simultaneously the response
of different variables and their relationship to physiological functions is
by phase plane profiles, i.e., curves of one dependent variable against
another. Moreover, such plots allow us also to represent and interpret
geometrically aspects of the model (e.g., activation curves) along with
the response trajectories. At a glance we can see if the model has one
or multiple steady states, and which stimuli might invoke switching between states, and where these steady states lie in relation to activation
and $i - v$ characteristics. Also, by plotting various dynamic variables
against each other we may justify certain simplifications of the model,
e.g., plotting m versus voltage for an Hodgkin and Huxley model might
reveal that m is well approximated by $m_\infty(V)$.

Phase plane analysis was used effectively by FitzHugh (1960, 1961,
1969) to understand various aspects of the Hodgkin and Huxley equations and the two-variable FitzHugh-Nagumo model. His review
(FitzHugh 1969) also defines some basic mathematical terminology of
nonlinear dynamics and supplements our presentation. For additional
mathematical introduction, we recommend the books by Edelstein-
Keshet (1988) and Waltman (1986).

5.3.1   The Geometry of Excitability

Let's begin by considering the Morris and Lecar model in the case where
there is a unique rest state and a threshold-like behavior for action potential generation. Figure 5.1A shows the voltage responses to brief
current pulses of different amplitudes. The peak voltage is graded, but
the variation occurs over a very narrow range of stimuli; in this case, as
in the standard Hodgkin and Huxley model, the threshold phenomenon
is not discrete, but rather, steeply graded. In fig. 5.1B these same responses are represented in the $v - w$ plane. The solution path in the
space of dependent variables is called a trajectory, and direction of motion along a trajectory is often indicated by an arrowhead. In fig. 5.1B,
the flow is generally counterclockwise. All the trajectories shown here
ultimately lead to the rest point: $v = \overline{v}, w = \overline{w} = w_\infty(\overline{v})$. One says that
the rest state is globally attracting. Each trajectory has a unique initial
point, a horizontal displacement from the rest point corresponding to
instantaneous depolarization by a brief current pulse. The trajectory
of an action potential shows the following features: an upstroke with
rapid increase in v (trajectory is moving rightward) and then the plateau

with a slower increase in w corresponding to the opening of more K^+
channels. When w is large enough, the downstroke in v occurs—the trajectory moves leftward rapidly. Finally, as w decreases the state point
returns to rest with a slow recovery from hyperpolarization.

In the phase plane, the slope of a trajectory at a given point is dw/dv,
which is just the ratio of dw/dt to dv/dt, and these quantities are evaluated from the righthand sides of the differential equations (eqs. 5.4–5.5).
(The program PHSPLAN has a command to plot short vectors that indicate the flow pattern generated by the equations. This allows a global
view of the flow without having to compute the trajectories.) Thus a
trajectory must be vertical or horizontal where $dv/dt = 0$ or $dw/dt = 0$,
respectively. These conditions:

$$0 = -\bar{g}_{Ca}\, m_\infty(v)\,(v - 1) - \bar{g}_K\, w\,(v - v_K) - \bar{g}_L\,(v - v_L) + i \qquad (5.9)$$

$$0 = \phi\,\frac{[w_\infty(v) - w]}{\tau_w(v)} \qquad (5.10)$$

define curves, the v and w nullclines, which are shown dashed in fig. 5.1B.
This provides a geometrical realization for where v and w can reach
their maximum and minimum values along a trajectory in the $v - w$
plane; notice how the trajectories cross the nullclines either vertically or
horizontally in fig. 5.1B. The w nullcline is simply the w activation curve,
$w = w_\infty(v)$. The v nullcline, from eq. 5.9, corresponds to v and w values
at which the instantaneous ionic current plus applied current is zero;
below the v nullcline, v is increasing, and above it, v is decreasing. The
cubic-like shape occurs because the approximation of rapid activation
($m = m_\infty(v)$) of the calcium current leads to an N-shaped *instantaneous*
$i - v$ relation, $i_{ion}(v, w)$ versus v with w fixed (eq. 5.6). Such an $i - v$
relation is effectively realized in an excitable membrane for which the
v-gated channels carrying inward current activate rapidly. For another
viewpoint of the v nullcline, which is motivated by the slower time scale
of w, suppose we fix w, say, at a moderate value. Then the three points
on the v nullcline at this w correspond to three pseudo-steady states; at
the low-v state, small outward and inward currents cancel, while at the
high-v state, both currents are larger but are again in balance. These
states are transiently visited during the plateau phase and the return-
to-rest phase of an action potential. Notice how the trajectory is near
the right and left branches of the v nullcline during these phases.

If ϕ were smaller still, then the phase plane trajectories (except when
near the v nullcline) would be nearly horizontal (since dw/dv would be
small). In this case, the action potential trajectory during the plateau

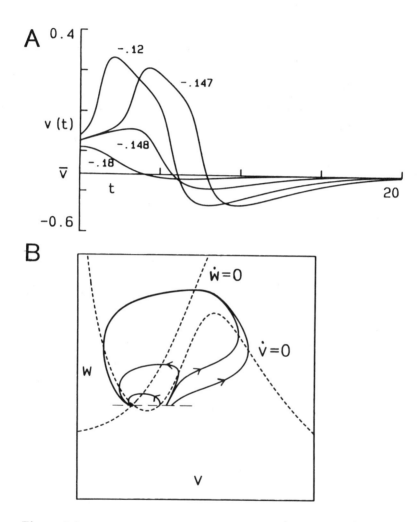

Figure 5.1
Response of the Morris and Lecar excitable system, eqs. 5.4–5.6, to brief current
pulse. For these parameters (Appendix 5.A), the model has a unique stable rest state:
$\bar{v} = -0.3173$, $\bar{w} = 0.1076$. Four different stimuli lead to instantaneous displacement
of v from $\bar{v}$ to v_o (values of v_o shown with curves). A shows time courses: v versus
t. Note intermediate-sized responses possible for some stimuli: threshold is graded;
firing occurs with finite latency. B shows trajectories in v-w phase plane; nullclines,
shown dashed, intersect only once. Effect of stimulus is to displace initial point
horizontally from rest (along long-dashed line).

and recovery phases would essentially cling to, and move slowly along, either the right or left branch of the v nullcline. The downstroke would occur at the knee of the v nullcline. The time course would be more like that of a cardiac action potential. Also, in the case of smaller ϕ, the threshold phenomenon would be extremely steep; the middle branch of the v nullcline would act as an approximate separatrix between sub- and super-threshold initial conditions. In contrast, for larger ϕ, the response amplitude is more graded. This theoretical conclusion led to an experimental demonstration for squid axon (Cole, Guttman, and Bezanilla 1970) that, at higher temperatures, the action potential does not behave in an "all-or-none" manner.

We remark that phase plane methodology applies to systems that are autonomous, i.e., in which there is no explicit time dependence in the equations. This means that the nullclines and flow field do not change with time. This could not be done if, for example, i were periodic in t; the treatment of periodic stimuli will be covered later. However, the phase plane method extends to cases where a step change in a parameter occurs. Then, the nullclines would change instantaneously, but not the current location of v and w. FitzHugh (1961) uses this trick to interpret anodal break excitation.

5.3.2 Oscillations Emerging with Non-Zero Frequency

In the phase plane treatment, the rest state of the model is realized as the intersection of the two nullclines; such steady-state solutions are also referred to as singular or equilibrium points. From the geometrical viewpoint, one sees how different parameter values could easily lead to multiple singular points—by changing the shapes and positions of the nullclines. In fig. 5.1, the unique singular point is attracting. Technically, we say it is asymptotically stable, i.e., for any nearby initial point the solution tends to the singular point as $t \to \infty$. In general, the local stability of a singular point can be determined by a simple algebraic criterion (Edelstein-Keshet 1988; Waltman 1986). The procedure is to linearize the differential equations and evaluate the partial derivatives at the singular point (this matrix of partial derivatives is called the Jacobian). Then one asks whether the exponential solutions to this constant coefficient system have any growing modes. If so, then the singular point is unstable; if all modes decay, then it is stable. For eqs. 5.4–5.6, the linearized equations that describe the behavior of small disturbances, $v \approx \overline{v} + x, w \approx \overline{w} + y$, from the singular point are

$$\frac{dx}{dt} = a\,x + b\,y \tag{5.11}$$

$$\frac{dy}{dt} = c\,x + d\,y \tag{5.12}$$

where

$$a = -\frac{\partial i_{ion}(v,w)}{\partial v} \tag{5.13}$$

$$b = -\frac{\partial i_{ion}(v,w)}{\partial w} \tag{5.14}$$

$$c = \frac{\phi}{\tau_w}\frac{dw_\infty}{dv} \tag{5.15}$$

$$d = -\frac{\phi}{\tau_w} \tag{5.16}$$

Solutions are of the form $e^{\lambda_1 t}, e^{\lambda_2 t}$ where λ_1 and λ_2 are the eigenvalues of the Jacobian matrix in eqs. 5.11–5.12; they are roots of the quadratic

$$\lambda^2 - (a+d)\lambda + (ad - bc) = 0 \tag{5.17}$$

For the parameters of fig. 5.1, the two eigenvalues are both real and negative.

As parameters are varied, the singular point may lose stability. In our example, the rest state could then no longer be maintained and the behavior of the system would change—it may fire repetitively or tend to a different steady state (if a stable one exists). Let us consider the effect of a steady applied current, and ask how repetitive firing arises in this model. We will apply linear stability theory to find values of i for which the steady state is unstable. First, we note that for eqs. 5.4–5.6, and for nerve membrane models of the general form (eqs. 5.1–5.2), a steady state solution $\overline{v}$ for a given i must satisfy $i = i_{ss}(\overline{v})$, where $i_{ss}(v)$ is the steady state $i - v$ relation of the model that is given by

$$i_{ss}(v) = i_{ion}(v, w_\infty(v)) \tag{5.18}$$

If i_{ss} is N-shaped (to be distinguished from the N-shaped instanta-neous $i - v$ relation, mentioned previously, for which w is held constant independent of v), then there will be three steady states for some range of i. However if i_{ss} is monotonic increasing with voltage, as for the case of fig. 5.1, then there is a unique $\overline{v}$ for each i, and moreover $(\overline{v}, \overline{w})$ cannot lose stability by having a single real eigenvalue pass through zero. (If zero were an eigenvalue, then eq. 5.17 would imply $ad - bc = 0$ which would further imply, from eqs. 5.13–5.17 and the definition 5.18, that $d\,i_{ss}/d\,v = 0$. This would contradict the assumed monotone behavior of

i_{ss} .) Therefore, destabilization can only occur by a complex conjugate pair of eigenvalues crossing the axis $Re\ \lambda = 0$ as i is varied through a critical value i_1. At such a transition, a periodic solution to eqs. 5.4–5.6 is born, and we have the onset of repetitive activity. This solution, for i close to i_1, is of small amplitude and frequency proportional to $Im\ \lambda$. Emergence of a periodic solution in this way is called a Hopf bifurcation (Edelstein-Keshet 1988; Waltman 1986).

From eqs. 5.11–5.12 or 5.17, we know that $\lambda_1 + \lambda_2 = a + d$. Thus, loss of stability occurs for the i whose corresponding $\overline{v}$ satisfies

$$\frac{\partial i_{ion}(v, w)}{\partial v} + \frac{\phi}{\tau_w} = 0 \tag{5.19}$$

The first term here is the slope of the instantaneous $i - v$ relation and the second is the rate of the recovery process; this condition also applies approximately to the Hodgkin and Huxley model (Rinzel 1978). From eq. 5.19 we conclude that loss of stability occurs (1) only if the *instantaneous $i - v$* relation has negative slope at $\overline{v}$; (2) when the destabilizing growth rate of v from this negative resistance just balances the recovery rate; and (3) only if recovery is sufficiently slow, i.e., if ϕ is small (low "temperature"). In fig. 5.2A, $\overline{v}$ is plotted versus i (this is the *steady state $i - v$* relation, but shown as voltage against i) and the region of instability is shown dashed.

Figure 5.2 also shows the maximum and minimum values of v for the oscillatory response. Just as a singular point can be unstable, so too can a periodic solution (Waltman 1986); unstable periodics are indicated by dashes. Here we see that the small amplitude periodic solution born from the loss in stability of $\overline{v}$ is itself unstable; it would not be directly observable. (In the phase plane, but not generally for higher-order systems, an unstable periodic orbit can be determined by integrating backwards in time.) Note that solutions along this branch depend continuously upon parameters and they gain stability at the turning point or knee. A stable periodic solution is called a *limit cycle*. The upper branch (solid) corresponds to the limit cycle of observed repetitive firing. The frequency increases with i over most of this branch (fig. 5.2B). At sufficiently large i repetitive firing ceases as $\overline{v}$ regains stability. The fig. 5.2A is referred to as a bifurcation diagram; it depicts steady-state and periodic solutions, and their stability, as functions of a parameter, and it shows where one branch bifurcates from another. Bifurcation theory allows one to characterize solution behavior analytically in the neighborhood of bifurcation points, e.g., the frequency of the emergent oscillation at the Hopf point is proportional to $|\ Im\ \lambda_{1,2}\ |$. When the periodic solutions that arise from

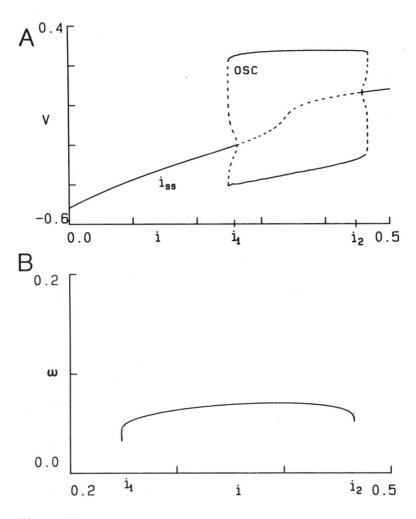

Figure 5.2
Repetitive firing in Morris and Lecar model for steady current. Bifurcation diagram
in A shows steady voltage $\overline{v}$ versus i (labeled i_{ss} , this curve is steady-state $i - v$ relation); instability indicated by dashes. Amplitude of periodic solutions (labeled "osc")
indicated by max and min values of v over one period. Repetitive firing represented
by solid portion of "osc" branch: stable solutions. Dashed portion (unstable periodic
solutions) continues smoothly from solid portion and meets i_{ss} with zero amplitude
(Hopf bifurcation). For these parameters, i_{ss} is monotone, and minimum firing frequency is non-zero (see B: frequency (ω) vs. i for stable oscillations). Parameters as
in fig. 5.1.

the Hopf bifurcation are unstable then, locally, the bifurcating branch bends back into the parameter region where the steady state is stable; this case is called a *subcritical* bifurcation. If the opposite occurs and the emergent oscillations are stable and "surround" an unstable steady state, then we say that the bifurcation is *supercritical*.

For a range of i values (between the Hopf point and the knee) this model exhibits bistability: a stable steady state and a stable oscillation coexist. Figure 5.3A illustrates the phase plane profile in such a case; a periodic response here appears as a closed orbit. The two attractors are separated by an unstable periodic orbit (not shown here). Initial values inside this orbit tend to the attracting steady state and a starting point outside of it will lead to the limit cycle of repetitive firing. A brief current pulse, whose phase and amplitude are in an appropriate range, can switch the system out of the oscillatory response back to the rest state. Such behavior has been seen for many models and observed, for example, in squid axon membrane (Guttman, Lewis, and Rinzel 1980). Time courses in fig. 5.3B illustrate the phenomenon. Bistable behavior of this sort could be exploited in order to turn on or turn off a pacemaker neuron with brief stimuli, i.e., a maintained stimulus would not be required to activate the pacemaker.

5.3.3   Oscillations Emerging with Zero Frequency

The Hopf bifurcation is one of a few generic mechanisms for the onset of oscillations in nonlinear differential equation models. In that case, the frequency at onset of repetitive activity has a well-defined, non-zero minimum. In contrast, some membranes and models (see, e.g., Connor, Walter, and McKown 1977) exhibit zero (i.e., arbitrarily low) frequency as they enter the oscillatory regime of behavior; Rall's model (see Goldstein and Rall 1974) also behaves this way. A basic feature in such systems is that i_{ss} versus v is N-shaped rather than monotonic as in the previous section. For eqs. 5.4–5.6 this occurs if the v-dependence of K^+ activation is translated rightward (see Appendix 5.A, and note value of v_3) so that the inward component of i_{ss} dominates over an intermediate v range. Thus, for some values of i, below the repetitive firing range, there are three singular points in the phase plane. We discuss this case, when the system is excitable, first. In fig. 5.4B we see the nullclines intersecting three times.

As determined by linear stability theory, the singular points are stable, unstable (a saddle), and unstable (spiral), respectively for the three increasingly larger values $\overline{v}$. The system is excitable with the lower $\overline{v}$ state being a globally attracting rest state: initial conditions near

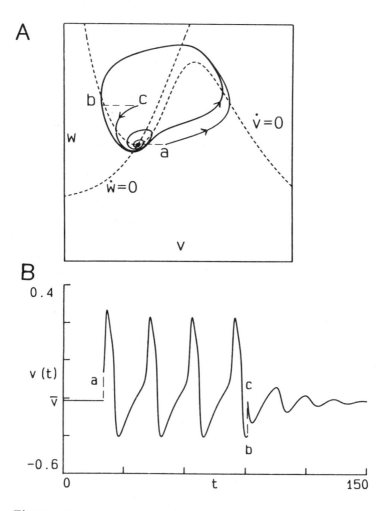

Figure 5.3
Bistability for steady current near threshold for repetitive firing. Morris and Lecar
model with parameters of figs. 5.1 and 5.2; $i = 0.25$. With i in "overlap" range of
fig. 5.2 near i_1, both a stable steady state $(\overline{v}, \overline{w})$ and a stable oscillation coexist. Initial
displacement with brief current pulse from $(\overline{v}, \overline{w})$ to point a leads to repetitive firing;
phase plane trajectory in A and v time course in B. Hyperpolarizing current pulse
during oscillation perturbs (v, w) from b to c and leads to annihilation of repetitive
firing.

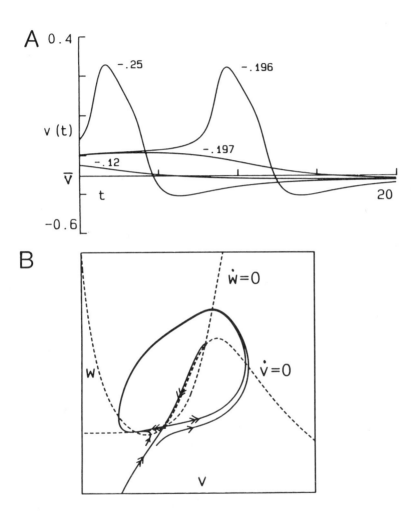

Figure 5.4
Excitability with three steady states and a distinct threshold; response to brief current pulse from unique stable rest state. Four different stimuli lead to instantaneous displacement of v from $\bar{v}$ to v_o (values of v_o shown with curves). A: Time courses: v versus t. B: Trajectories in v-w phase plane for two cases from A: $v_o = -0.12, -0.25$; note that starting points are slightly earlier in time to show more of trajectory through $(v_o, \bar{w})$. Nullclines, shown dashed, intersect three times. Double arrowheads indicate the stable and unstable manifolds of saddle point. Here (compare with fig. 5.1) firing can occur with infinite latency; threshold is strict and corresponds to separatrix (saddle point's stable manifold); intermediate-sized responses are not possible. Parameters as in preceding figures except $g_{Ca} = 1.0$, $v_3 = 0.1$, $v_4 = 0.145$, $\phi = 1/3$, and $i = 0.07$.

it lead to a prompt decay to rest, while larger stimuli lead to an action potential—a long trajectory about the phase plane. The phase plane portrait moreover reveals that this case of excitability indeed has a distinct threshold that is due to the presence of the saddle point. To understand this we note that associated with the saddle are a unique pair of incoming trajectories (double arrowheads), corresponding to the negative eigenvalue of the Jacobian matrix; together these represent the *stable manifold*. Corresponding to the positive eigenvalue are a pair of trajectories (double arrowheads) that enter the saddle as $t \rightarrow -\infty$; these are the *unstable manifold*. PHSPLAN has a command that generates these manifolds. The stable manifold defines a separatrix curve in the phase plane that sharply distinguishes sub- from super-threshold initial conditions. For initial conditions near the threshold separatrix there is a long latency before firing or decaying as a subthreshold response (see fig. 5.4A). This is because the trajectory starts close to (but not exactly on) the stable manifold and so the solution comes very near the saddle singular point (where it moves very slowly) before taking off. Note, the action potential trajectory follows along the unstable manifold, which passes around the unstable spiral and eventually tends to the rest point. Such a trajectory that joins two singular points is called a heteroclinic orbit. The other branch of the unstable manifold is also a heteroclinic orbit from the saddle to the rest point. This heteroclinic pair forces any trajectory that begins outside it to remain outside it—thus preserving the amplitude of the action potential. In this case we do not find graded responses for any brief current pulses from the rest state.

This case also provides a counterexample to a common misconception in which it is believed that if there are three steady states then the "outer" two are stable while the "middle" one is unstable. In fact, in some parameter regimes this model has three singular points, none of which is stable.

Next we tune up i and ask when repetitive firing occurs. Because i_{ss} is N-shaped we know that the lower and middle $\bar{v}$ move toward each other as i increases, and there is a critical value i_1 where they meet. In the phase plane, this means that the rest point and the saddle coalesce and then disappear; this is called a *saddle-node bifurcation*. Moreover, the heteroclinic pair become a single closed loop, a limit cycle, which for i just above i_1 has very long period (fig. 5.5). Thus, in this parameter regime, the transition to repetitive firing is marked by arbitrarily low frequency (fig. 5.6B). For i near the critical current, the frequency is proportional to $\sqrt{i - i_1}$. When $i = i_1$ the limit cycle has infinite period; it is called a *homoclinic orbit*—it begins and ends on a singular point.

In this case, the singular point is degenerate, a saddle node, with one zero eigenvalue, and the homoclinic is also said to be degenerate. This behavior is generic and this type of zero-frequency onset occurs over a range of parameters. We emphasize, as did Connor *et al.*, (1977), that this mechanism allows arbitrarily low firing rates without relying on channel activation rates which are slow. The value i_1 is determined by evaluating i_{ss} at the value of v for which $di_{ss}/dv = 0$, and this latter condition is equivalent to having the determinant $ad - bc$ of the Jacobian matrix equal zero.

The global picture of repetitive firing is shown in the bifurcation diagram of fig. 5.6A, with frequency versus i in fig. 5.6B. The branch of steady states (unstable shown dashed) form the S-shaped curve, and the oscillatory solutions are represented by the forked curve whose open end begins at $i = i_1$. As i increases beyond i_1 the peak-to-peak amplitude on the stable (repetitive firing) branch decreases and frequency generally increases. The family of periodic solutions terminates at $i = i_2$ via a subcritical Hopf bifurcation. Except for i in a small interval of this upper range, this system is monostable. Annihilation of repetitive firing as in fig. 5.3 cannot be carried out for i near i_1 in this case.

5.3.4   More Bistability and Bursting

It is important to realize that the behavior of the solutions (bifurcation diagrams) we have described depend on other parameters in the model. The temperature parameter ϕ is particularly convenient, with useful interpretative value, for additional parametric tuning. This parameter, since it plays no role in i_{ss} , does not affect the values along the S-shaped curve of steady states in fig. 5.6, or the corresponding curve in fig. 5.2. The stability of a steady state does however depend on ϕ. As is seen from eq. 5.19, when ϕ is large, oscillatory destablization is precluded; Hopf bifurcation from a steady state only occurs when the time scales of v and w are comparable. Thus for large ϕ both the upper and lower branches of the S curve are stable; the middle branch is of course unstable. This system is bistable. In this large-ϕ limit, the kinetics of the K^+ system are so fast (essentially instantaneous with $w = w_\infty(v)$) that the model reduces to one dynamic variable, v. Then stability is determined only by the slope of i_{ss} so the two "outer" states are stable and the "middle" is unstable. This simple example also shows that sometimes a model can be conveniently reduced to a lower dimension when there are significant time scale differences between variables.

For intermediate values of ϕ, the dynamics of both v and w influence stability and the upper branch is unstable for a certain range of i.

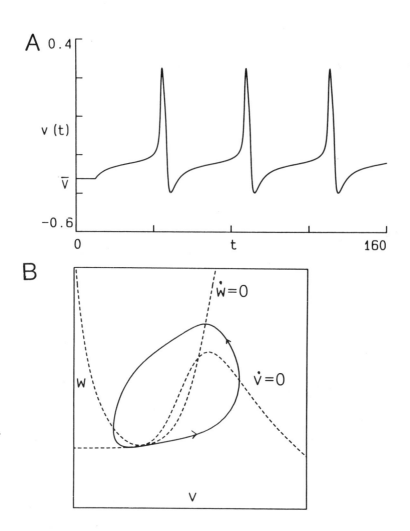

Figure 5.5
Onset of repetitive firing with arbitrarily low frequency for constant current. Parameters as in fig. 5.4 with current stepped to $i = 0.085$, just above value for which stable rest state and threshold saddle point coalesce. Time course in A and v-w phase plane in B. Note that most of interspike interval is spent with trajectory moving very slowly in region of phase plane where rest state/saddle coalescence occurred.

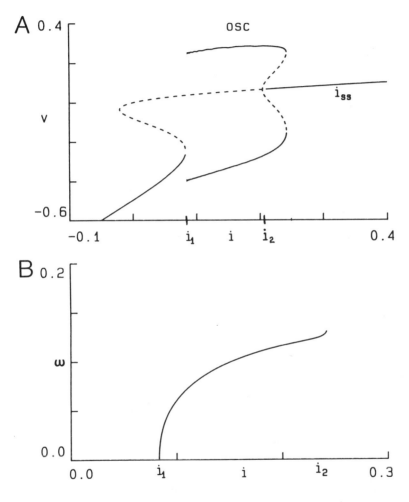

Figure 5.6
Multiple steady states and periodic solutions for steady current when i_{ss} relation is
N-shaped. Bifurcation diagram in A; solid indicates stable solution and dashed for
unstable. Parameters as in figs. 5.4 and 5.5. In spite of coexistent states, system is
monostable for each $i < i_2$. Onset of repetitive firing occurs for $i = i_1$, where stable
rest state and saddle coalesce, and with zero frequency; corresponds, in fig. 5.4, to
unstable manifolds of saddle forming a closed orbit. Branch "osc" becomes unstable at "turning point," just beyond i_2, and terminates via Hopf bifurcation at i_2.
Frequency (ω) of stable periodic solutions versus i shown in B.

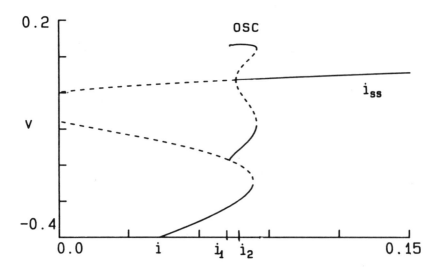

Figure 5.7
Bifurcation diagram as in fig. 5.6 but for $\phi = 1.15$. Note magnified scale. Here, "osc" branch emanates at i_1, before coalescence of rest state and saddle. For much larger ϕ, "osc" branch would not exist and high-v steady state would be stable for each i. Note "ss" branch is identical in shape to that in fig. 5.6; ϕ only affects stability of steady states.

Figure 5.7 shows a case (parameters slightly different from examples above) in which a branch of periodic solutions emerges via (subcritical) Hopf bifurcation along the upper branch and then terminates when the limit cycle makes contact with the saddle (middle branch of S curve); we might say when the oscillating v just meets the threshold. At this point ($i = i_1$) the periodic solution is lost with infinite period. This situation of a homoclinic orbit differs from that in fig. 5.6 because here the homoclinic connection is not made at the S curve's knee; this is not a degenerate homoclinic orbit. Also, here the frequency tends to zero like $1/log(i-i_1)$, rather than as the square root in the preceding section. Another difference from the previous example is that this case exhibits multistability for i between i_1 and the lower knee of the S; there is a stable steady state at a lower value of $\overline{v}$ and a stable oscillation around a higher $\overline{v}$ (which itself may be stable or unstable). Figure 5.8A gives the phase plane profile for such a case, and fig. 5.8B illustrates how the response may be switched between two stable states with brief current pulses. The Hodgkin and Huxley model, adjusted for higher than normal external potassium, exhibits similar behavior (Rinzel 1985).

This example of multistability is important as it also forms the basis for a general class of bursting phenomena. Consider what would be observed if i were very slowly swept back and forth through the overlap range. The response would exhibit alternating phases of high-v spike-like oscillations and near-steady-state behavior at low-v, i.e., bursting with a trajectory in the $i - v$ plane as indicated in fig. 5.9B. However, this example relies on external control, the imposed oscillating i, to generate the bursting behavior. It would be an appropriate model for a "follower" cell rather than for an autonomous or endogenous burster. For the latter case, the slowly changing variable should be coupled bidirectionally to (i.e., it affects and is affected by) the membrane dynamics. In many cases, intracellular free calcium concentration, $[Ca^E2+]_i$, plays the role of this slowly changing variable. Voltage-gated Ca^{2+} channels provide the source for $[Ca^E2+]_i$, which then feeds back to the membrane to turn on an outward current (e.g., Ca^{2+}-activated K^+ current) or perhaps inactivate the inward Ca^{2+} current (see the previous chapter). Such a model has been proposed to explain the electrical activity of insulin-secreting pancreatic β cells in the presence of steady glucose (Chay and Keizer 1983).

Here we illustrate the underlying basis of such endogenous bursting by exploiting the structure of fig. 5.7 and by adding i as a dynamic dependent variable to our model (eqs. 5.4–5.6). A very simple dynamics will suffice—it merely guarantees that i changes slowly and that i is decreasing when the membrane is in the high-v oscillating mode but increasing when the membrane is in the low-voltage steady-state mode. The long dashed curve in fig. 5.8 represents a nullcline for i that satisfies the latter goal and is incorporated into the following equation for i:

$$\frac{di}{dt} = \epsilon[(v^* - v) - \alpha i] \qquad (5.20)$$

Here, ϵ is small to guarantee that i is a slow variable. Although we do not force the physiological interpretation of $i(t)$ for this illustration, i may be viewed as a slow current that, at steady state, is outward for $v > v^*$ and inward for $v < v^*$. The autonomous burst pattern for the three-variable model, eqs. 5.4–5.6 and 5.20, is shown in fig. 5.9A. Its projection onto the $i - v$ plane appears in fig. 5.9B. This type of square-wave bursting, as also seen in the β-cell system (and analyzed in this way by Atwater and Rinzel [1986]), is to be contrasted with parabolic bursting (Rinzel and Lee 1987), which seems to depend on there being

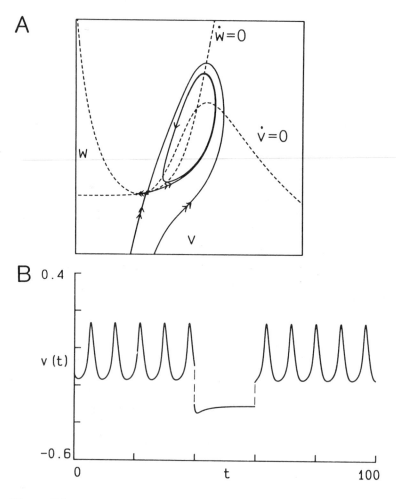

Figure 5.8
Bistability, high-v stable oscillation coexists with low-v stable steady state, for a case
of N-shaped i_{ss} . Parameters as in fig. 5.7 with $i\,(=0.075)$ slightly greater than i_1.
Phase plane A: shows oscillation as closed orbit around high-v steady state; stable
manifolds of saddle shown with double arrowheads. B: Brief current pulses cause
switching between stable states.

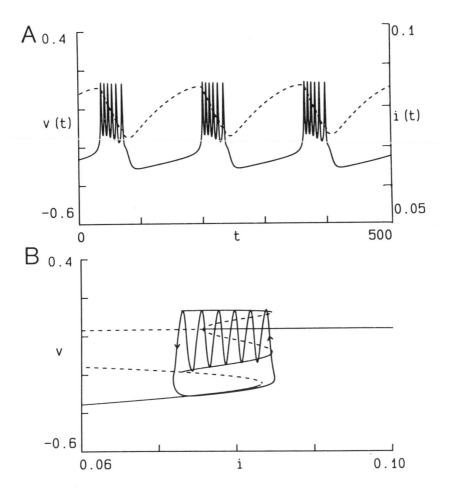

Figure 5.9
Bursting oscillation arises when i becomes autonomous slow variable and spike-generating dynamics are bistable as in fig. 5.8. Morris and Lecar model is appended by eq. 5.20 with parameters: $v^* = -0.22$, $\epsilon = 0.002$, $\alpha = 0$. A: time courses of voltage and i show that i slowly decreases when (v, w) are in high-v oscillatory state and slowly increases when (v, w) are in low-v steady state. B: projection of burst pattern onto $i - v$ plane with bifurcation diagram of fig. 5.7 shows that trajectory alternately tracks the two coexistent attractors of fast dynamics with rapid transitions when either attractor coalesces with threshold saddle point.

at least two slow variables and which does not require that the dynamics for the faster variables exhibit bistability as seen in fig. 5.7.

Here again we have understood the complex nonlinear dynamics by exploiting the significantly different time scales of variables to dissect the model. First, we treat the slow variable as a parameter and determine the attracting states of the fast dynamics. Then we superimpose the slow dynamics to see how the trajectory of the full system slowly tracks along the attracting branches of the fast subsystem. Rapid transitions can occur when branches terminate abruptly (e.g., at turning points).

We emphasize that even such a simple three-variable model can exhibit the complex behavior of bursting oscillations. Moreover, because of this simplicity and the geometric viewpoint we offer, the role of each of the three variables is clear. Finally, this model is sufficiently robust that in certain parameter ranges it appears to exhibit chaotic behavior (not shown here, but which can be seen for parameters as in fig. 5.9 but with $\epsilon = 0.009$ and $v^* = -0.12$. For an introduction to the concepts of deterministic chaos for autonomous as well as periodically forced nonlinear systems see Glass and Mackey (1988).

5.4   Phase Resetting and Phase Locking of Oscillators

We now turn our attention to a brief description of forced and coupled neural oscillators. This is in general a very difficult problem and we will only touch on it briefly. Before treating a specific example, it is useful to discuss certain important aspects of oscillators. We say that a periodic solution to an autonomous (time does not explicitly appear in the righthand side) differential equation is (*orbitally*) asymptotically stable if perturbations from the oscillation return to the oscillation as $t \to \infty$. The difference between asymptotic stability of an oscillation and that of a steady-state solution is that for the oscillation the time course may exhibit a shift. That is, we do not expect the solution of the perturbed oscillation to be the same as the unperturbed (see fig. 5.10A). This shift is due to the time-translation invariance of the periodic solution. Indeed, in phase space, the periodic trajectory is unchanged by translation in time. This shift that accompanies the perturbation of the limit cycle can be exploited in order to understand the behavior of the oscillator under external forcing. Suppose that an oscillator has a period, say T. We may let $t = 0$ correspond to the time of peak value of one of the oscillating variables, so that at $t = T$ we are back to the peak. Given that we lie on the periodic solution, if some t is specified then we know precisely the state of each oscillating variable. This allows us to introduce the notion of *phase* of the periodic solution. Let $\theta = t/T$ define the phase of the periodic solution so that $\theta = 0, 1, 2, \ldots$ all define the same point on the periodic solution. For example, if $\theta = 8.5$ then we are halfway through the cycle of the oscillator.

With the notion of phase defined, we now examine how a perturbation shifts the phase of the oscillator. In fig. 5.10A, we show the voltage time course for the Morris-Lecar system in the oscillating regime. At a fixed time, say t, after the voltage peak, we apply a brief depolarizing current pulse. This shifts the time of the next peak and this shift remains for all time (the solid curve is the perturbed oscillation and the dashed is the unperturbed—in this case the time for the next peak is shortened). If the time of the next peak is shortened from the natural time, we say that the stimulus has advanced the phase. If the time of the next peak is lengthened then we have delayed the phase. Let T_1 denote the time of the next peak. Then the phase shift is $(T - T_1)/T$, and T_1 depends on the time t or the phase $\theta = t/T$ at which the stimulus is applied. Thus, we can define a phase shift $\Delta(\theta) \equiv (T - T_1(\theta))/T$. The graph of this function is called the *phase response curve* for the oscillator. If $\Delta(\theta)$ is positive then the perturbation advances the phase and the peak will occur sooner. On the other hand, if $\Delta(\theta)$ is negative then the phase is delayed and the next peak will occur later. We can easily compute this function numerically and the same idea can be used to analyze an experimental system. Moreover, this curve can be used as a rough approximation of how the oscillator will be affected by repeated perturbation (periodic forcing) with the same current pulse. More complete descriptions and numerous examples of phase models and phase response curves can be found in Winfree (1980) and Glass and Mackey (1988).

In fig. 5.10B, we show a typical phase response curve for the Morris and Lecar model computed for both a depolarizing stimulus (solid line) and a hyperpolarizing stimulus (dashed line). The stimulus consists of a current pulse of magnitude 1.0 applied for 0.1 time units at different times after the voltage peak. The time of the next spike is determined and this yields the phase response curve as above. The figure agrees with our intuition; if the depolarizing stimulus comes while $v(t)$ is increasing (i.e., during the upstroke or slow depolarization of recovery), the peak will occur earlier and we will see a phase advance. If the stimulus occurs while $v(t)$ is decreasing (i.e., during the downstroke), there will be a delay. The opposite occurs for hyperpolarizing stimuli. The curves show that it is difficult to delay the onset of an action potential

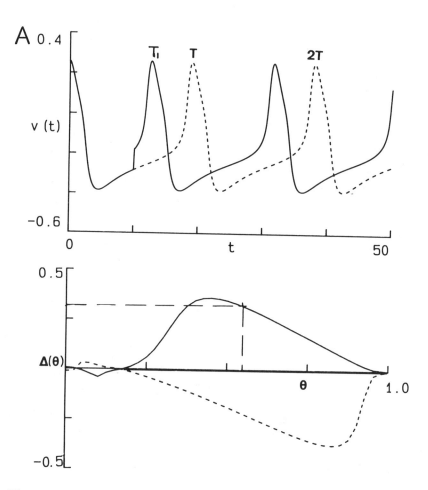

Figure 5.10
Phase resetting of a Morris-Lecar oscillator. Parameters as in figs. 5.4–5.6, with $i = 0.095$. A: a brief depolarizing stimulus can shorten the onset to the next spike and thus advance the phase. B: phase response curve (PRC) for stimulus at different times. The current pulse lasts 0.1 time units and has an amplitude of ±1.0. The solid curve indicates the phase response curve for a depolarizing stimulus and the dashed curve for a hyperpolarizing stimulus. The darkened axis indicates the regime where the voltage is increasing; generally, depolarizing stimuli lead to phase advance ($\Delta > 0$) in this range. The small cross on the depolarizing phase response curve refers to the experiment performed in fig. 5.11.

with a depolarizing stimulus or advance it with a hyperpolarizing one. For different sets of parameters, these curves may change. As we have seen in the previous section, it is sometimes possible to completely stop the oscillation if a stimulus is given at the right time. In this case, the phase response curve is no longer defined; nearby phases can then have arbitrarily long latencies before firing.

We now show how this function can be used to analyze a periodically forced oscillator. Suppose that every P time units a current pulse is applied to the cell. Let θ_n denote the phase at the time of the nth stimulus. This stimulus will either advance or delay the onset of the next peak depending on the phase at which the stimulus occurs. In any case, the new phase after time P and just before the next stimulus will be $\theta_n + \Delta(\theta_n) + P/T$. To understand this, first consider the case where there is no stimulus. Then after time P the oscillator will advance P/T in phase. But the stimulus advances or delays the phase by an amount $\Delta(\theta_n)$ so that this is just added to the unperturbed phase. This results in an equation for the new phase just before the next stimulus:

$$\theta_{n+1} = \theta_n + \Delta(\theta_n) + P/T \qquad (5.21)$$

This difference equation can be solved numerically. Here we will consider the natural question of whether the periodic stimulus can entrain the voltage oscillation. That is, we ask whether there is a periodic solution to this forced neural oscillation. In general, a periodic solution is one for which there are M voltage spikes for N stimuli where M and N are positive integers. When such a solution exists, we have what is known as *M:N phase locking*.

Finding *M:1* phase-locked solutions is quite easy. We require the oscillator to undergo M oscillations per stimulus period. In terms of eq. 5.21 this means we seek a solution that satisfies

$$\theta + M = \theta + \Delta(\theta) + P/T \qquad (5.22)$$

for some value of θ. For if such a solution exists and if the solution is stable (to be defined below), then if we start near θ, we can iterate eq. 5.21 and end up back at θ. This θ is the locking phase just before the next stimulus and since it doesn't change from stimulus to stimulus, the resulting solution must be periodic. Obviously, a necessary condition for a solution to eq. 5.22 is that $M - P/T$ lie between the maximum and minimum of $\Delta(\theta)$, i.e., we must solve

$$M - P/T = \Delta(\theta) \qquad (5.23)$$

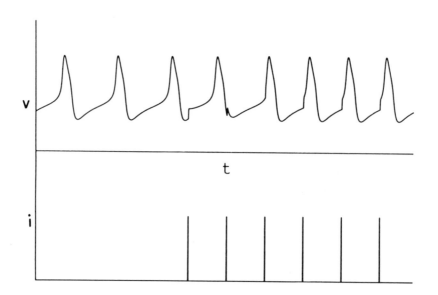

Figure 5.11
Phase locking (1:1) of the Morris-Lecar model subjected to a repeated short current pulse with period 13.5 time units. The period of the unperturbed oscillator is 19.0. The measured locking time of the stimulus after the peak is 11.2. This is exactly as predicted from solving eq. 5.23 (cross on the phase response curve in fig. 5.10B).

Having solved this, we need to determine the stability of the solution. For equations of the form of eq. 5.21 a necessary and sufficient condition for θ to be a stable solution is that $-2 < \Delta'(\theta) < 0$. Since $\Delta(\theta)$ is periodic and continuous there will in general be two solutions to eq. 5.23 (see fig. 5.10B), but only one of them will occur where $\Delta(\theta)$ has a negative slope, so that there will be a unique stable solution. We must also worry about whether the negative slope is too steep (i.e., more negative than -2); for small stimuli, this will never be the case—stability is assured. When $\Delta'(\theta) < -2$ (instability), very complex behavior can occur such as chaos (e.g., see Glass and Mackey 1988). The case of $M{:}N$ phase locking where $N > 1$ is more difficult to explain, so we will not consider it here. It is clear that if the stimulus is weak, the magnitude of $\Delta(\theta)$ will also be small so that $M - P/T$ must be small in order to achieve $M : 1$ locking. On the other hand if the stimulus is too strong, then we must be concerned with the stability of the locked solution. We note that in a sense eq. 5.21 is only valid for stimuli that are weak compared to the strength of attraction of the limit cycle, since for stronger stimuli it will take the solution more than a single oscillation to return to points close to the original cycle. The phase response curve in fig. 5.10B shows that, when the stimulus is depolarizing, it is easier to advance the Morris-Lecar oscillator and thus force it at a higher frequency than it is to force it at a lower frequency. For hyperpolarizing stimuli, we can more easily drive it at frequencies lower than the natural frequency (the counter results are possible but for small ranges of parameters; also, see Perkel, Schulman, Bullock, Moore, and Segundo 1964).

To illustrate these concepts, we have periodically stimulated the Morris-Lecar model (natural period of 19.0) with the same brief depolarizing current pulse repeated every 13.5 time units. Figure 5.11 shows that the oscillation is quickly entrained to the new higher frequency. Equation 5.23 allows us to predict the time after the voltage peak that the stimulus will occur for 1:1 phase locking. From the phase response curve we can see that $\Delta(\theta) = 1 - 13.5/19$ corresponds to two values of θ, one stable (cross in fig. 5.10B), $\theta = 0.591$, and the other unstable. Thus the locking time after the voltage peak, i.e., when the stimulus occurs, is predicted from the phase response curve to be $t = T \cdot \theta = 11.2$. This is exactly the shift observed in fig. 5.11.

The technique illustrated here is useful for analyzing the behavior of a single oscillator when forced with a short pulsatile stimulus. For more continuous types of forcing, such as an applied sinusoidal current, other techniques must be used. We will not go into the various methods, but note that most of them depend on certain approximations. Among these are very weak forcing (Ermentrout 1981) and simplifying approximations to the oscillator dynamics, e.g., the singular limit of very small ϕ (Grasman 1987) or integrate-and-fire models (Glass and Mackey 1988).

Coupled oscillators present problems similar to those in the previous paragraph and again certain approximations must be made in order to analyze their behavior. For two weakly coupled oscillators it is possible to reduce the many-dimensional problem to a single algebraic equation for the phase shift between the two. This method is described by Ermentrout (1981) and exploited in modeling of large numbers of coupled physiological oscillators by Ermentrout and Kopell (1984) and Kopell (1988). As with the sinusoidally forced case, there are analogous methods for coupled oscillators. Some of these methods are described by Grasman (1987).

5.5   Summary and Beyond

We have introduced and used some of the basic concepts of the qualititative theory of differential equations to describe the dynamic repertoire of a representative model of excitability. We believe that a geometrical treatment, as in the phase plane, gives one an opportunity to see more clearly and appreciate the underlying qualitative structure of models. One can see which initial conditions, e.g., as the result of a brief perturbing stimulus, will lie in the domain of attraction of any particular stable steady state or limit cycle. This is especially helpful for the design of experiments to switch a multistable system from one mode to another. Analytic methods are also important—for determining and interpreting the stability of solutions (e.g., eq. 5.19 for the Hopf bifurcation) and for approximating aspects of the solution behavior (e.g., eq. 5.22 for phase locking). Another useful conceptual device is the bifurcation diagram by which we have provided compact descriptions of the system attractors. In each of our illustrations, the bifurcation parameter was i, and in this case the steady-state $i - v$ relation appeared explicitly in the diagram. Any parameter can be used in such considerations, such as channel density or synaptic weight as in the Wilson-Cowan network model.

With regard to implementation of models, there are sophisticated software packages and subroutines available nowadays that help make theoretical experimentation and analysis a real-time endeavor; the "tooling-up" time is greatly reduced. Programs like PHSPLAN incorporate a mix of numerical integration and analytic formulation (linear stability analysis—carried out numerically) with graphical representation, all in an interactive framework (the numerical methods employed by PHSPLAN are described in Appendix 5.B). To set up and get running the Morris-Lecar model should take less than 15 minutes. Although we have primarily used PHSPLAN here for the two-variable model, it can also deal with higher order systems (like the bursting model of section 5.3.4). Stability of steady states can be computed, and time courses plotted interactively. The generalization of nullclines to surfaces is not available computationally, but two-variable projections of trajectories from the higher-order phase space can be insightful (e.g., fig. 5.9). A widely distributed program that we have also found valuable for dissecting nonlinear systems is AUTO (Doedel 1981) which automatically generates bifurcation diagrams (as in figs. 5.2, 5.6, and 5.7; see Appendix 5.B). For the evaluation and algebraic manipulation of analytic prescriptions (e.g., lengthy perturbation and bifurcation formulas), many modelers have used symbol manipulation programs like REDUCE or MACSYMA with success; see Rand and Armbruster (1987). In the use of numerical packages we advise that one be generally familiar with the methods being employed, and with their limitations. It is not so uncommon to pose a problem that seems to just miss the criteria for suitablity of a given technique—and one should be careful to recognize the symptoms of breakdown of the particular method being used.

In the course of our presentation we have illustrated, for a membrane model, some qualitative differences in threshold behavior when the steady-state current-voltage relation is monotonic or N-shaped. In the former case, action potential size may be graded, although generally quite steeply with stimulus strength, and latency for firing is finite. In the latter case, there is a true (saddle point) threshold for action potentials, latency may be arbitrarily long, and intermediate-sized responses are not possible. Correspondingly, for a steady stimulus, the monotonic case leads to onset of oscillations with a well-defined, non-zero frequency (Hopf bifurcation), and with possibly small amplitude (supercritical). In contrast, in the N-shaped case repetitive firing first appears with zero frequency (homoclinic bifurcation). These features are consistent with some of those used by Hodgkin (1948) to distinguish axons with different repetitive firing properties, Class II and Class I, respectively. Moreover, our treatment has shown that even a relatively simple model can express either behavior, as well as a rich variety of other dynamic responses, in different parameter regimes. This latter point was also made by Morris and Lecar, 1981, in their study to account for a wide range of experimentally observed behaviors in barnacle muscle with a membrane model having only two non-inactivating conductances.

Finally, we emphasize the value of using idealized, but biophysically reasonable, models in order to capture the essence of system behavior. If models are more detailed than necessary then identification of critical elements is often obscured by too many possibilities. On the other hand, if justified by adequate biophysical data, more detailed models are valuable for quantitative comparison with experiments. Thus the modeler should be mindful and appreciative of these two different approaches: which one is chosen depends on the types of questions being asked and how much is known about the underlying physiology.

The address of John Rinzel is Mathematical Research Branch, NIDDK, National Institutes of Health, Bethesda, Maryland 20892. G. B. Ermentrout's address is Department of Mathematics, University of Pittsburgh, Pittsburgh, Pennsylvania 15260. His research was partially supported by NSF grant DMS 87–01405. Readers who are interested in obtaining PHSPLAN should contact G.B. Ermentrout via electronic mail at phase@pittvms.bitnet.

Appendix 5.A: Morris-Lecar Equations

The dimensionless differential equations and v-dependent functions are

$$\frac{dv}{dt} = -\overline{g}_{Ca}\, m_\infty(v)\,(v - 1) - \overline{g}_K\, w\,(v - v_K) - \overline{g}_L\,(v - v_L) + i \qquad (5.24)$$

$$\frac{dw}{dt} = \phi\,\frac{[w_\infty(v) - w]}{\tau_w(v)} \qquad (5.25)$$

where

$$m_\infty(v) = 0.5 * [1 + \tanh\{(v - v_1)/v_2\}] \qquad (5.26)$$

$$w_\infty(v) = 0.5 * [1 + \tanh\{(v - v_3)/v_4\}] \qquad (5.27)$$

and

$$\tau_w(v) = 1/\cosh\{(v - v_3)/(2 * v_4)\} \qquad (5.28)$$

For figs. 5.1–5.3, we use the parameters $v_1 = -0.01$, $v_2 = 0.15$, $v_3 = 0$, $v_4 = 0.3$, $\overline{g}_{Ca} = 1.1$, $\overline{g}_K = 2.0$, $\overline{g}_L = 0.5$, $v_K = -0.7$, $v_L = -0.5$, and $\phi = 0.2$. These same parameters are used for figs. 5.4–5.6, with the following exceptions: $v_3 = 0.1$, $v_4 = 0.145$, $\overline{g}_{Ca} = 1.0$, and $\phi = 1/3$. With regard to the nondimensionalization of eqs. 5.4–5.5, this latter set corresponds to fig. 11 of Morris and Lecar (1981) when we use $\overline{G}_{ref} = \overline{G}_{Ca} = 4\ mS/cm^2$. In this case, with $C = 20\,\mu F/cm^2$, we would have a reference time scale $\tau = 5\,msec$, and $\phi = \tau\overline{\lambda}_W = 1/3$ for the Morris-Lecar value $\overline{\lambda}_W = 1/15$.

Appendix 5.B: Numerical Methods

Most of the figures shown in this chapter were produced by numerically solving the Morris-Lecar equations. We have used a program PHSPLAN written by G.B. Ermentrout that uses a variety of numerical integration methods to solve the equations on an IBM PC-compatible. Most of these numerical methods are discussed in depth in chapter 13. In this appendix, we briefly discuss some of the numerical algorithms pertinent to PHSPLAN. For the most part, we have used a fourth-order predictor-corrector method (Adams) that uses a fixed step size. This method has the same order of accuracy as the familiar Runge-Kutta method but requires half as many evaluations of the right-hand side of the equations, thus it is faster. This method must be started, and Runge-Kutta serves that purpose.

For many nerve models, there are widely varying time scales; some variables change very rapidly while others remain virtually constant. For equations of this type, fixed time step methods are very slow since the time step must be chosen to be very small for accuracy in the regions of rapid change. More importantly, even in regions where the solution may be changing slowly (e.g., the silent phase of a burst, or the plateau or recovery phase of a cardiac action potential) many variable time step methods would not be able to take large steps because they are not numerically stable (Press, Flannery, Teukolsky, and Vetterling 1986); even though the fast variables are equilibrated, and at pseudo-steady state the integration algorithm still "feels" their rapid time scale. Problems that have dramatically different time scales are called "stiff" and require a more sophisticated approach. The most widely used class of methods, due to Gear, is stable and able to adjust automatically the time step. PHSPLAN has this option and it was used to solve the "bursting" equations, eqs. 5.4–5.6 and 5.20, where the current variable i changes very slowly with time.

For the Morris-Lecar model, the nullclines can be found explicitly by solving each of the equations for w as a function of voltage. But this is generally not easy, so that numerical techniques are in order. All of the phase plane pictures were found by numerically computing the nullclines. The method we have used is to search first for a point on the nullcline (by successive approximations). Once we find a point on the nullcline, a path-following method is used to trace the nullcline until the path leaves a particular window or the user intervenes.

Singular points are found using Newton's method with a numerically computed Jacobian. Once a steady state is found, the Jacobian is computed and the QR algorithm is used to find the eigenvalues. These determine the stability of the singular point.

For certain steady states in the Morris-Lecar model, we want to find special trajectories called the unstable and stable manifolds. This is done by computing an eigenvector for a particular eigenvalue (the eigenvectors are tangent to these manifolds) by inverse iteration. Once the eigenvector is known, the equations are integrated (either forward or backward in time) with initial conditions that are on the eigenvector and slightly off the singular point.

The qualitative behavior of higher-dimensional systems as a parameter is varied can be understood and described compactly by determining the bifurcation diagrams. A program called AUTO (Doedel 1981) was used in this chapter to trace, essentially automatically, the bifurcation curves as the parameter i is varied. This program is able to find all steady states and periodic solutions regardless of their stability. The characteristics of stability, eigenvalues for steady states and Floquet exponents for periodic solutions, are computed along with the frequencies of periodic solutions. Two parameter bifurcation diagrams (similar to fig. 12 in Morris and Lecar 1981) that indicate where steady states and where iodic solutions exist and where they gain or lose stability can also be computed by AUTO.

A general and practical reference to many of the above numerical methods, which also leads to more literature, is Press et al. (1986).

CHAPTER 6

Reconstruction of Small Neural Networks

PETER A. GETTING

6.1   Introduction

The small nervous systems of invertebrates have been used extensively
to study the cellular and synaptic basis for neural network organization and operation. In these systems, the neural networks controlling
specific behaviors contain relatively few neurons, many of which can be
identified as individuals from animal to animal, thus permitting neural
circuits to be described in detail on a cell-by-cell, synapse-by-synapse
basis (for review see Selverston 1985). From the study of these systems
it has become evident that the operation of neural networks depends
upon the interaction of diverse cellular, synaptic, and network properties. Cellular properties include such features as how each neuron summates synaptic inputs and how it generates an output spike pattern.
The firing properties (input/output relationship) for different neurons
or classes of neurons appear to be unique and under modulatory control
(see Getting 1989; Harris-Warrick 1988; Kaczmarek and Levitan 1988).
Synaptic properties include characteristics such as sign, strength, time
course, and mechanism of transmission, all of which influence the nature
of information transfer from one cell to another (see Getting 1989). Finally, the pattern of connectivity within a network defines permissible
interactions and provides the substrate for network operation. How do
cellular and synaptic mechanisms interact with the pattern of connectivity within a neural network to give rise to a behaviorally important
output pattern? One approach to this question is to use pharmacological, electrophysiological, and lesion techniques to manipulate cellular,
synaptic, and connectivity properties experimentally. These techniques,
although powerful, have their limitations in that only some of the potentially important cellular or synaptic properties are accessible for manipulation. For example, it is difficult to alter selectively the strength or
time course of a single synaptic connection. A complementary approach
is to construct a model network preserving biologically important cellular and synaptic mechanisms and to use the model network to probe

the role of these mechanisms in network operation. The success of such a reconstruction approach, however, depends critically upon how well the model network replicates mechanisms operating in the real system. This chapter outlines and discusses one approach for the reconstruction of small neural networks.

The reconstruction scheme presented in this chapter is applicable to many neural networks, but I have chosen to illustrate how this approach can be implemented by the simulation of the network underlying escape swimming of the mollusc *Tritonia diomedea*. When touched by the tube feet of predatory starfish, *Tritonia* escapes by making a series of 2–20 alternating dorsal and ventral flection movements. The alternating burst pattern underlying the swim is produced by a central pattern generator (CPG) network consisting of at least 14 interneurons, each of which synapses directly onto motor neurons to form the final motor output pattern (for review see Getting 1983c). The interneurons of the CPG can be grouped into three classes, called dorsal swim interneurons (DSI), ventral swim interneurons (VSI), and cerebral cell 2 (C2). Figure 6.1A shows the burst pattern produced by the three major interneuron groups within the CPG during a swim. In response to a transient input (bar) signaling the presence of a predator, the CPG network generates a pattern of alternating bursts in the DSI and VSI with the C2 bursts overlapping the transition from a DSI to a VSI burst. The pattern of synaptic connectivity between the 14 interneurons is complex (Getting 1981, 1983b), but it has been postulated that the basis for oscillation within the CPG network can be represented by reciprocal inhibition between the DSI and VSI, paralleled by delayed excitation from DSI to C2. A simplified network representing the CPG is shown in fig. 6.1 in two forms, as a "ball-and-stick" model familiar to neurobiologists (fig. 6.1B) and as a connection matrix (fig. 6.1C). The network contains synapses that mediate either excitation or inhibition as well as a multiaction connection (C2 to DSI) that mediates two actions, an initial period of excitation followed by a prolonged inhibition. Reciprocal inhibition is mediated by the direct inhibitory connections between DSI and VSI. It has been proposed that the delayed excitation in parallel with the reciprocal inhibition is controlled by multiple mechanisms, some synaptic and some intrinsic to the neurons (Getting 1981, 1983b), but how these different mechanisms contribute to pattern generation remains unknown. To test whether this network could form the basis for the generation of the swim pattern, the network was reconstructed replicating not only the pattern of connectivity but also the diverse properties of the various cells and

synapses. A complementary approach using associative network models
is presented in the next chapter.

6.2 Model

Reconstruction of the swim CPG network shown in fig. 6.1B proceeded
in three major steps. First, the input/output relationship for each neuron was defined by specifying passive membrane properties and repetitive firing characteristics. Second, the time course and strength of each
synaptic action was stipulated. Finally, the network was assembled and
provided with an appropriate input corresponding to normal sensory
activation. At each step parameters were chosen so that the behavior
of the model matched comparable experimental data. Once parameters
were assigned they were no longer free parameters, and they could not
be changed at subsequent steps. This general procedure helped to insure
that the final set of parameters matched experimental data at the cellular and synaptic levels. It also insured that the parameters were chosen
on criteria other than the ability of the assembled network to produce
the observed swim pattern.

6.2.1   Reconstruction of Single Neurons

Reconstruction of single neurons requires the replication of both passive
and active membrane properties. Passive properties reflect the geometry
of the cell and how current flows within the cell (see chapters 2 and 3).
Although the CPG interneurons have long axons with many neuropilar
processes, simultaneous intracellular recording from the cell body and
from a neuropilar process indicates that these cells are largely isopotential and can be modeled as a single compartment (Getting 1983a).
Figure 6.2A shows the equivalent electrical circuit used to simulate a single neuron. Passive membrane properties were modeled by a resistance,
R_N, corresponding to the measured input resistance of the soma, in series with a battery, E_r, representing the resting potential, paralleled by
the cell capacitance, C_N. The value of C_N was determined by dividing
the measured time constant of the cell by R_N, because the membrane potential trajectory in response to a hyperpolarizing constant current step
was fit well by a single exponential (Getting 1983a). For other systems,
it may be necessary to use multiple compartments to represent passive
properties, and techniques are available for calibrating compartmental
models (see chapters 2 and 3; also Edwards and Mulloney 1984).

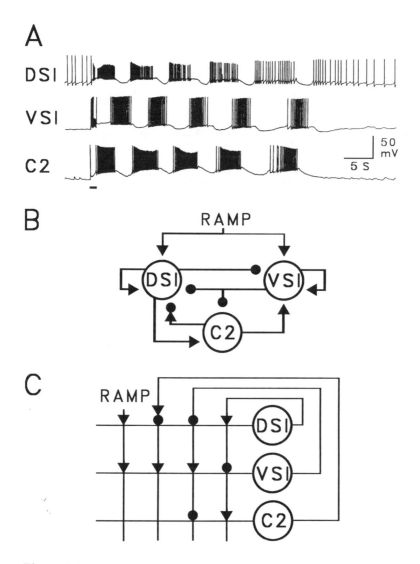

Figure 6.1
(A) Simultaneous intracellular recording from a DSI, a VSI, and a C2 showing the
normal interneuron burst pattern underlying a swim. The swim was initiated by electrical stimulation (10 Hz) of a peripheral nerve during the bar below the C2 trace.
(B) Ball-and-stick diagram of the proposed CPG network. (C) Connection matrix
representing the same network as shown in B. Symbols: triangles—excitatory connections; filled circles—inhibitory connections; mixed symbols—multiaction synapse
mediating a sequence of both excitation and inhibition.

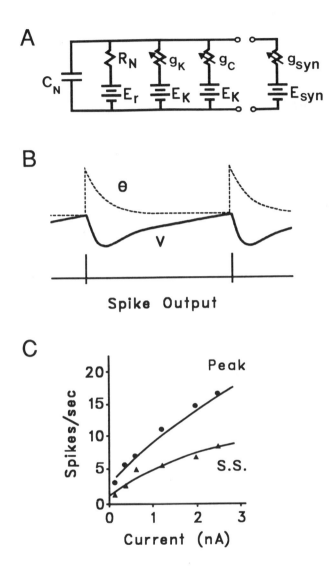

Figure 6.2
(A) Equivalent electrical circuit for a single neuron, including the time-dependent conductances (g_K and g_C) underlying the spike afterpotential. Also shown is a single synaptic conductance, g_{syn}. Additional synaptic conductances were added for each connection. (B) Time course of membrane potential (V_m) and threshold (θ) during repetitive firing. (C) Representative frequency-current (f-I) plot for a DSI neuron, showing the initial peak and the final steady-state (S.S.) spike frequency in response to long constant current pulses.

Active membrane properties of neurons are determined by multiple voltage- and time-dependent ionic currents (as discussed in chapter 4). A full kinetic description of a single voltage-dependent ionic current requires the specification of approximately 15–20 parameters most of which can be measured only by detailed voltage clamp experiments. Since the active membrane properties of a single neuron may depend upon the presence of many ionic currents (five or more for molluscan neurons), reproduction of repetitive firing characteristics by a full kinetic description of all the ionic currents presents a formidable problem in parameter specification, not to mention computational complexity. Although the computational power necessary for such a simulation is readily available today, detailed voltage clamp data are only available for very few cases; therefore the specification of an appropriate set of parameters becomes largely a matter of conjecture and subject to error. An alternative approach is to consider what features these ionic currents impart to the firing characteristics of a particular cell type and to reproduce those features by computationally simpler schemes.

One such scheme is an integrate-and-fire model based upon the idea that a neuron summates inputs impinging upon it and fires a spike whenever the membrane potential exceeds a threshold level (θ). After each spike, threshold is elevated and then allowed to decay towards an asymptotic level. Only three variables are necessary to specify threshold: the asymptotic level (θ_∞), the level to which threshold is elevated after a spike (θ_o), and the decay time constant (τ_θ). Models based upon this idea will produce repetitive firing upon depolarization, but low frequency firing can be attained only if τ_θ is long, a condition that is biologically unrealistic.

For molluscan neurons, the time between spikes is determined largely by the activation of three distinct potassium currents that contribute to the time course of the afterpotential following each spike. These currents are known as the delayed rectifier (I_K), the transient A-current (I_A), and a calcium-activated potassium current (I_C) (see chapter 4). Because these currents are voltage- or calcium-dependent, they become activated by the voltage transient, and subsequent Ca entry, during each action potential. If, for simplicity, we consider each action potential to be essentially alike, then the time course and magnitude of the potassium conductances underlying the afterpotential can be approximated by voltage-independent conductances with fixed time courses. The effects of the two potassium currents, I_K and I_C, were mimicked by the activation of time-dependent but voltage-independent conductances associated with a battery of -80 mV, corresponding to the

potassium reversal potential (E_K). The current for I_K was given by
$I_K(V_m, t) = \overline{g}_K \cdot g_K(t) \cdot (V_m(t) - E_K)$ where $\overline{g}_K$ scales the conductance
and the time course is given by $g_K(t) = (t/\tau_K)e^{-t/\tau_K}$. The calcium-
activated current, I_C, however, is known to activate quickly upon the
entry of calcium but to decay slowly as calcium is cleared from the cytoplasm (Meech 1978). The time course of this conductance was described
by $g_C(t) = (\tau_d/(\tau_d - \tau_o)) \cdot (e^{-t/\tau_d} - e^{-t/\tau_o})$, where τ_o and τ_d are the onset and decay time constants respectively. The transient current, I_A, is
largely inactivated at potentials more positive than $-45\ mV$. Since the
bursts in DSI and C2 occur in this voltage range, I_A was not considered
important in determining the repetitive firing properties for these two
cell types. Figure 6.2B shows diagramatically the time course of membrane potential and threshold during repetitive firing. When $V_m = \theta$,
a spike occurs and sets into motion a sequence of events. Threshold is
instantaneously elevated and subsequently decays. The two potassium
conductances, g_K and g_C, are activated to produce an afterpotential
with two components, an initial portion regulated by g_K and a slow
return of membrane potential controlled by g_C.

The repetitive firing properties for each cell type were determined
experimentally by injecting prolonged constant-current pulses and measuring the frequency and time course of the resultant spike train. A
distinct feature of DSI and C2 is the presence of spike frequency adaptation, a decrease in spike frequency despite a maintained depolarization. Repetitive firing properties were quantified by constructing spike
frequency (f) versus injected current (I) plots as illustrated in fig. 6.2C
for a DSI. Two curves are shown representing the peak frequency at
the beginning of the spike train and the steady-state (S.S.) frequency at
the end of a 5–10 sec current pulse. The repetitive firing properties of
the model neurons were matched to the observed f-I plot for each cell
type by adjusting the parameters for θ, I_K, and I_C. Because the time
course of I_C is long compared to the first interspike interval, the shape
of the f-I plot for peak frequency is determined primarily by the parameters for threshold (three parameters) and those for I_K (two parameters).
Asymptotic threshold, θ_∞, was measured directly as the membrane potential at which the first spike was fired when the cell was depolarized
from below threshold. The remaining four parameters (θ_o, τ_θ, $\overline{g}_K$, τ_K)
were estimated from the time course of the refractory period and the
early portion of the spike afterpotential. The estimated values were adjusted further until the peak firing curve was reproduced. Once the peak
f-I curve was matched, the three parameters ($\overline{g}_C$, τ_o, τ_d) describing g_C
were adjusted to match the steady-state f-I plot and the time course of

adaptation. To simplify parameter specification, τ_o for g_C was set equal to the τ_K, thus only two free parameters (τ_d, $\overline{g}_C$) were adjusted to replicate adaptation. The solid lines in the f-I plot of fig. 6.2C represent the output of the model while the data points show values measured from the real neuron.

The VSI presented a somewhat more difficult situation. The average rest potential of VSI is -55 mV and is in the voltage range where the transient current I_A will be activated by depolarizations. The activation of I_A causes a prolonged delay between the beginning of a depolarization and the first spike (fig. 6.3A). The delay can be as long as several hundred milliseconds in vertebrate neurons (Dekin, Getting, and Johnson 1987) and 3–4 sec in molluscan neurons (Getting 1983b). In order to reproduce the delay in excitation caused by I_A, it was necessary to simulate the voltage and time dependence of g_A by a kinetic model similar to that used by Connor and Stevens (1971). The current was given by $I_A(V_m, t) = \overline{g}_A \cdot m(V_m, t) \cdot h(V_m, t) \cdot (V_m(t) - E_K)$, where $\overline{g}_A$ is the maximum conductance, m and h are independent activation and inactivation variables respectively, and E_K is the potassium reversal potential. The voltage and time dependence of m and h were estimated from voltage clamp experiments performed on VSI (Getting 1983b). For simplicity, the time constants for m and h were made constant, independent of voltage, and were determined from the time course of the current under voltage clamp. The magnitude of $I_A(\overline{g}_A)$ was set to produce delays comparable to those of the real VSI (fig. 6.3B). The model for VSI, therefore, was a hybrid containing the fixed time course currents, I_K and I_C, along with a voltage- and time-dependent current, I_A.

6.2.2   Reconstruction of Synaptic Potentials

Postsynaptic potentials (PSP) were considered to be generated by the binding of a transmitter substance and the subsequent opening of synaptic channels. Synaptic current was given by $I_{syn}(V_m, t) = \overline{g}_{syn} \cdot g_{syn}(t) \cdot (V_m(t) - E_{syn})$, where $\overline{g}_{syn}$ scales synaptic strength, $g_{syn}(t)$ gives the time course of the underlying conductance, and E_{syn} is the synaptic reversal potential. Synaptic conductance, $g_{syn}(t)$, was activated each time a specified presynaptic neuron fired a spike. The general form of $g_{syn}(t)$ was $g_{syn}(t) = (\tau_d/(\tau_d - \tau_o)) \cdot (e^{-t/\tau_d} - e^{-t/\tau_o})$, where τ_o and τ_d represent the onset and decay time constants respectively. Synaptic strength and the time course were specified separately because they were based upon different types of data from the real system.

The time course of the PSP produced by each synapse was measured using dual intracellular recording under conditions that allowed only

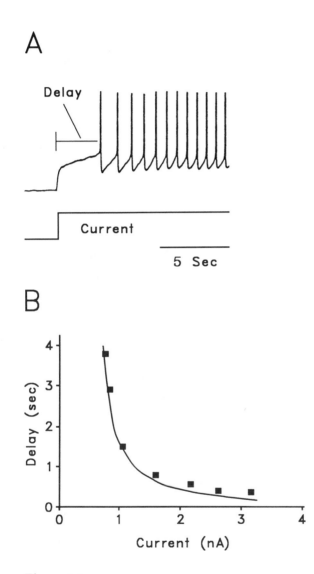

Figure 6.3
(A) Prolonged delay in the onset of firing of VSI caused by the activation of I_A
with depolarization. The upper trace shows an intracellular recording from VSI in
response to a step-current injection. At this level of current, the delay measured 3 *sec*.
(B) Plot of the delay versus injected current for a typical VSI. The points represent
data collected from the real neuron, the line shows comparable delays produced by
a simulated VSI.

monosynaptic connections to be expressed (Getting 1981, 1983b). These data were used to select the appropriate values for τ_o and τ_d. The graphs of fig. 6.4, which were generated from the equations for $g_{syn}(t)$, can be helpful for selecting initial values for τ_o and τ_d. The first step is to determine the PSP shape parameter, which is obtained by dividing the PSP fall time by the rise time, where rise time and fall time are measured as the time from 50% of peak amplitude to the peak level (fig. 6.4A). Using the graph of fig. 6.4B, the normalized rise time (N.R.T.) as a fraction of τ_o can be determined by the intersection of the curve with a vertical line drawn at the measured shape parameter. The onset time constant, τ_o, is obtained by dividing the measured rise time (in milliseconds) by the normalized rise time. Once the shape parameter and τ_o are known, the decay time constant, τ_d, can be obtained from the ratio of time constants shown in the graph of fig. 6.4C. The curves of fig. 6.4 were derived from the time course of the conductance change underlying a PSP, but the voltage waveform of a measured PSP depends additionally upon the time constant of the cell. If the time course of the PSP is long relative to the time constant of the cell, which is the case for most of the PSPs within the *Tritonia diomedea* swim CPG, then the voltage waveform of the PSP reflects the time course of the underlying conductance. If the falling phase of the PSP has a time course comparable to the time constant of the cell, then the values for τ_o and τ_d obtained by applying the graphs of fig. 6.4 to the PSP waveform will be too large and smaller values should be tried. In either case, the graphs of fig. 6.4 provide reasonable starting values which usually will need additional adjustment to obtain agreement between the time course of the simulated and real PSPs.

Figure 6.5 shows a comparison of recorded and simulated PSPs for two of the monosynaptic connections within the central pattern generator network. The amplitudes of the PSPs have been normalized to illustrate the similarity in their time course. The connection from C2 to DSI (fig. 6.5b) is a multiaction PSP having two components, an initial depolarizing component that reverses sign to become a long-lasting hyperpolarization. The multiaction PSP was modeled by using two pathways from the presynaptic to the postsynaptic neuron, one mediating the excitatory effect and the other mediating the inhibitory component. Synaptic reversal potentials, E_{syn}, were chosen from measured values for *Tritonia* synapses ($+10\ mV$ for EPSPs, $-60\ mV$ for chloride-dependent IPSPs, and $-80\ mV$ for potassium mediated IPSPs) (Hume and Getting 1982).

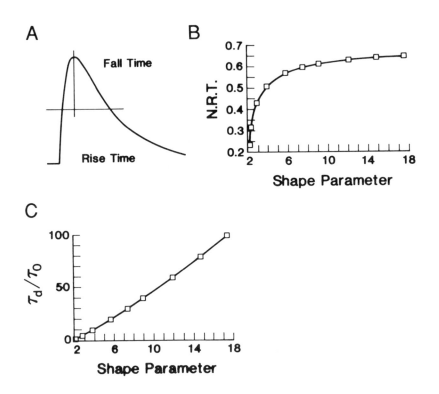

Figure 6.4
Graphs used for the determination of τ_o and τ_d. (A) Measurement of PSP rise and fall times used to calculate the shape parameter. (B) Graph of normalized rise time (N.R.T.) as a fraction of τ_o versus PSP shape parameter. (C) Ratio of time constants (τ_d/τ_o) versus PSP shape parameter.

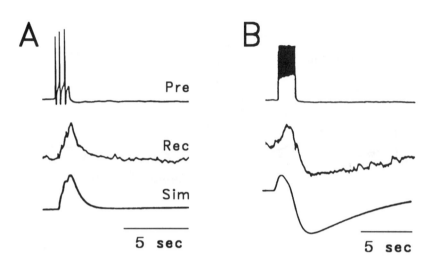

Figure 6.5
Comparison of the time courses for recorded and simulated PSPs. The upper trace (Pre) shows the presynaptic activity used to evoke the PSP, the middle trace (Rec) is the observed PSP, and the bottom trace (Sim) shows the corresponding simulated PSP generated by the model. (A) Monosynaptic EPSP from one DSI to another DSI. (B) Monosynaptic multiaction PSP from C2 to DSI.

Synaptic strength, $\overline{g}_{syn}$, is the most difficult parameter to specify. Strength can be set by matching the amplitude of the recorded and simulated PSP, but doing so does not guarantee that activating the synapse in the model will have the same effectiveness as in the real system. In order to isolate monosynaptic PSPs, it is sometimes necessary to change the ionic environmemt (Getting 1981), introducing the possibility that PSP amplitude may be altered. In addition, the model neurons use an integrate-and-fire scheme to produce repetitive firing whereas the real neurons use voltage- and time-dependent conductances; therefore, the model neurons may require a different synaptic strength to produce an equivalent change in firing pattern. Finally, the network of fig. 6.1B represents the condensation of several neurons of a common pool into a single model neuron (e.g., there are six DSI, two C2, and four VSI); thus the strength of the connections from a single model neuron would have to be stronger than reflected by an individual monosynaptic connection. As an alternative, synaptic strength can be adjusted to approximate the observed functional interactions between the interneuron pools. Functional interactions can be defined by the change in postsynaptic firing pattern resulting from a specified presynaptic spike train. Experimentally one interneuron (or several members of a group) were driven by current injection to produce a known level of activity and the resultant change in firing rate of its postsynaptic targets observed (Getting 1981, 1983b). The basal firing rate of the postsynaptic cell could be biased to various levels by constant current injection in order to observe the effectiveness of the synapse at different postsynaptic activity levels. Repeating similar experiments on pairs of the model cells allowed synaptic strength, $\overline{g}_{syn}$, to be adjusted so as to approximate the observed functional interactions.

6.3   Results

Two issues will be addressed in this section. First, how well does the behavior of the simulated network match the real system? Second, can the simulation be used to gain insight into how the network operates?

Once an initial set of synaptic strengths was assigned for pairs of neurons, the network of fig. 6.1B was assembled and provided with an input to mimic normal sensory activation. Swimming is initiated by a transient sensory stimulus lasting only 1–3 sec. This input, however, gives rise to a prolonged depolarization that is largest during the stimulus and decays as the swim progresses. Voltage clamp experiments have shown that the ramp depolarization is distributed primarily to DSI and to a lesser extent VSI (Getting and Dekin 1985a). The ramp depolarization was simulated by an extrinsic synaptic input to the DSI with a τ_o of 25 $msec$ and a τ_d of 15 sec, thus giving rise to a long-lasting depolarization. This input fiber was activated for 1 sec at 10 Hz to mimic sensory input.

With only minor adjustment of the initial synaptic strengths, the simulated network produced an oscillatory burst pattern remarkably similar to the swim pattern (fig. 6.6A). In the absence of a sensory input the real swim network is stable, with DSI firing spontaneously at less than 1–2 $spikes/sec$ and both C2 and VSI silent. In the simulated network it was necessary to inject a small hyperpolarizing current (-0.2 nA) into DSI to keep the network stable in this configuration. The hyperpolarizing current represents an inhibitory effect normally mediated by a tonically active cell not included in the simulated network (Getting and Dekin 1985b). When the input fiber was transiently activated (bar below C2 trace), a 4-cycle burst pattern was produced with a normal sequence of alternation between DSI and VSI and C2 overlapping the transition from a DSI to VSI burst. In addition, the range of cycle periods produced by the simulation closely matched that observed for real swims (4–7.5 sec for simulations, 3.5–8 sec for swims). During a typical swim, cycle period is shortest in the beginning and becomes longer as the swim progresses. The increase in cycle period, however, is not evenly distributed throughout a cycle but occurs mainly by an increase in the time from the end of a VSI burst to the beginning of the next C2 burst—a time called D_r (Lennard, Getting, and Hume 1980). The simulated swim also displayed an asymmetric increase in cycle period with D_r, accounting for 70–85% of the increase, which compares favorably to real swims in which D_r accounts for approximately 80%.

Another test of a simulated network is whether it behaves appropriately under a variety of conditions not originally considered in the formulation of the network. One feature of the real swim network is that tonic depolarization of C2 by constant current injection results in pattern generation (Getting 1977). Figure 6.6B shows that tonic depolarization of C2 in the simulated network also results in the generation of a coordinated burst pattern. The parallels between the behavior of the model and real swim network suggest that the simulated network provides a reasonable description of the biological system.

One of the powers of simulated networks is that all parameters are accessible for manipulation; thus "experiments" can be performed on the model system that are either impossible or difficult to control in liv-

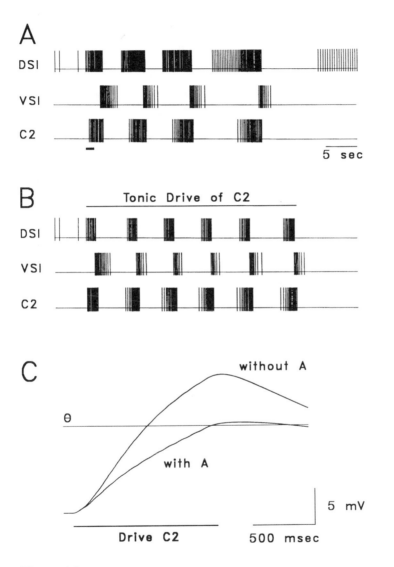

Figure 6.6
(A) Control burst pattern produced by the simulated network in response to a
transient (10 Hz for 1 sec) activation of the input fiber to DSI (stimulus duration
marked by the bar below C2 trace). (B) Tonic depolarization of C2 in the simulated
network resulted in pattern generation. (C) Simulated effect of I_A on the time course
of EPSP summation in VSI. A summated EPSP was generated in VSI by driving the
presynaptic C2 neuron at a constant frequency of 10 $spikes/sec$, with and without
I_A present in the postsynaptic VSI. The spike threshold level of VSI is shown by the
line labeled θ.

ing systems. Multiple mechanisms have been suggested for delaying the excitation from DSI through C2 to VSI. One of these is the presence of I_A in the VSI. Theoretically, depolarization of VSI by excitatory input from C2 would activate I_A, which would tend to oppose the depolarizing effect of the synaptic input. With time, however, I_A would inactivate and free VSI to respond to the full strength of the synaptic drive. Unfortunately, it has not been possible to test this hypothesis directly in the living system because no method is available to block I_A in only VSI without also affecting other cells or processes. In the simulated network, however, I_A can be removed while keeping all other properties constant. Because g_A is not fully inactivated at rest potential in VSI, it contributes to the resting input resistance. Therefore, setting g_A to zero also necessitated adjustment of R_N to maintain the same input resistance. In the absence of I_A, the network produced an oscillatory burst pattern with appropriate coordination (DSI–C2–VSI burst order) and similar cycle periods (range 4.0–7.5 sec). However, the same stimulus resulted in 5 rather than 4 cycles. I_A, therefore, does not appear to be necessary for pattern generation but does contribute to the proper timing of bursts within a cycle. When I_A is removed the delay from the onset of a C2 burst to the beginning of the VSI burst is significantly reduced. In fact I_A in the model accounts for 25–35% (approximately 500 $msec$) of the delay in excitation from C2 to VSI. The remainder of the delay results from the time required for summation of the C2 EPSP to reach the high threshold of VSI. The effect of I_A on the time course of summation of EPSPs in VSI is illustrated in fig. 6.6C. For a constant firing rate in C2 of 10 $spikes/sec$, the EPSP in VSI reaches threshold about 450 $msec$ later in the presence of I_A than without I_A. The transient potassium current, therefore, appears to mediate a significant portion of the delay in excitation of VSI.

Another distinctive cellular feature of DSI and C2 is the presence of spike frequency adaptation mediated by I_C. How does this intrinsic cellular property contribute to pattern generation? As with I_A, pharmacological agents are not available to block I_C in living systems without altering other properties. In the model network, removal of adaptation from both DSI and C2 by setting g_C to zero resulted in a dramatic change in the swim pattern produced by the simulated network. In response to the same stimulus, the network produced 10 rather than 4 cycles. In addition, cycle period remained relatively constant in the range of 3.9–4.8 sec rather than showing the usual progression from 4 sec at the beginning to 8 sec at the end of a swim. Removal of both I_A and I_C did not cause a significant alteration in the expressed pattern above that produced by the removal of I_C alone. Alterations in synaptic properties also result in changes in the expressed rhythm, including changes in cycle period, burst timing, and burst structure. Considering the large number of possible synaptic modifications, however, the detailed consequences of these alterations are beyond the scope of this chapter.

In conclusion, the production of an appropriate swim pattern appears to depend upon the interaction of network connectivity and the intrinsic properties of the cells involved. Removal of both adaptation and delayed excitation mediated by I_A did not abolish the generation of an oscillatory pattern with the correct order of bursting within a cycle; thus it would appear that the basis for pattern generation by this system is embodied in the pattern of synaptic connectivity. Important timing information is, however, imparted by the intrinsic membrane properties of the neurons. Spike frequency adaptation plays an important role in regulating cycle period and in determining the number of cycles produced. The transient potassium current, I_A, contributes to delaying excitation of VSI, thus prolonging the time of coactive firing between DSI and C2. The inclusion of both these cellular properties appears necessary to produce the normal swim pattern.

6.4   Discussion

The simulation scheme as presented allows a number of general conclusions to be drawn about the adequacy of this form of network reconstruction. First, the ability to reproduce the f-I plots for all three cell types suggests that an integrate-and-fire model can adequately simulate the repetitive firing characteristics of real neurons only when additional features are added. To reproduce the f-I plots for each cell type, it was necessary to incorporate into each neuron two conductances (g_K and g_C) to mimic the effects of the spike afterpotential. The model was also capable of reproducing delayed excitation by the inclusion of a kinetic description for I_A. The kinetic description was necessary because the activation (and inactivation) of this current is dependent upon membrane voltage in the subthreshold range. Kinetic descriptions for other currents were not deemed necessary because their major action was to influence repetitive firing, rather than summation of synaptic input.

Synaptic current was generated by a time-dependent conductance increase in association with a reversal potential. The model, in its present form, does not include conductance decrease synapses, facilitation, or depression, but if necessary these features could be added easily. Using conductance changes to generate synaptic current reproduces two important properties of synaptic interactions, the membrane potential change of a PSP and a change in input conductance, both of which play important roles in integration. The potential change of a PSP is important to bring the membrane potential either closer to threshold or farther from threshold, but the magnitude of the potential change does not necessarily reflect the strength of the connection. For example, an inhibitory synapse with a reversal potential close to rest potential may produce only a small IPSP but the underlying conductance change can be large and can mediate a powerful form of inhibition by shunting other synaptic currents. The magnitude of the conductance change influences not only the size of the PSP generated but also the magnitude of other concurrent PSPs, thus leading to nonlinear spatial summation. To reproduce the actions of synapses accurately, it is necessary to incorporate both the membrane potential and conductance changes.

One of the most difficult tasks associated with any reconstruction is parameter assignment. By avoiding kinetic descriptions of ionic currents except where absolutely necessary (I_A), the number of parameters can be kept to a minimum. A particularly notable feature of this simulation scheme is that most of the experimental data needed to specify parameters can be collected by intracellular recording and current clamp techniques. These include passive membrane properties, f-I plots, and synaptic time course. Only in the case of the subthreshold, voltage-dependent current (I_A) was voltage clamp data necessary. Nevertheless, faithful reconstruction does require detailed knowledge of the constituent neurons and synapses. For small systems this may be done on a cell-by-cell basis, as was presented for the *Tritonia* system. In larger systems, neurons can usually be categorized into groups, classes, or types that share similar properties (e.g., Dekin et al. 1987). For these systems it may not be necessary to know the properties of each cell in detail but only the properties (and distribution) for each class; thus large networks could be simulated by relatively few cell types.

Another troublesome aspect of parameter specification centers around the uniqueness of the set selected. With so many parameters it may be possible to generate a desired output pattern using many different sets of parameters. For the *Tritonia* reconstruction most of the parameters were set on criteria other than the ability of the simulated network to produce the swim pattern; thus the pattern generated represents a true emergent property of the network not insured by the selection of cellular or synaptic parameters. The uniqueness of parameters is difficult to assess. At each step in the current simulation, parameters were selected to match experimental data and then were fixed. In subsequent steps involving the processes governed by these parameters, alteration of already set parameters was not allowed but only of new parameters. This procedure insured that the final set of parameters matched all the experimental data. The procedure, however, does not guarantee a unique set of parameters. For example, if a cellular property was involved in many steps of the simulation, an error in setting the parameters for that property could have profound effects upon the selection of parameters for other processes at subsequent steps. One way of assessing the quality of parameter specification is to look at the robustness of the network, that is, the sensitivity of the operation of the network to variation in parameters. In biological systems, cellular and synaptic properties can vary considerably from animal to animal but the system still functions appropriately. Any reconstruction that depends heavily upon close parameter tolerance should be suspect. The reconstructed swim network is particularly robust. Spike frequency adaptation or delayed excitation can be removed completely and the network continues to produce a coordinated oscillatory pattern. In addition synaptic strengths can be varied by at least ±50% without loss of pattern generation. Under any of these conditions, the details of the pattern produced may change but the ability of the network to sustain oscillation remains.

Most of this chapter has dealt with how a simulated network can be built from experimental data, but what about the reverse? Can simulation assist in suggesting or designing experimental approaches? A previous simulation of the *Tritonia* swim network demonstrated that a different network based upon a different class of VSI was also capable of producing the observed swim pattern (Getting 1983a), but this simulated network failed to generate a pattern when C2 was tonically depolarized. The inability of the previously simulated network to reproduce this aspect of the real system, along with several other mismatches in network behavior, led to the discovery of a second type of VSI and illustrates the value of interplay between simulation and experiment. Reconstructed networks can, therefore, provide one way for assessing the sufficiency of current knowledge in understanding network operation, although caution should be exercised because additional mechanisms that were not incorporated into the model may be operational in the biological system. Although a simulated network can reproduce the function of a neural network, there may not be sufficient grounds to conclude that the biological system necessarily operates by the same mechanisms or principles.

Does the *Tritonia* swim generator represent a general scheme for the generation of rhythmical patterned activity? Experimental manipulation of the swim network and its simulation suggests that the existence of patterned output from this network is heavily dependent upon synaptic interaction among the interneurons (Getting, Lennard, and Hume 1980). The simulation presented here suggests further that intrinsic cellular properties such as spike frequency adaptation and delayed excitation may serve primarily to confer appropriate timing and coordination but may not be necessary for pattern generation. Comparative studies of mechanisms for pattern generation in other systems, however, have revealed that the existence of patterned activity resides in the intrinsic properties of "burster" neurons. In these systems synaptic connectivity serves to coordinate and shape the final pattern (for review see Getting 1988a). It would be misleading, therefore, to conclude that synaptic connectivity necessarily plays a major role in pattern generation in all systems, even though in some model networks connectivity may be capable of pattern generation. The relative dependence upon connectivity as a basis for pattern generation appears to depend on the nature of the behavior being controlled (see Getting 1988). Continuously active rhythmic systems seem to rely heavily upon intrinsic cellular bursting properties while brief, episodic behaviors such as *Tritonia* swimming may be based in network oscillators.

Peter Getting thanks Dr. Donald Perkel for kindly making his simulation programs, MICKEY and MANUEL, available to him and for providing helpful suggestions during the development of the *Tritonia* swim network simulation. Special thanks go to David Lawrence for writing the current simulation program called MARIO. Peter Getting was supported by NIH research grant NS17328. His address is Department of Physiology and Biophysics, University of Iowa, Iowa City, Iowa 52242.

Appendix 6.A: Computer Implementation

Early simulations of the *Tritonia* swim network were implemented by a program called MANUEL written by Dr. Donald Perkel at the University of California, Irvine. More recent simulations use a program called MARIO devised by David Lawrence and myself. MARIO is written in Turbo PASCAL and runs on an IBM PC/AT-type machine with 640 K memory and an EGA graphics board. In its present form MARIO is capable of simulating 16–25 neurons with up to 4 voltage-dependent currents per neuron and a total of 300 connections. The program is organized into two sections. The first section is used to specify properties of the individual cells and synapses, while the second section sets up what manipulations are to be applied to the network, what variables are to be recorded, and how the simulation is to be run. As the simulation is running, a graphics screen displays the spike activity and membrane potential of specified cells or axons. Run time increases with the complexity of the network (how many neurons, voltage-dependent currents, and connections). Simulation of the control swim shown in fig. 6.6A required about 30 *min* running on an IBM PC-type machine with an 8 *mHz* clock. The simulated swim network of fig. 6.1B had 3 cells, 1 voltage-dependent conductance, and a total of 19 synaptic connections. The number of connections exceeds the number of pathways shown in fig. 6.1B because many of the synapses mediate PSPs with multiple components, each of which was simulated by a separate connection. The count of connections also includes the 2 connections per cell mediating I_K and I_C.

Appendix 6.B: Detailed Equations

The following equations describe the simulation implemented by the program MARIO. Time is measured in milliseconds.

For each cell, the membrane potential is described by

$$C_N \frac{dV_m(t)}{dt} = -I_{leak}(V_m) - I_{syn}(V_m, t) - I_{act}(V_m, t) - I_{stim}(t)$$

where V_m = membrane potential (mV)
$\quad C_N$ = membrane capacitance (nF)
$\quad I_{leak}$ = leak current (nA)
$\quad I_{syn}$ = individual synaptic current (nA)
$\quad I_{act}$ = intrinsic voltage-dependent current (nA)
$\quad I_{stim}$ = externally applied currents (nA)

Leakage Current

$$I_{leak} = \frac{V_m - E_r}{R_N}$$

$\quad E_r$ = resting potential (mV)
$\quad R_N$ = input resistance $(M\Omega)$

Synaptic Current

$$I_{syn} = \overline{g}_{syn} \cdot g_{syn}(t)(V_m - E_{syn})$$

$\quad \overline{g}_{syn}$ = maximum conductance for a given synapse (μS)
$\quad E_{syn}$ = synaptic reversal potential (mV)
$\quad g_{syn}(t)$ = synaptic conductance time course

$$g_{syn}(t) = \frac{\tau_d}{\tau_d - \tau_o} \sum_{i=1}^{N} \left(e^{(t_i - t)/\tau_d} - e^{(t_i - t)/\tau_o} \right)$$

$\quad \tau_o$ = onset time constant $(msec)$
$\quad \tau_d$ = decay time constant $(msec)$
$\quad N$ = number of presynaptic spikes before time t
$\quad t_i$ = time of ith presynaptic spike $(msec)$

Intrinsic Voltage-Dependent Current

$$I_{act} = \overline{g}_{act} m^x h(V_m - E_{act})$$

$\quad \overline{g}_{act}$ = maximum conductance (μS)
$\quad m$ = activation parameter
$\quad x$ = exponent on activation parameter
$\quad h$ = inactivation parameter
$\quad E_{act}$ = reversal potential of active process (mV)

$$\frac{dm}{dt} = \frac{m_\infty - m}{\tau_m}$$

$$m_\infty = \frac{1}{\left[1 + e^{(V_m+B)/C}\right]} \quad \text{steady} - \text{state activation}$$

B = shift parameter (mV)
C = shape parameter (mV)
τ_m = activation time constant ($msec$)

$$\frac{dh}{dt} = \frac{h_\infty - h}{\tau_h}$$

$$h_\infty = \frac{1}{\left[1 + e^{(V_m+B)/C}\right]} \quad \text{steady} - \text{state inactivation}$$

B = shift parameter (mV)
C = shape parameter (mV)
τ_h = inactivation time constant ($msec$)

Threshold

$$\theta(t) = \theta_\infty + (\theta_o - \theta_\infty)e^{(t_x-t)/\tau_\theta}$$

θ_∞ = steady-state threshold (mV)
θ_o = threshold value immediately after a spike (mV)
t_x = time of last spike in cell ($msec$)
τ_θ = threshold time constant ($msec$)

External Current

Externally applied currents (I_{stim}) can be applied to any cell at any time with any waveform.

Parameter Values

Cellular parameters:

Cell	R_N	C_N	E_r	θ_∞	θ_o	τ_θ
DSI	30	4.17	-40	-48	0	50
VSI	15	6.13	-55	-43	-30	10
C2	12	4.17	-50	-30	-10	100

The currents I_K and I_C were simulated as a recurrent synapse connecting back onto the cell of origin. Specification of the parameters for I_K and I_C, therefore, takes the form of synaptic parameters.

Cell	$\overline{g}_{syn}$	τ_o	τ_d	E_{syn}
DSI				
I_K	0.25	20	20	-80
I_C	0.00223	20	5000	-80
VSI				
I_K	0.08	5	5	-80
I_C	0.0075	5	400	-80
C2				
I_K	0.033	40	40	-80
I_C	0.00083	40	10000	-80

The intrinsic voltage-dependent I_A of VSI was described by:

$\overline{g}_A = 1.287$

$x = 1$

$m_\infty;\ \ B = 40, C = -5.5$

$h_\infty;\ \ B = 68, C = 6.7$

$\tau_m = 10$

$\tau_h = 760$

Synaptic parameters:

Pre	Post	PSP	$\overline{g}_{syn}$	τ_o	τ_d	E_{syn}
RAMP	DSI	EPSP	0.012	25	15000	10
DSI	DSI	EPSP	0.001	100	500	10
DSI	DSI	EPSP	0.001	2000	2000	10
VSI	DSI	IPSP	0.6	150	150	-80
C2	DSI	EPSP	0.045	400	400	10
C2	DSI	IPSP	0.0015	400	5000	-80
VSI	VSI	EPSP	0.000025	750	3000	10
DSI	VSI	IPSP	0.003	80	800	-80
C2	VSI	EPSP	0.003	100	1500	10
DSI	C2	EPSP	0.02	200	800	10
DSI	C2	EPSP	0.00001	200	2000	10
VSI	C2	IPSP	0.07	400	400	-80
VSI	C2	IPSP	0.000008	400	2000	-80

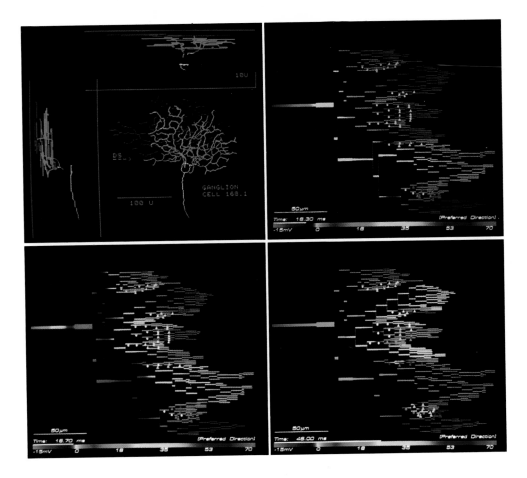

PLATE I. Intracellular potential in a computer-reconstructed cell in
the presence of massive synaptic input. The upper left image shows a
three-dimensional computer rendering of an HRP-injected, ON-OFF directional selective retinal ganglion cell (from Amthor, Oyster and Taka-
hashi, 1984). The colors distinguish different layers of dendrites. An
electrical cable model was then constructed from the anatomical data,
using SPICE. The dendrites are passive, while the cell body contains
a Hodgkin-Huxley type of nonlinearity. The voltage scale is relative to
the cell's resting potential. In the simulation shown, a bar moves from
the bottom toward the top through the cell's receptive field. In the
upper right image, the bar has just activated the excitatory synapses
(triangles). The amplitude of the conductance change is also given by
the color bar, that is, no conductance change has occurred at a gray
synapse while a red synapse is maximally activated. A fraction of a
msec later, the resulting EPSP has triggered an action potential at the
soma (lower left image). In the bottom right figure, activation of the
inhibitory synapses of the shunting type (circles) leads to a reduction of
the local EPSP in the bottom part of the dendritic tree, without leading
to a hyperpolarization. From O'Donnell, Koch and Poggio (1985). See
Chapter 3.

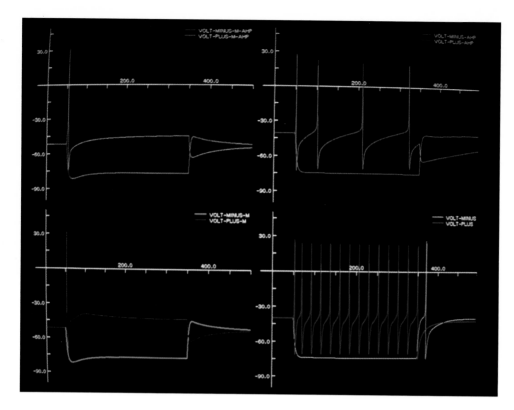

PLATE II. Roles of two potassium currents in controlling cellular adaptation. The response of a type "B" bullfrog sympathetic ganglion cell is shown during long-lasting (300 $msec$) injections of depolarizing (1.25 nA) and hyperpolarizing (-1.25 nA) current steps. The response of the cell during its adapted state is indicated in the upper left panel. The next two panels illustrate the cellular response if either the non-inactivating voltage-dependent potassium current I_M (upper right) or the calcium-dependent, voltage-independent potassium current I_{AHP} (lower left) is blocked. Adaptation is practically absent if both of these currents are blocked simultaneously (lower right). Notice the anodal break spike at the end of the hyperpolarizing input. Spike frequency adaptation is characteristic of many nerve cells. VOLT-MINUS and VOLT-PLUS refer to the voltage trace in response to the positive or negative current injections. See Chapter 4.

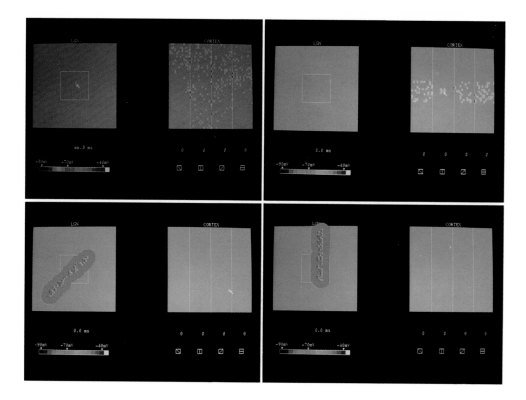

PLATE III. Structural features of the simulated cat visual cortex. The 48 by 48 array of cells in the lateral geniculate nucleus is illustrated in the left part of each of the four panels and the 48 by 48 array of cells in layer IVc of striate cortex on the right side. Each geniculate cell projects to a large number (about 220) of cortical cells (upper left panel). A typical cortical interneuron (arrow in the lower left panel) inhibits a large number of other cortical neurons. The cortex module measures 1.2 *mm* on each side, about the dimension of a hypercolumn in the cat. Cells are grouped into four orientation columns. The receptive field of two such cells is plotted in the two bottom panels. They correspond to simple cells with a 1:3 to 1:4 aspect ratio and a width of about 0.5°. See Chapter 10.

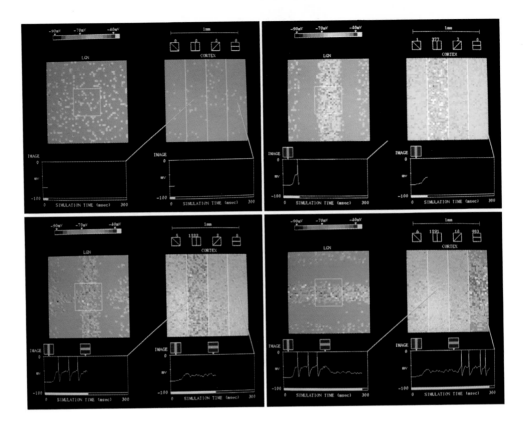

PLATE IV. The response of the visual cortex model to different stimuli. Cortical inhibition has been inactivated during this run. Thus, cortical cells acquire orientation selectivity via a Hubel and Wiesel (1962) type of feedforward circuit. The color of each cell indicates its membrane potential (see the color bar; action potentials are in white). Insets show the intracellular potential of two cortical neurons in the vertical and horizontal orientation columns. The response of the model to a homogeneous field of view is illustrated in the upper left panel. Cellular activity is due to random firing (at 10 Hz) in the retinal fibers. After 20 $msec$, a vertical bar is projected onto the retina (not shown), and both the geniculate and the vertical orientation column in cortex respond vigorously. After a further 130 $msec$, the vertical bar is rotated into a horizontal position. The numbers above the orientation columns represent the number of action potentials in that particular column. See Chapter 10.

CHAPTER 7

Associative Network Models for Central Pattern Generators

DAVID KLEINFELD and HAIM SOMPOLINSKY

7.1 Introduction

The collective properties of highly interconnected networks of model neurons have been the focus of much theoretical analysis. Recent work on this topic involves networks whose dynamics are governed by a cooperative relaxation process (e.g., Hopfield 1982, 1984; Peretto 1984; Amit, Gutfreund, and Sompolinsky 1985a, 1985b; Gardner 1988). Starting from an initial state, these networks will relax to one of a select number of stable states. The stable states are local minima of a suitable "energy" function. Network models of this form have been used for associative memory (Hopfield 1982) and for solving certain optimization problems (Hopfield and Tank 1986). The final, stable states represent the retrieved information or the optimized configuration.

Despite some very suggestive analogies between the network models and biological computational processes, their application in biology is unclear. The difficulty in relating the models to experimental observations reflects, in part, the difficulty in identifying a cooperative relaxational process in large, complex nervous systems. Similarities between associative memory networks and central nervous functions, such as place learning in the hippocampus (e.g., O'Keefe 1983), olfaction (Gelperin, Hopfield, and Tank 1985; Haberly 1985; Baird 1986) and visual processing (Koch, Marroquin, and Yuille 1986; Wang, Mathur, and Koch 1989) have been proposed. Yet the models remain untested at the level of neurophysiology.

In this chapter we study an associative network model whose collective outputs consist of temporally coherent patterns of linear or cyclic sequences of states (Sompolinsky and Kanter 1986; Kleinfeld 1986; Kleinfeld and Sompolinsky 1988). This model and its extensions may have a variety of implications for the learning and recall of temporally ordered information. Our objective in the present work is to draw a connection between the properties of the model and biological nervous systems that produce fixed patterns of neural outputs. In particular, we focus on a class of biological systems known as central pattern generators.

Central pattern generators (CPGs) control the muscles involved in executing well-defined rhythmic behaviors, such as breathing, chewing, walking, swimming, and scratching. Some networks forming CPGs are anatomically well localized and may contain small numbers of neurons. Their output consists of coherent, oscillatory patterns. These features make CPGs strong candidates for studying the relation between the collective output properties of a biological network and its underlying circuitry.

A number of basic principles about CPGs have emerged from studies on a wide variety of rhythmic behaviors (for review, see Delcomyn 1980; Kristan 1980; Roberts and Roberts 1983; Cohen, Rossignol, and Grillner 1986; Selverston and Moulins 1986):

1. A rhythmic neural output can occur in the absence of sensory feedback from the muscles and structures controlled by the CPG, and in the absence of control by higher neural centers. These features are clearly demonstrated with "spinal" preparations (e.g., Grillner 1975), i.e., isolated segments of spinal cord. The output activity of the motor neurons in these preparations is similar to the rhythmic firing pattern observed in the intact animal.

2. Some CPGs function without a pacemaker cell, i.e., a single neuron whose firing rate determines the output period of the network. This implies that the rhythmic output is a collective property of the network. Examples include the CPG that controls swimming in the mollusc *Tritonia diomedea* (Getting 1981, and chapter 6) and possibly the CPGs that control flight in the locust (Wilson 1961; Robertson and Pearson 1985) and swimming in the leech (Stent, Kristan, Friesen, Ort, Poon, and Calabrese 1978; Weeks 1981).

3. The same set of motor neurons can be involved in a variety of rhythmic behaviors in an animal. This suggests that a CPG may be capable of producing multiple patterns of rhythmic outputs. Further, animals can rapidly switch between rhythmic behaviors and may blend different rhythms together (e.g., Stein, Camp, Robertson, and Mortin 1986).

4. The output of the CPG can be modulated by external inputs, such as feedback from proprioceptors and from higher neural centers.

For example, modulation is used both to turn on and off the CPG and to control the period of its rhythm.

The dynamic properties of several CPGs have been analyzed by performing detailed simulations of specific circuits. Simulation techniques have been used in the study of the lobster pyloric and gastric mill rhythms (Perkel 1965; Hartline 1979) and the swim rhythm in *Tritonia* (Getting 1983a, and chapter 6). This approach often involves simulating the equations that describe the dynamics of the neurons in the CPG, e.g., Hodgkin and Huxley-like equations (Hodgkin and Huxley 1952), using the known biophysical parameters for each neuron and the synaptic connections between neurons. Detailed simulations have been useful for determining the completeness of a set of measurements of a CPG (e.g., Getting 1983a, 1983b). A complementary approach for understanding the biological mechanisms responsible for pattern formation is to compare the properties of CPGs with those of simple network models (for a discussion of this approach, see Selverston 1980).

The smallest circuit that can produce a rhythmic output consists of two neurons coupled by reciprocal inhibitory synaptic connections (Harmon 1964; Reiss 1964). If both neurons are tonically excited and contain a mechanism for synaptic fatigue, they will alternately produce a bursting output. The period of the output oscillation is proportional to the time scale of the fatigue. The two-neuron oscillator and networks of coupled two-neuron oscillators provided an early basis for understanding some aspects of the motor system controlling flight in the locust (Wilson and Waldron 1968).

A generalization of the two-neuron oscillator was made by Kling and Szekély (1968). They studied networks containing closed loops of neurons connected by inhibitory synapses. This topology results in recurrent, cyclic inhibitory pathways that allow the networks to produce a rich set of oscillatory patterns. These networks have been used, although with limited success, as a basis for understanding the CPG controlling the swim rhythm in the leech (Friesen and Stent 1977).

The mechanism of recurrent cyclic inhibition can be extended to arbitrarily large networks. However, certain features of these networks make them inappropriate as general models of CPGs. All of the synaptic connections in a loop are inhibitory; this precludes the use of loops for modeling CPGs that also contain excitatory synapses. The loops rely on a specific cyclic topology of their connections in order to function. Finally, simulations have indicated that each loop is capable of producing only a *single* stable output pattern (Kling and Szekély 1968).

Several other network models have been studied as candidates for CPGs (Harth, Lewis, and Csermely 1975; Glass and Young 1979; Thompson 1982; Kopell 1986). A mechanism for the generation of multiple, coherent patterns by highly interconnected networks is, however, lacking in these models.

In this chapter we present a general model for producing rhythmic patterns in associative neural network models. The network consists of highly interconnected model neurons whose essential feature is a non-linear relation between their inputs and their firing rate. The form of the output patterns is encoded in the strength of the synaptic connections between pairs of neurons. Rhythmic output emerges as a collective property of the network.

Many of the structural and dynamic properties of our model are similar to those observed in CPGs. The network can produce rhythmic output in the absence of external feedback. It can naturally produce multiple stable patterns of rhythmic outputs. Well-defined mechanisms exist for modulating the output period of the patterns and for switching between individual patterns. Both excitatory and inhibitory synapses are typically present. Thus the model may serve as a formal framework for understanding some biological systems that produce rhythmic output.

We compare the predictions of our model with Getting's detailed measurements on the CPG controlling the swim rhythm in *Tritonia* (Getting 1981, 1983a, 1983b; chapter 6). This CPG contains a small number of neurons and produces a single rhythmic output pattern. Yet the comparison will serve to highlight many features of the model and to assess its applicability to biological systems.

7.2   The Model

The present model is an extension of Hopfield's model of associative memory (Hopfield 1982, 1984). We consider a network that contains N interconnected model neurons. The output of each neuron, $V_i(t)$, varies between zero (quiescent) and unity (maximum firing rate). The state of the network is specified by the output activity of all of its neurons. It is represented by $V(t) = \{V_i(t)\}_{i=1}^N$.

A pattern is defined as a temporal sequence of a subset of all possible output states. The states, $V^\mu = \{V_i^\mu\}_{i=1}^N$, comprising this subset are referred to as the *embedded* states. For example, a pattern of length r consists of the sequence

$$V^1 \to V^2 \to V^3 \to \cdots \to V^{r-1} \to V^r$$

where each state V^μ is an embedded state. For the case of a cyclic sequence, of relevance for modeling CPGs, $V^r = V^1$. The networks can produce multiple patterns; we define $V^{\mu,\nu}$ as the μth embedded state in the νth pattern.

We consider patterns in which the output activity of the model neurons alternates between a relatively low firing rate and a relatively high rate. The precise form of this activity depends upon the detailed characteristics of the neurons. We therefore assume for simplicity that the output of each neuron, while the network is in an embedded state, alternates between quiescence and its maximum firing rate. Each component $V_i^{\mu,\nu}$ of the embedded states is thus given by either 0 or $+1$. This assumption allows us to focus on properties of the networks that result specifically from the form of the connections between neurons.

In the remainder of this chapter we first define the rules for encoding the output patterns in the synaptic connections. Next we describe the dynamics of the network, followed by a description of its general properties. Some of these properties are illustrated by numerical examples.

7.2.1   Synaptic Connections and Their Response Time

The desired output patterns are encoded in the form of the synaptic connections between the model neurons. We define the synaptic connection between the jth presynaptic neuron and the ith postsynaptic neuron as T_{ij}. A central feature of the present model is that each connection T_{ij} is *functionally* separated into two components, denoted T_{ij}^S and T_{ij}^L. The two components are hypothesized to have different characteristic response times. The synaptic connections T_{ij}^S act on the shorter of the two time scales. This time scale, τ_S, determines the time required for the network to settle in each of the embedded states. The synaptic connections denoted T_{ij}^L act on the longer of the two times. This time scale, $\tau_L(\tau_L \gg \tau_S)$, sets the time for the onset of the transitions between consecutive states in the pattern. Thus the duration of an individual state in a pattern will be $\sim \tau_L$, while the transitions between states occur on the faster time scale of τ_S.

The role of the connection strengths T_{ij}^S is to stabilize the network in an embedded state, until a transition to the next state occurs. This is achieved by defining the T_{ij} in terms of a formal version of the Hebb (1949) learning rule (see also Hopfield 1982), i.e.,

$$T_{ij}^S = \frac{J_0}{N} \sum_{\nu=1}^q \sum_{\mu=1}^r (2V_i^{\mu,\nu} - 1)(2V_j^{\mu,\nu} - 1), \qquad i \neq j, \; J_0 > 0 \qquad (7.1)$$

where q is the total number of patterns, $r = r(\nu)$ is the length of the νth pattern, and $T_{ii}^S = 0$. The prefactor J_0/N ensures that the magnitude of the total synaptic input is of order J_0. The variable $(2V_i^{\mu,\nu} - 1)$ has a value of either -1 (quiescent) or $+1$ (maximally firing) so that inhibitory as well as excitatory synapses are formed.

The role of the connection strengths T_{ij}^L is to induce transitions from the μth embedded state to the μ+1th state. Thus we define

$$T_{ij}^L = \lambda \frac{J_0}{N} \sum_{\nu=1}^q \sum_{\mu=1}^{r-1} (2V_i^{\mu+1,\nu} - 1)(2V_j^{\mu,\nu} - 1), \qquad i \neq j, \; \lambda > 0 \qquad (7.2)$$

where λ is a scaling parameter for the transition strength and $T_{ii}^L = 0$. We will discuss the constraints on λ in a later section. For the case of cyclic patterns, $V^{r,\nu} = V^{1,\nu}$. Note that the T_{ij}^L synapses, which depend on the consecutive output activity of the neurons, are asymmetric ($T_{ij}^L \neq T_{ji}^L$), while the T_{ij}^S synapses, which depend only on the activity within the individual states, are symmetric.

The rule for forming the T_{ij}^L synapses (eq. 7.2) encodes transitions between pairs of embedded states. This allows the network to generate patterns that involve unambiguous transitions between states. The permissible patterns correspond either to linear sequences (fig. 7.1A), cyclic sequences (fig. 7.1B) or sequences *down* a tree structure (fig. 7.1C). Several different patterns, as well as isolated, stable states, can be embedded in the same network. Patterns that involve ambiguous transitions, such as when two patterns share the same embedded state, cannot be reliably produced by the present network. This includes patterns that involve transitions *up* a tree. We will return to this issue in section 7.4.

The rules defined by eqs. 7.1 and 7.2 for forming the synaptic components are applicable only when the overlaps between the embedded states are small, i.e.,

$$\frac{1}{N} \sum_{j=1}^N (2V_j^{\mu,\nu} - 1)(2V_j^{\mu',\nu'} - 1) \simeq 0 \quad \text{for} \quad (\mu,\nu) \neq (\mu',\nu') \qquad (7.3)$$

and when, on average, half of the neurons are active in each of the embedded states, i.e.,

$$\frac{1}{N} \sum_{j=1}^N (2V_j^{\mu,\nu} - 1) \simeq 0 \qquad (7.4)$$

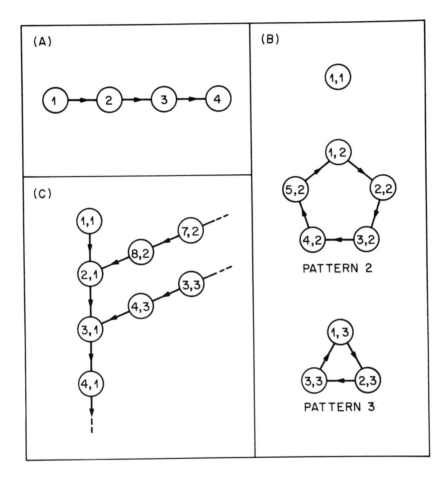

Figure 7.1
State diagrams of the different topologies of patterns that can be produced by the
model network. Circles correspond to stable outputs, i.e., embedded states, and
arrows correspond to the transitions between these states. (A) A linear sequence of
embedded states. The network will remain in the final state, V^4, after completing
the sequence. (B) Cyclic sequences of embedded states. Two cyclic patterns, along
with an isolated stable state, $V^{1,1}$, are shown. This arrangement of patterns was
used in the simulation shown in fig. 7.6. (C) A tree structure, in which two or more
sequences ultimately share the same set of embedded states.

These relations will be satisfied if the embedded states are approximately orthogonal to each other. For a large network, eqs. 7.3 and 7.4 are satisfied if the embedded states are chosen from a random sample; the average overlap in this case is $\sim \sqrt{1/N}$. Alternative rules, appropriate for embedding states that have a high degree of overlap, are described in Appendix 7.A.

Synaptic Inputs   The integrated synaptic input to each model neuron is assumed to be a *linear* summation of the outputs of the presynaptic neurons. The total synaptic input to the ith neuron via the fast components of the synapses , $h_i^S(t)$, is

$$h_i^S(t) = \sum_{j=1}^{N} T_{ij}^S V_j(t) \tag{7.5}$$

The total synaptic input via the slow components, $h_i^L(t)$, is

$$h_i^L(t) = \sum_{j=1}^{N} T_{ij}^L \overline{V_j(t)} \tag{7.6}$$

where $\overline{V_j(t)}$ is the time-averaged output of the neuron, i.e.,

$$\overline{V_i(t)} = \int_0^\infty V_i(t - t')\, w(t')\, dt' \tag{7.7}$$

The synaptic response function $w(t)$ for the slow, T_{ij}^L, components is a non-negative function that is normalized to unity, i.e.,

$$\int_0^\infty w(t)\, dt = 1 \tag{7.8}$$

and characterized by a mean time constant τ_L, i.e.,

$$\int_0^\infty t\, w(t)\, dt = \tau_L. \tag{7.9}$$

The inputs $h_i^L(t)$ correspond to a weighted average over the histories of the neural activities, with a characteristic averaging time of τ_L. An example of the time course of a postsynaptic response to a short presynaptic stimulus is illustrated in fig. 7.2.

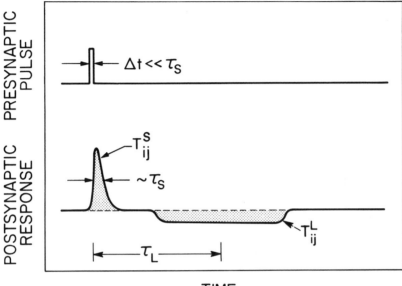

Figure 7.2
Illustration of a two-component synaptic connection from the jth to the ith neuron. The components are resolved following a short pulse ($\Delta t \ll \tau_S$) of activity in the presynaptic neuron. The area (shaded region) under the fast synaptic response is equal to T_{ij}^S (eq. 7.1); in this example T_{ij}^S is taken to be excitatory. The area (shaded region) under the slow synaptic response is equal to T_{ij}^L; in this example T_{ij}^L is taken to be inhibitory. The ratio of these areas, averaged over all pairs of synapses, equals the transition strength λ (eqs. 7.2 and 7.10). The time course of the slow synaptic response corresponds to the response function $w(t)$ (eq. 7.6); it has a time constant of τ_L.

7.2.2   Network Dynamics

Before we define the detailed dynamics of the network, we present a qualitative description in terms of the time dependence of the neural inputs. For simplicity of notation we consider a network that produces a single pattern. Immediately after a transition from the μ–1th embedded state to the μth state, the output of the network is $V(t) = V^\mu$, and the time-averaged output is $\overline{V(t)} \simeq V^{\mu-1}$. The inputs via the fast synaptic components are (eq. 7.5)

$$
\begin{aligned}
h_i^S(t) &= \sum_{j=1}^{N} T_{ij}^S V_j^\mu \\
&= \frac{J_0}{2} \sum_{\eta=1}^{r} (2V_i^\eta - 1) \left(\frac{1}{N} \sum_{j=1}^{N} (2V_j^\eta - 1)(2V_j^\mu - 1) \right. \\
&\qquad\qquad \left. + \frac{1}{N} \sum_{j=1}^{N} (2V_j^\eta - 1) \right) \\
&\simeq \frac{J_0}{2} (2V_i^\mu - 1)
\end{aligned}
$$

where we used eqs. 7.1–7.4. The synaptic input $h_i^S(t)$ is negative, i.e., inhibitory, if $V_i^\nu = 0$ (quiescent) and is positive, i.e., excitatory, if $V_i^\nu = 1$ (maximally firing). The inputs via the slow synaptic components are (eqs. 7.6 and 7.7)

$$
h_i^L(t) = \sum_{j=1}^{N} T_{ij}^L V_j^{\mu-1} \simeq \lambda \frac{J_0}{2} (2V_i^\mu - 1)
$$

Thus both $h^S(t)$ and $h^L(t)$ tend to stabilize the network in its current state. With increasing time, $\overline{V(t)}$ gradually shifts away from $V^{\mu-1}$ and toward the current state V^μ. This shift generates an increasingly large component of $h^L(t)$ that is conjugate to $V^{\mu+1}$. After the network has remained in the state V^μ for an interval $\sim \tau_L$, the inputs become

$$
h_i^S(t) = \sum_{j=1}^{N} T_{ij}^S V_j^\mu \simeq \frac{J_0}{2} (2V_i^\mu - 1)
$$

and

$$h_i^L(t) = \sum_{j=1}^{N} T_{ij}^L V_j^{\mu-1} \simeq \lambda \frac{J_0}{2}(2V_i^{\mu+1} - 1)$$

The new values of $h_i^L(t)$ tend to drive the network toward the state $V^{\mu+1}$. For sufficiently large values of λ ($\lambda \gtrsim 1$) the network makes a rapid transition to the $\mu+1$th embedded state.

A persistent sequential output pattern does not emerge if the T_{ij}^S and T_{ij}^L synaptic components act on the same time scale (i.e., $\tau_S \simeq \tau_L$). The transitions occur too frequently to allow the network to settle in an embedded state, resulting in an irregular output pattern that quickly dephases.

Detailed Dynamics   The dynamic evolution of the network is described by the equations

$$\begin{aligned}
\tau_S \frac{du_i(t)}{dt} + u_i(t) &= h_i^S(t) + h_i^L(t) + I_{stim_i} \\
&= \sum_{j=1}^{N} \left(T_{ij}^S V_j(t) + T_{ij}^L \overline{V_j(t)} \right) + I_{stim_i} \qquad (7.10)
\end{aligned}$$

where $u_i(t)$ is the net input to the ith neuron and I_{stim_i} represents an external input to the ith neuron. The equivalent electrical circuit described by these equations is shown schematically in fig. 7.3.

The output of a model neuron, $V_i(t)$, is related to its net input, $u_i(t)$, by a nonlinear gain function

$$V_i(t) = g\left[u_i(t) - \theta_i\right] \qquad (7.11)$$

where θ_i is defined as the mean operating level of the neuron.[1] The dynamic features of the network do not depend on the details of the gain function;[2] fig. 7.4 illustrates an appropriate form (e.g., Fuortes and Mantegazzini 1962). Note that the output of a neuron is most sensitive to changes in its input when $u_i(t) \simeq \theta_i$.

---

[1] This definition is more precise than the usual description in the literature on associative neural network models, in which θ_i is equated with the threshold level of a neuron. The later designation, however, is in discord with the neurobiological definition of the threshold level as the minimum input required to elicit a non-zero firing rate. The two definitions are equal only for neurons operating in the high-gain limit (see eq. 7.14).

[2] More generally, we require only that the postsynaptic response of a neuron is nonlinear. This can occur even if the firing frequency of the presynaptic neuron is a linear function of its input current.

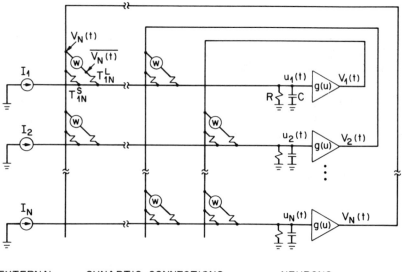

EXTERNAL   SYNAPTIC CONNECTIONS   NEURONS
INPUTS

Figure 7.3
Schematic representation of the circuit diagram for the model network. Neurons
are represented by saturating amplifiers (triangles; eq. 7.11) with a charging time
of $\tau^N = RC$, where R represents the *net* input resistance of the neuron. Synaptic
connections between each pair of neurons are represented by conductances (—⌁—)
proportional to T_{ij}^S (fast synaptic components; eq. 7.1) or T_{ij}^L (slow synaptic components; eq. 7.2). The response function of the slow synapses, $w(t)$ (circles; eqs. 7.7 to
7.9) has a characteristic time constant of τ_L. The fast response time of the network,
τ_S, corresponds to the larger of τ^N or the time constant of the fast synapses. The
detailed dynamics of the network are described by eq. 7.10.

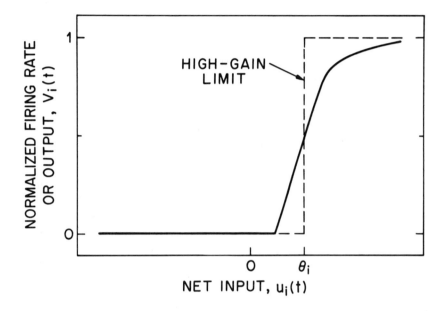

Figure 7.4
Schematic representation of a saturating gain function for a neuron. This function relates the output, or firing frequency of a neuron, $V_i(t)$, to the value of the net input, $u_i(t)$, and the mean operating level, θ_i (eq. 7.11). The output of a neuron is most sensitive to changes in its inputs when $u_i(t) \simeq \theta_i$ (eqs. 7.12 and 7.13).

The temporal relation between the fast and slow synaptic inputs, $h_i^S(t)$ and $h_i^L(t)$, respectively, the total input to the neuron, $u_i(t)$, and the output of the neuron, $V_i(t)$, are illustrated later in fig. 7.6B. The calculations leading to this figure are described later.

The biological interpretation of the short time constant (τ_S) in eq. 7.10 depends on the relative values of the response time, τ^S, of the *fast* synapses compared with the charging time, τ^N, of the neurons. In general, τ_S should be identified with the longest of the two time constants τ^N and τ^S. The emergence of patterns in our networks relies only on the time separation of τ_S and τ_L, i.e., $\tau_S \ll \tau_L$. In practice, a separation of time scales by a factor of approximately four or more is sufficient.

Output Period   In the present model the time spent by the network in each embedded state is constant. This time is $t_0 \sim \tau_L$, while the time spent making the transition between two states is $\sim \tau_S$. Thus the period of a cyclic pattern comprised of r states will be $\simeq r \cdot t_0$. The time t_0 is a monotonically decreasing function of the transition strength λ. The precise value of t_0 depends on the value of λ, on the detailed form of the synaptic response function, $w(t)$, and on the length of the pattern. Expressions for t_0, valid for the special case of a very long sequence and for the case of biphasic oscillations, are given in Appendixes 7.B and 7.C.

Neuron Operating Levels   In order that the patterns embedded in the T_{ij}^S and the T_{ij}^L synapses emerge as stable outputs of the network, the mean operating value of each neuron must be adjusted so that its output is maximally sensitive to changes in its input. This implies that the difference between the mean operating level of a neuron and the net input to that neuron, averaged over all its possible values, is small. This difference is denoted by $\Delta\theta_i$, where

$$
\begin{aligned}
\Delta\theta_i &= \theta_i - \frac{1}{2}\left[h_i^S(V_j(t)_{max}) + h_i^S(V_j(t)_{min})\right. \\
&\qquad \left. + h_i^L(V_j(t)_{max}) + h_i^L(V_j(t)_{min})\right] - I_{stim_i}(t) \qquad (7.12) \\
&= \theta_i - \frac{1}{2}\sum_{j=1}^{N}\left(T_{ij}^S + T_{ij}^L\right) - I_{stim_i}(t)
\end{aligned}
$$

We require that

$$\Delta\theta_i \simeq 0 \qquad (7.13)$$

More precisely, $\Delta\theta_i$ must be small compared to the typical value of the synaptic inputs present while the network is producing a pattern, i.e.,

$\Delta\theta_i \ll J_0$. A similar constraint holds for other associative networks (Little 1974; Hopfield 1982; Bruce, Gardner, and Wallace 1986).

High-Gain Limit The analysis of the dynamic properties of the network is simplified in the limiting case of a network containing two-state model neurons (McCulloch and Pitts 1943). These neurons are either quiescent or fully active, i.e., $V_i(t) = 0, +1$ (fig. 7.4). In this limit the analog circuit equations (eqs. 7.10 and 7.11) are replaced by the difference equations, or update rules,

$$
\begin{aligned}
V_i(t + \delta t) &= stp\left[h_i^S(t) + h_i^L(t) - \theta_i\right] \qquad (7.14)\\
&= stp\left[\frac{1}{2}\sum_{j=1}^{N}\left(T_{ij}^S\left(2V_j(t) - 1\right) + T_{ij}^L\left(2\overline{V_j(t)} - 1\right)\right)\right]
\end{aligned}
$$

where the step function, $stp(x)$, is defined by

$$
stp(x) = \begin{cases} +1; & x > 0 \\ 0; & x \le 0 \end{cases}
$$

In eq. 7.14 we assumed $\Delta\theta_i = 0$ with $I_{stim_i} = 0$ (eq. 7.13).

The update rules (eq. 7.14) can be implemented either synchronously or asynchronously. In synchronous updating the output of every neuron is changed simultaneously; in this case $\delta t = \tau_S$. In asynchronous updating a neuron is selected at random and its output is updated. In this case τ_S should be identified with the mean update time of the entire network and $\delta t = \tau_S/N$. Asynchronous updating more closely resembles the dynamic behavior of the analog network (eqs. 7.10 and 7.11) and may also provide a more realistic representation of biological systems.

The effect of stochastic noise can be incorporated into the model by replacing the deterministic update rules (eq. 7.14) with probabilistic update rules. A useful example of such rules is given by

$$
P[V_i(t + \tau_S) = 1] = \frac{1}{1 + exp[-2\beta(h_i^L(t) + h_i^S(t) - \theta_i)]} \qquad (7.15)
$$

where $P(V_i = 1)$ is the probability that the ith neuron is firing (Little 1974). The parameter $1/\beta$ plays the role of temperature. It is a measure of the level of stochastic noise in the network; e.g., noise caused by rapid fluctuations in the strength of the synapses (e.g., Dionne 1984). In the limit $\beta \to \infty$ we recover eq. 7.14.

7.2.3   Adiabatically Varying Energy Function

It has been useful to describe the properties of some associative neural
networks in terms of an energy function (Hopfield 1982, 1984; Cohen and
Grossberg 1983; Amit et al. 1985a). Strictly speaking, such a function
does not exist in our network. The stable outputs do *not* correspond
to states that are local minima of an energy function. Nevertheless,
we can describe the dynamics of our model in terms of a relaxational
process to a local minimum of an adiabatically varying energy function.
The parameters of this function depend on the history of the network.
The relaxation process occurs on the fast time scale of τ_S, while the
underlying energy landscape changes on the slower time scale of τ_L. An
appropriate energy function for our network is:

$$
E = -\frac{1}{2} \sum_{i=1}^{N} \sum_{j=1}^{N} (2V_i - 1) \, T_{ij}^{S} \, (2V_j - 1)
$$

$$
- \sum_{i=1}^{N} (2V_i - 1) \left(2h_i^{L}(t) - \sum_{j=1}^{N} T_{ij}^{L} \right) \tag{7.16}
$$

In writing eq. 7.16 we assumed for simplicity that the outputs of the
neurons are close to saturation; this corresponds to the high-gain limit
(eq. 7.14). The first term in eq. 7.16 is identical to the energy function
of the Hopfield's associative network (Hopfield 1982). The embedded
states, $V^{\mu,\nu}$, are robust minima of this term. The second term in the
energy (eq. 7.16) is a field term that varies with the slow time dependence
of $h^L(t)$ (eqs. 7.6–7.9).

The time dependence of the energy landscape is illustrated by the
surfaces shown in fig. 7.5. Each cross-point on a surface corresponds
to a state of the network. The minima in the surface correspond to the
embedded states V^{μ} and $V^{\mu+1}$. The "distance" between two cross-points
is equal to the number of neurons whose output is different between the
two corresponding states. The path between the states V^{μ} and $V^{\mu+1}$
passes through a set of unstable, intermediate states that are present
only during a transition.

After the network has settled into the μth embedded state the field
term, $h^L(t)$, initially acts to stabilize the network in this state (fig. 7.5A).
As the value of $h^L(t)$ evolves, the energy minimum at the current state
in the pattern weakens while that at the next state, $V^{\mu+1}$, grows deeper
(fig. 7.5B). Eventually the minimum at V^{μ} disappears and the network
makes a rapid transition to the state $V^{\mu+1}$ (fig. 7.5C).

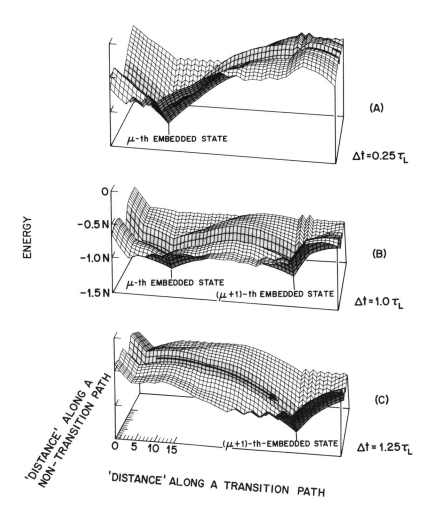

Figure 7.5
The time dependence of the adiabatic energy function for a network operating in the high-gain limit (eq. 7.16). A network containing 64 neurons was constructed to produce a cyclic pattern among seven (orthogonal) embedded states (eqs. 7.1, 7.2, 7.7, 7.12 with $\Delta\theta_i = 0$, and 7.14). The slow synaptic response was $w(t) = 1/\tau_L$ for $\tau_L/2 < t < 3\tau_L/2$ and $w(t) = 0$, otherwise with $\tau_L = 20\tau_S$ and $\lambda = 2$. To form the energy surface we defined a plane in the output space of the network in terms of a path that runs along the output sequence, i.e., $\cdots \rightarrow V^{\mu-1} \rightarrow V^{\mu} \rightarrow V^{\mu+1} \rightarrow \cdots$, and a path that runs approximately orthogonal to this sequence. Each of the cross-points on this plane corresponds to a possible output state of the network. (A) The energy values after the network has made a transition to the μth state. The delayed output corresponds to $\overline{V(t)} \simeq V^{\mu-1}$. The field term in the energy (eq. 7.16) has deepened the minimum at the μth embedded state at the expense of the minimum at the $\mu-1$th state (not shown) and the $\mu+1$th state. (B) The energy values after the delayed output has changed to $\overline{V(t)} \simeq 0.5V^{\mu-1} + 0.5V^{\mu}$. The field term contributes equally to the minima at the μth and the $\mu+1$th embedded states. (C) The energy values after the field term has completely removed the minimum at the μth embedded state, causing the network to make a transition to the $\mu+1$th state. The time spent in each state, $t_0 = 1.25\tau_L$, is in accord with theory.

The existence of an approximate energy function suggests that the output patterns are robust against moderate levels of static and dynamic noise in the network. In the case of stochastic noise (see eq. 7.16), the dynamics of the network are governed by an adiabatically varying free-energy function with a "temperature," $1/\beta$, determined by the amplitude of the noise.

7.2.4 Numerical Simulations and Additional Properties of the Model

A number of general features of the model were examined by numerical simulations and analytical techniques. Simulations were performed using eqs. 7.7 and 7.10 and the gain function

$$V_i(t) = \frac{1}{1 + exp[-2G\left(u_i(t) - \theta_i\right)]} \tag{7.17}$$

where G is the gain constant. The form of the gain function was chosen because of its similarity to the form of the stochastic update rules (cf. eqs. 7.15 and 7.17). Note, however, that the gain function is part of an analog system of equations (eq. 7.10) that describes *deterministic* dynamics.

Example: A Network with Multiple Patterns   To illustrate some of the properties of the model we simulated a network consisting of 100 neurons with nine randomly selected embedded states. These states were arranged as a single isolated state, a cyclic pattern among five states, and a cyclic pattern among three states (fig. 7.1B). We chose a delayed, uniform-averaging function for the slow synaptic response, i.e.,

$$w(t) = \begin{cases} \frac{1}{\tau_L} & \frac{1}{2}\tau_L < t < \frac{3}{2}\tau_L \\ 0 & \text{otherwise} \end{cases}$$

with $\tau_L = 20\tau_S$ and took $\lambda = 2$ (eq. 7.2) and $G^{-1} = J_0/4$ (eq. 7.17). The connection strengths were formed according to eqs. 7.1 and 7.2, and the analog network equations (eqs. 7.7, 7.10, and 7.17, and eq. 7.12 with $\Delta\theta = 0$) were approximated using finite difference methods (Appendix 7.D). We interpreted the values for the neuronal outputs, $V_i(t)$, as the probability that the ith neuron fired in the interval τ_S. These probabilities were used to construct the firing patterns for each neuron.

Figure 7.6A shows the firing pattern obtained from the output of 8 of the 100 neurons; the remainder of the neurons exhibited a similar firing pattern. The network was initially in the isolated, stable state $V^{1,1}$. At time t_1 an external input $I_{stim}(t_1)$, with duration $\Delta t = \tau_L$, was applied to drive the network into state $V^{1,2}$ of the (ν=2)th pattern. At the later time t_2 a second external input $I_{stim}(t_2)$ was applied to drive the network into a state in the (ν=3)th pattern. The appearance of stable patterns after each input illustrates how the same network can produce multiple output patterns.

Figure 7.6B illustrates the temporal relation between the synaptic inputs to the (i=8)th neuron, $h_8^S(t)$ and $h_8^L(t)$, the net input $u_8(t)$, and the output $V_8(t)$; these values coincide with the output marked by the box in fig. 7.6A. The peak values of $h_8^L(t)$ are approximately twice the amplitude of the peak values of $h_8^S(t)$ because of the choice $\lambda = 2$.

In the above simulation the output of each neuron is either quiescent or firing near its maximum rate. This feature of the output behavior results from the saturation characteristics of the gain function (eq. 7.17) chosen for this example. Other choices for a gain function can lead to stable output patterns in which the firing rate of the neurons does not saturate in each of the embedded states.

Maximum Number of Embedded States   A network can contain several patterns. The total number of embedded states in these patterns, p, is

$$p = \sum_{v=1}^{q} r(\nu) \tag{7.18}$$

(eqs. 7.1 and 7.2). The value of p is limited to

$$p < \alpha_c N \tag{7.19}$$

where the coefficient α_c depends on the length and topology of the embedded patterns, the transition strength λ, and the form of the slow synaptic response function $w(t)$. When $w(t)$ is given by a simple time delay, i.e., $w(t) = \delta(t - \tau_L)$, the value of the coefficient is $\alpha_c \simeq 0.3$ ($\lambda = 1$ to 2). This value is larger than the value $\alpha_c = 0.14$ for Hopfield's associative memory (Amit et al. 1985b; Crisanti, Amit, and Gutfreund 1986; see also Gutfreund and Mézard 1988). When $w(t)$ is represented by a smoothly varying function of time, the value of the coefficient is reduced to $\alpha_c \lesssim 0.1$.

The input to each neuron will contain a static noise term of order $\sqrt{p/N}$ when the number of embedded states is close to its maximum value. This noise may enhance the transitions between the embedded states. This enhancement, in turn, will reduce the minimum value of the transition strength necessary to generate patterns to a value $\lambda \lesssim 1$.

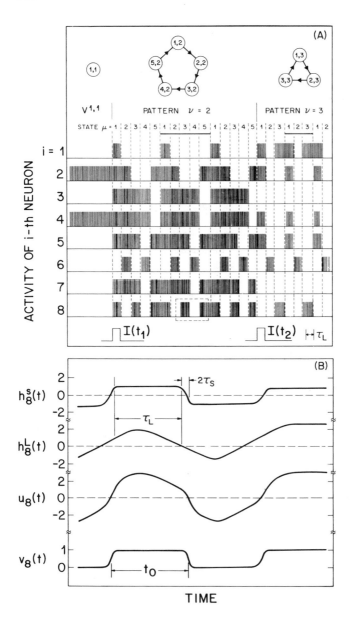

Figure 7.6
Simulation of a network containing 100 neurons with nine embedded states; see text
for details. The heavy lines at the top of the figure correspond to the output period
of each pattern. (A) The firing pattern calculated from the outputs $V_i(t)$ of 8 of
the 100 neurons. The network was initialized in state $V^{1,2}$. At time t_1 an external
input $I_{stim}(t_1)$ was applied for a time τ_L. This input drove the network into state
$V^{2,1}$ and thus initiated the $(\nu=2)$th pattern. Similarly, the external input $I_{stim}(t_2)$
was applied at time t_2 to drive the network into state $V^{1,3}$ and initiate the $(\nu=3)$th
pattern. (B) Details of the dynamic behavior of the $(i=8)$th neuron for the period
of time delineated by the box in (A). Shown are the inputs from the fast synaptic
components, $h_8^S(t)$, the inputs from the slow synaptic components, $h_8^L(t)$, the net
synaptic input, $u_8(t)$, and the output of the neuron, $V_8(t)$.

Eliminating Synaptic Connections   The model we described assumes the existence of synaptic connections between all pairs of neurons.
Biological networks may contain a much smaller set of connections either intrinsically or as a result of damage or disease. Will our network
function with a reduced set of connections?

The performance of the network model is only marginally affected
when up to 50% of the fast components of the synaptic connections (T_{ij}^S)
are eliminated at random. The main effect of eliminating a fraction,
c^S, of these components is to proportionately decrease the maximum
number of states that can be embedded in the network (see eq. 7.18).
Eliminating the slow components of the synaptic connections (T_{ij}^L) has a
relatively small effect on this number (except for the case of $w(t) \simeq \delta(t -
\tau_L)$). However, random elimination of a fraction, c^L, of the T_{ij}^L synapses
will decrease the ability of the network to make a transition between
the embedded states. This decrease can be offset by a compensating
increase in the value of λ. The effective transition strength, λ^{eff}, in this
case is

$$\lambda^{eff} \simeq \lambda \frac{1 - c^L}{1 - c^S} \tag{7.20}$$

The value of λ^{eff} must be greater than 1, implying that

$$\lambda \gtrsim \frac{1 - c^S}{1 - c^L}$$

Analog Versus Two-State Neurons   The analog character of the
model neurons does not play a major role in our network, as it does not
in Hopfield's network (Hopfield 1984). Patterns are reliably generated
when the gain of the neuron, G in eq. 7.17, is chosen to be larger than a
critical value, G_c. The value of G_c^{-1} is approximately equal to the value
of the typical net input to the neuron, i.e., $G_c^{-1} \simeq J_0$. Its precise value
depends on both the number of embedded states and on the topology
of the patterns. At moderate values of gain, $G \gtrsim G_c$, the transitions
between the embedded states are enhanced. This reduces the minimum
value of the transition strength to $\lambda < 1$, similar to the effect found
using two-state neurons with the stochastic update rules (eq. 7.15).

7.2.5   Biphasic Oscillations

A particularly simple pattern is one that oscillates between an embedded
state $V^\mu = \{V_i^\mu\}_{i=1}^N$ and its antiphase, $(1 - V^\mu)$, in which the quiescent
neurons are now firing and vice versa. Multiple patterns of this form

can be embedded in our network. The resulting synaptic strengths are (eqs. 7.1 and 7.2)

$$T_{ij}^S = \frac{J_0}{N} \sum_{\mu=1}^{q} (2V_i^{\mu} - 1)(2V_j^{\mu} - 1), \quad i \neq j, \ J_0 > 0 \qquad (7.21)$$

and

$$T_{ij}^L = \lambda \frac{J_0}{N} \sum_{\mu=1}^{q} [2(1 - V_i^{\nu}) - 1](2V_j^{\mu} - 1) = -\lambda T_{ij}^S, \quad i \neq j, \ \lambda \geq 1 \ (7.22)$$

where k is the number of patterns and $T_{ii}^S = T_{ii}^L = 0$.

Although the synaptic components T_{ij}^L are, in general, asymmetric (i.e., $T_{ji}^L \neq T_{ij}^L$) they are symmetric for the special case of biphasic oscillations (cf. eqs. 7.2 and 7.21). The relation $T_{ij}^L = -\lambda T_{ij}^S$ implies that the connections between each pair of neurons correspond either to short-term reciprocal inhibition followed by delayed excitation, or to short-term reciprocal excitation followed by delayed inhibition. Note that even in this case, the symmetry in both the T_{ij}^S and the T_{ij}^L components may be broken, e.g., by eliminating synaptic connections, without strongly affecting the output behavior of the network.

In Appendix 7.C we derive an analytical expression (eq. 7.40) that relates the duration of each state, t_0, to the slow synaptic response time, τ_L, the transition strength, λ, and the form of the synaptic response function, $w(t)$. We use this expression to calculate the dependence of t_0 on λ for a number of response functions (Table 7.3).

7.3   Central Pattern Generator in Tritonia

In this section we draw a connection between our model and detailed measurements on the central pattern generator controlling the swim rhythm in the mollusc *Tritonia diomedea*. A description of the swim rhythm can be found in the previous chapter.

The CPG in *Tritonia* consists of four neural groups, denoted by VSI-A, VSI-B, C2, and DSI. [3] The VSI neurons are the ventral swim in-

---

[3] There are three DSI neurons connected to each other by strong, fast-acting excitatory connections. Following Getting (1981), we group all three as a single neuron. The role of the DSI neurons as single neurons pertains to the turning on and off of the cyclic response (Getting and Dekin 1985), a topic we do not consider in detail. The fast, excitatory interaction among the DSI neurons may be incorporated by including a nonzero self-coupling term, i.e., T_{22}^S, into the model. An analysis shows that the inclusion of this term has a relatively minor effect on the output of the network (Kleinfeld and Sompolinsky 1988).

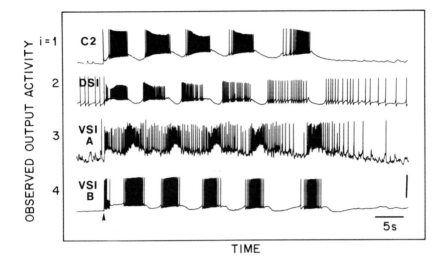

Figure 7.7
The output activity simultaneously measured from a C2, DSI, VSI-A, and VSI-B
neuron in an isolated brain preparation from *Tritonia*. These neurons comprise the
CPG that controls the escape swim sequence. Their output corresponds to $V_1(t)$,
$V_2(t)$, $V_3(t)$, and $V_4(t)$, respectively, in the analysis presented in section 7.3. The
arrow indicates the initiation of the sequence. Note that in the present work we are
concerned only with the oscillatory behavior of the CPG, and not with the gradual
dephasing that leads to its turning off. Vertical bar: 50 mV for C2, DSI, and VSI-B
and 25 mV for VSI-A. Adapted from Getting (1983b).

terneurons, C2 is a cerebral neuron, and DSI represents the dorsal swim
interneurons. The observed output pattern consists of bursting output
from VSI-A and VSI-B neurons alternating with bursts from the C2 and
DSI neurons (figs. 7.7, 6.1A). The time interval between consecutive action potentials within a bursting state is ~ 0.01 *sec* to 0.1 *sec*, and the
duration of each state is, on average, approximately 5 *sec*.

Of primary importance is Getting's observation that some of the
synaptic connections have components that act on two different time
scales. For example, the synaptic input to C2 from DSI shows a rapid excitatory response followed by a much slower inhibitory response (figs. 7.8,
6.5B). The observed form of the synaptic response in *Tritonia* suggests
that there is an analogy between the mechanism for oscillations in our
theory and the biological mechanism for oscillations in this CPG.

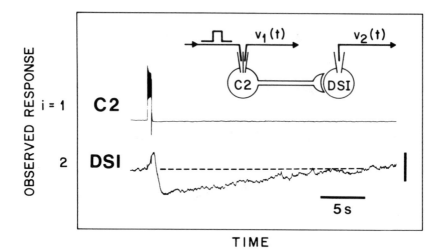

Figure 7.8
An example of the synaptic interaction between two neurons in the CPG in *Trito-*
nia. Shown is the presynaptic activity measured in the C2 neuron, $v_1(t)$, and the
postsynaptic response measured in a DSI neuron, $v_2(t)$, as the result of a short pulse
of current injected into C2. The measurement was performed under conditions that
insured that only monosynaptic connections contributed to the observation. The
observed response applies to two out of the three DSI neurons (DSI_B and DSI_C);
the other DSI neuron (DSI_A) exhibits only a slow response. The area under the
initial, positive-going response corresponds roughly to T_{21}^S; that under the slowly
decaying response corresponds to T_{21}^L. The time dependence of the slow decay corresponds to the time dependence of the slow synaptic response function, $w(t)$. Vertical
bar: 40 mV for C2 and 2 mV for DSI. Adapted from Getting (1981).

The focus of our analysis is to determine if the properties of the CPG in *Tritonia* support the mechanism we propose for generating patterns. Specifically, we ask:

1. Are the observed synaptic strengths consistent with those calculated from the form of the observed output states?

2. Are the simple update rules (eq. 7.14) sufficient to demonstrate the emergence of an oscillatory output that qualitatively resembles the observed pattern?

3. Is the period of the observed output pattern accounted for in terms of the magnitude and form of the observed slow synaptic response?

4. Are the observed operating levels of the neurons consistent with the constraint that their output is maximally sensitive to changes in their net synaptic input (eq. 7.13)?

It is important to emphasize that we are not attempting to reproduce accurately all of the details of the output behavior of *Tritonia*. For this one would necessarily include the detailed biophysical properties of the neurons and their synaptic connections, as was discussed in chapter 6.

7.3.1 Synaptic Connections

The observed output sequences will be approximated by an oscillation between a state V^+ and its antiphase $V^- \equiv (1 - V^+)$, where

$$V^+ = \begin{pmatrix} \text{activity of} & C2 \\ & DSI \\ & VSI - A \\ & VSI - B \end{pmatrix} = \begin{pmatrix} +1 \\ +1 \\ 0 \\ 0 \end{pmatrix} \text{ and}$$

$$V^- = \begin{pmatrix} 0 \\ 0 \\ +1 \\ +1 \end{pmatrix} \tag{7.23}$$

These states are used as the stable embedded states in our model. The short-term connection strengths T_{ij}^S, and the long-term connection strengths T_{ij}^L, deduced from the outputs V^+ and V^- (eqs. 7.21 to 7.23), are shown in table 7.1. Note that these matrices contain *all* possible connections that can be present between pairs of neurons.

How do the predicted synaptic strengths compare with the observed values? The strength of a synaptic connection is proportional to the

Fast Synaptic Components, T_{ij}^S	Slow Synaptic Components, T_{ij}^L
Theory $\dfrac{J_0}{4}\begin{pmatrix}0 & +1 & -1 & -1\\ +1 & 0 & -1 & -1\\ -1 & -1 & 0 & +1\\ -1 & -1 & +1 & 0\end{pmatrix}$	$j = 1\ \ 2\ \ 3\ \ 4$ $\lambda\dfrac{J_0}{4}\begin{pmatrix}0 & -1 & +1 & +1\\ -1 & 0 & +1 & +1\\ +1 & +1 & 0 & -1\\ +1 & +1 & -1 & 0\end{pmatrix}\begin{matrix}i = 1\\2\\3\\4\end{matrix}$
Observed[a] $\dfrac{J_0}{4}\begin{pmatrix}0 & +1 & \bullet & -1\\ +1 & 0 & -1 & -1\\ -1 & -1 & 0 & +1\\ \bullet & -1 & \bullet & 0\end{pmatrix}$	$C\ \ D\ \ VA\ \ VB\ ^{pre}\!/_{post}$ $\lambda\dfrac{J_0}{4}\begin{pmatrix}0 & \bullet & \bullet & \bullet\\ -1 & 0 & \bullet & \bullet\\ +1 & +1 & -0 & \bullet\\ +1 & \bullet & \bullet & -0\end{pmatrix}\begin{matrix}C\\D\\VA\\VB\end{matrix}$

(a) Abstracted from the data of Getting (1981, 1983b); see text for details. Dots (●) indicate synaptic connections that are not present in *Tritonia*; their value is taken to be zero for purposes of calculation [*e.g.*, Eqs. (3.3) to (3.5)].

Table 7.1
Synaptic connection strengths for *Tritonia*.

time integral of the conductance changes induced in the postsynaptic neuron by a short ($t < \tau_S$) pulse of activity in the presynaptic neuron. These integrals can be *estimated* from measurements of the potentials induced in the postsynaptic neuron by a short ($t < \tau_S$) burst of action potentials in the presynaptic neuron. The action potentials in the post-synaptic neurons must be suppressed so that only direct interactions, i.e., monosynaptic pathways, contribute to the observed response.

The strength of the observed synaptic components T_{ij}^S and T_{ij}^L were estimated from the pairwise measurements reported by Getting (1981, 1983b, Appendix 6.B) (e.g., fig. 7.8). We grouped the data according to the time scale of the observed synaptic response. Synaptic components that decayed on a time scale less than 1 *sec* were designated as fast, whereas synaptic components that decayed on a time scale substantially greater than 1 *sec* were designated as slow. For this simple system we need only consider the *sign* of the measured response, and thus detailed variations between the values of the individual T_{ij}^S connection strengths and between the T_{ij}^L connection strengths were neglected. We did not include synaptic components whose strengths were considerably weak in comparison with the other components. For example, the observed synaptic connection from C2 to DSI (fig. 7.8) was parameterized by the values $T_{21}^S = T_0/4$ and $T_{21}^L = -\lambda T_0/4$.

The complete set of connection strengths T_{ij}^S and T_{ij}^L that we abstracted from Getting's data are summarized in table 7.1; note that theoretically possible connections that are not present in *Tritonia* are taken as zeros. This set was also used to construct the equivalent circuit shown in fig. 7.9. Ambiguities in our assignment of the connection strengths will be discussed at the end of this section.

The observed transition strength, λ (eq. 7.2), was determined by calculating the average magnitude of the fast synaptic components relative to that of the slow components. This determination contains a large uncertainty, in part because of the difficulty in separating the fast and slow contributions to the measured synaptic response. We roughly estimate

$$\lambda = 5 \text{ to } 10 \tag{7.24}$$

The signs of the experimentally observed synaptic strengths match those of the theoretically predicted strengths (table 7.1). Three of the possible twelve synaptic connections show both a short-term and a long-term response. Connections $(i, j) = (3, 1)$ and $(i, j) = (3, 2)$ both show short-term inhibition followed by a long-term excitation, while connection $(i, j) = (2, 1)$ shows short-term excitation followed by long-term

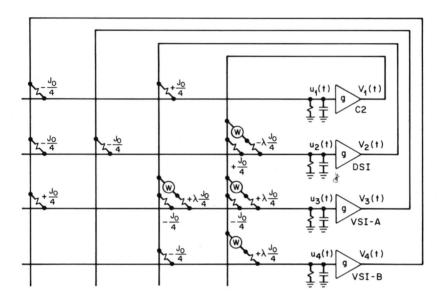

Figure 7.9
Schematic representation of the equivalent circuit for the analog network model describing the CPG in *Tritonia*; symbols as in fig. 7.3. The synaptic strengths contained in this circuit correspond to the observed connections T_{ij}^S and T_{ij}^L (table 7.1).

inhibition. The form of these three connections illustrates how the sign of the net synaptic input to a neuron can change over time.

7.3.2   Network Dynamics

We now examine whether the observed network parameters in *Tritonia* indeed give rise to rhythmic output in the network model. We begin our analysis with a simplified model that accents the role of the observed synaptic connections in generating stable oscillations. For this simplified analysis we use two-state neurons with synchronous update rules (eq. 7.14 with $\delta t = \tau_s$) and a delta function delay for the slow synaptic response function, i.e., $w(t) = \delta(t - \tau_L)$. A more detailed analysis, using analog model neurons and a smooth synaptic response function, is presented later.

Immediately after the network has stabilized in the embedded state V^+, the output of the ith neuron is $V_i(t) = V_i^+$, but the delayed output is $\overline{V_i(t)} = V_i(t - \tau_L) = V_i^-$. The output of the ith neuron after the next update is

$$
\begin{aligned}
V_i(t + \tau_S) &= stp\left[\frac{1}{2}\sum_{j=1}^{4} T_{ij}^S\left(2V_j^+ - 1\right) + T_{ij}^L\left(2V_j^- - 1\right)\right] \quad (7.25)\\[2mm]
&= stp\left[\frac{J_0}{8}\begin{pmatrix} 0 & +1 & 0 & -1 \\ +1 & 0 & -1 & -1 \\ -1 & -1 & 0 & +1 \\ 0 & -1 & 0 & 0 \end{pmatrix}\begin{pmatrix} +1 \\ +1 \\ -1 \\ -1 \end{pmatrix}\right.\\[2mm]
&\qquad\left. +\lambda\frac{J_0}{8}\begin{pmatrix} 0 & 0 & 0 & 0 \\ -1 & 0 & 0 & 0 \\ +1 & +1 & 0 & 0 \\ +1 & 0 & 0 & 0 \end{pmatrix}\begin{pmatrix} -1 \\ -1 \\ +1 \\ +1 \end{pmatrix}\right]\\[2mm]
&= stp\left[\frac{J_0}{8}\begin{pmatrix} 2 \\ 3+\lambda \\ -3-2\lambda \\ -1-\lambda \end{pmatrix}\right] = \begin{pmatrix} +1 \\ +1 \\ 0 \\ 0 \end{pmatrix} \quad \text{for} \quad \lambda > 0\\[2mm]
&= V_i^+
\end{aligned}
$$

Thus the output of the network is stable on the time scale of τ_S. After the network has remained in the state V^+ for a time τ_L, the delayed output changes to $\overline{V(t + \tau_L)} = V(t) = V^+$. The output of the ith neuron after the next update is

$$V_i(t + \tau_L + \tau_S) \;=\; stp\left[\frac{1}{2}\sum_{j=1}^{4} T_{ij}^S \left(2V_j^+ - 1\right) + T_{ij}^L \left(2V_j^+ - 1\right)\right] \quad (7.26)$$

$$=\; stp\left[\frac{J_0}{8}\begin{pmatrix} 2 \\ 3 - \lambda \\ -3 + 2\lambda \\ -1 + \lambda \end{pmatrix}\right] = \begin{pmatrix} +1 \\ 0 \\ +1 \\ +1 \end{pmatrix} \quad \text{for } \lambda > 3$$

The network is now in a mixed, unstable state. Using this new value for the current state in the update procedure gives

$$V_i(t + \tau_L + 2\tau_S) \;=\; stp\left[\frac{1}{2}\sum_{j=1}^{4} T_{ij}^S \left(2V_j(t + \tau_L + \tau_S) - 1\right)\right.$$

$$\left. + T_{ij}^L \left(2V_j^+ - 1\right)\right] \quad (7.27)$$

$$=\; stp\left[\frac{J_0}{8}\begin{pmatrix} -2 \\ -1 - \lambda \\ 1 + 2\lambda \\ 1 + \lambda \end{pmatrix}\right] = \begin{pmatrix} 0 \\ 0 \\ +1 \\ +1 \end{pmatrix}$$

$$=\; V_i^-$$

The network has now completed a transition from the state V^+ to the state V^-. It will remain in this state for a time $t_0 \simeq \tau_L$, after which the cycle will repeat itself. The output of the network will oscillate only if the transition strength is $\lambda > 3$ (eq. 7.26). This value is consistent with the observed value (eq. 7.24) of $\lambda = 5$ to 10.

The simplified analysis presented above suggests that the observed connection strengths can give rise to rhythmic output in the model network. We now examine the steady-state behavior of the network model for *Tritonia* (fig. 7.9) using analog dynamics and a synaptic response function that is a smooth function of time. The observed form of the response function, $w(t)$, is approximated by an exponential, i.e.,

$$w(t) = \begin{cases} \frac{1}{\tau_L}e^{-t/\tau_L} & 0 \le t < \infty \\ 0 & \text{otherwise} \end{cases}$$

The analog equations (eqs. 7.7, 7.10, and 7.17, and eq. 7.12 with $\Delta\theta_i = 0$) were simulated (Appendix 7.D) using the observed connection strengths

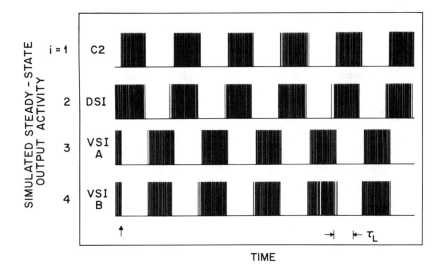

Figure 7.10
Simulated output activity from the analog network model describing the CPG in *Tritonia* (fig. 7.9). The arrows indicate the start of the simulated output from the initial states $V(t < 0) = \overline{V(t < 0)} = (\ 0\ 1\ 1\ 1\ )^T$. The network equations were simultated using the observed values of T_{ij}^S and T_{ij}^L; see text for details.

T_{ij}^S and T_{ij}^L (table 7.1), the above form for $w(t)$, $\tau_L = 10\tau_S$, and $G^{-1} = J_0/10$ for the gain parameter (eq. 7.17). Stable oscillations of the form described by the previous simplified analysis (eqs. 7.25 to 7.27) were observed. The output activity for the transition strength $\lambda = 10$ is shown in fig. 7.10.

The period observed for the output of the CPG in *Tritonia* is $2t_0 = 6\ sec$ to $10\ sec$ (fig. 7.7), while the time constant for the slow synaptic response (eq. 7.9) lies in the range $\tau_L = 2\ sec$ to $5\ sec$ (Appendix 6.B). Is this value for the period accounted for by the model? As discussed in the previous section, the predicted value for t_0 depends on the values of τ_L and λ and on the form of the response function $w(t)$. In Table 7.3 we give an analytic expression for t_0 appropriate for the above weighting function, from which we find $2t_0 = 1\ sec$ to $4\ sec$ for values of τ_L in the range $2\ sec$ to $5\ sec$ and λ in the range 5 to 10. However, this estimate of $2t_0$ may be inaccurate; the effective value of the λ should be significantly smaller than the observed value because of the relatively

large number of T_{ij}^L connections that are absent. We checked this point
by simulating the analog equations for the network (see above) with
different values for λ; the dependence of $2t_0$ on λ is shown in fig. 7.11. As
expected, the theoretical range of values for the duration was longer, i.e.,
we calculated $2t_0 = 5$ sec to 20 sec. The estimate compares favorably
with the experimentally observed range $2t_0 = 6$ sec to 10 sec ($2t_0 =$
$2.5\tau_L \simeq 5$ sec to 12 sec for $\lambda = 10$; fig. 7.10).

7.3.3   Neuron Operating Levels

We now consider the issue of the mean operating level of each neuron,
θ_i. As discussed in section 7.2, the mean operating levels should obey
the relation given by eq. 7.13 in order that the firing rate of each neuron
is most sensitive to changes in the value of its input. For *Tritonia*, this
relation becomes

$$\theta_i \simeq I_{stim_i} + \frac{1}{2} \sum_{j=1}^{4} \left(T_{ij}^S + T_{ij}^L \right) = I_{stim_i} + \frac{J_0}{8} \begin{pmatrix} 0 \\ -1 - \lambda \\ -1 + 2\lambda \\ -1 + \lambda \end{pmatrix} \qquad (7.28)$$

with $\lambda = 5$ to 10. We first consider the DSI neuron ($i = 2$): eq. 7.28 implies either that this neuron should be in a tonically excited state when
it is functionally isolated from its synaptic inputs ($\theta_2 < 0$), or that this
neuron requires an external excitatory input for the CPG to be active
($I_{stim_i} > 0$). A combination of both of these features is observed *in
vivo* (Getting 1983a; Getting and Dekin 1985). The DSI neurons fire
tonically, although at a reduced rate, in isolation (Getting 1983a). Activation of the CPG in *Tritonia* requires an effective excitatory input to
the DSI neurons (Getting and Dekin 1985). After this input is removed
the output from the CPG gradually dephases and the CPG becomes
inactive. We next consider the VSI neurons. In the absence of synaptic
inputs and external inputs, the output of VSI-B is expected to be quiescent ($\theta_4 > 0$). This result is in agreement with observation (Getting
1983b).

The problematic neuron is VSI-A, which is not known to receive an
external input while the CPG is producing oscillatory output. Thus,
according to eq. 7.28, VSI-A should have a positive operating level. In
practice, VSI-A exhibits a weak tonic output when it is functionally isolated (Getting 1983a). Violation of eq. 7.28 suggests, by the arguments
of section 7.2, that the oscillations in the output of VSI-A will be less
robust than those of the other neurons. This conclusion is consistent
with the observed outputs, i.e., the relative change in the firing rate of

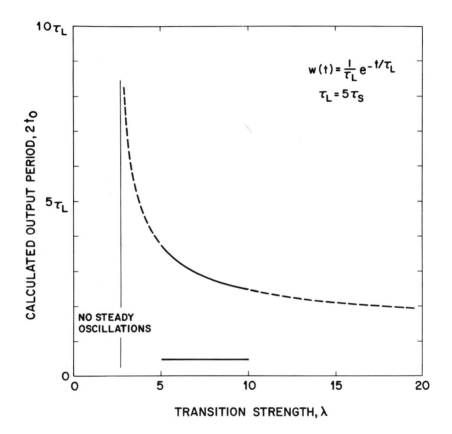

Figure 7.11
The output period, $2t_0$, of the analog network model for *Tritonia* (fig. 7.9) as a function of the average transition strength λ. A period of $2t_0 \simeq 6$ *sec* to 10 *sec*, roughly equivalent to $2\tau_L \lesssim 2t_0 \lesssim 5\tau_L$, corresponds to the period observed in *Tritonia* (fig. 7.7). The solid line delimits the range of values for λ estimated from the measured connection strengths (e.g., fig. 7.8). For a value of λ near 10, the period deduced from the model is in accord with the observed period. The spectrum $2t_0(\lambda)$ was determined by simulating the network equations using the observed values of T_{ij}^S and T_{ij}^L; see text for details.

VSI-A during the oscillations is smaller than that of the other neurons in the CPG (fig. 7.7). Note also that this neuron is weakly coupled to other neurons in the network (table 7.1). Hence VSI-A is expected to play a relatively minor role in the CPG, as noted previously (Getting and Dekin 1985).

7.3.4   Reexamination of the Connection Strengths

We consider in detail several assumptions that were made in assigning the T_{ij}^S and T_{ij}^L synaptic strengths. The connection from DSI to C2 exhibits short-term excitation followed by a much weaker long-term excitation. We ignored the weak long-term effect; thus $T_{12}^S = +J_0/4$ and $T_{12}^L = 0$. A similar choice was made for the inhibitory connection from VSI-B to the DSI, i.e., $T_{24}^S = -J_0/4$ and $T_{24}^L = 0$. Both of these relatively weak long-term components are believed to contribute primarily to the turning off of the CPG (Getting, unpublished), an effect we do not consider at present.

The synaptic connection from the DSI to VSI-A exhibits two short-term responses as well as a long-term response. Short-term inhibition is preceded by a relatively shorter period of excitation, with the pair followed by long-term excitation. We ignored the initial excitation and assigned $T_{32}^S = -J_0/4$ and $T_{32}^L = +\lambda J_0/4$. A different choice for the sign of T_{32}^S does *not* significantly affect the output pattern of the network.

The synaptic coupling between VSI-A and VSI-B could not be measured under conditions that suppressed possible indirect interactions, i.e., polysynaptic pathways, between these neurons (Getting 1983b). Externally exciting VSI-B caused VSI-A to fire weakly; we assigned $T_{34}^S = +J_0/4$ and $T_{34}^L = 0$. Externally exciting VSI-A caused a slow depolarization in VSI-B, but did not cause it to fire. We chose $T_{43}^S = T_{43}^L = 0$, but one cannot rule out the possibility $T_{21}^S = 0$ and $T_{21}^L > 0$. An analysis of the network dynamics, similar to that performed above (eqs. 7.25 to 7.27), shows that stable oscillations persist as long as T_{43}^L is weaker (by approximately 25% or more) than the other slow synaptic components.

7.4   Discussion

7.4.1   Properties of the Model

We have presented an associative neural network model that is capable of generating patterns of linear sequences or cyclic sequences of states. The patterns are stored in synaptic connections that have two components. One component, with a fast response time, stabilizes the individual states that comprise a pattern. The second component, with a slow response time, triggers the transitions between the consecutive states in a pattern.

The present model for generating output patterns has several attractive structural and functional features. It describes pattern generation in arbitrarily large, highly interconnected networks. The model does not necessarily rely on specific organization of the connections (e.g., a ring-like organization). The synaptic connections are not symmetric and the network can contain both excitatory and inhibitory synapses.

The distributed nature of the network and the inherent feedback between neurons endows the network with a high robustness. Removing at random as many as half of the synaptic connections does not affect the generation of patterns, except for reducing the number of states that can be embedded, i.e., used to form patterns, in the network. The patterns are stable to moderate levels of stochastic noise. An individual pattern can be accessed in an associative manner, such as by an input that only partially resembles one of the embedded states in the pattern. Finally, the model employs a simple relation between the output patterns and the synaptic connections.

The network can produce multiple patterns of different lengths and topologies. Neither the embedded states nor the patterns need to have any specific structure. In fact, the model works optimally with patterns of random, uncorrelated states. The number of states that can be embedded in the network scales linearly with the number of neurons in the network.

The present model does not use pacemaking cells or a system clock to generate patterns. Rather, the sequential output results from the interplay between fast synaptic components, which stabilize the embedded states, and slow synaptic components, which trigger the transitions. The detailed form of the slow synaptic response function is not critical. It can be either a sharp function of time, such as a delta function delay, or a smooth function, such as a low-pass filter. In particular, the form of the slow synaptic response may fluctuate from one synapse to another. The network will function properly so long as most of the slow components have roughly the same time constant.

Amari (1972), Fukushima (1973), and Kohonen (1980) have proposed models for generating temporal patterns in which *all* of the synaptic connections are formed according to rules similar to the rule we use to form the *slow* synaptic components (eq. 7.2). In contrast to the model we present, these models function as finite state machines in which the

existence of temporal patterns is dependent upon an internal synchro-
nizing clock and on synaptic delays that are sharp functions of time.[4]

Initiation of a Pattern   A particular output pattern can be selected
by an external input, I_{stim_i} (eq. 7.10 and fig. 7.3). This input must
place the network in an initial state that has a substantial overlap with
one of the embedded states in the desired pattern. The network will
rapidly relax to this embedded state and subsequently proceed to generate the full pattern. The external input need be present only for a brief
time, $\Delta t \stackrel{<}{\sim} \tau_L$, if the mean operating levels of the neurons are properly
matched to their average synaptic input (eq. 7.13). Otherwise, lasting
inputs may be required to maintain the output pattern.

A variety of mechanisms exist for terminating a cyclic output sequence. A direct way is to use an external input to drive the network
into a state that is not part of the pattern (fig. 7.1B). Similarly, raising
the mean operating level, θ_i, of the majority of the neurons will halt the
output. An indirect way of ending a pattern is to change the value of
the transition strength, λ, to a value outside the range of stability (see
Appendixes 7.B and 7.C). The output will gradually dephase until the
pattern has effectively decayed. A similar decay will occur for an output
pattern that is initiated in a network in which the number of embedded
states is above its maximum value (α_c, see eq. 7.18).

Modulation of the Output Period   The output period of a pattern
is proportional to t_0, the time spent by the network in each state. This
time scales linearly with the time constant, τ_L, of the slow synaptic
response, but is a decreasing function of the transition strength, λ.[5]
Thus a change in either τ_L or λ will induce a substantial change in the
output period. The value of t_0, and thus the period, is fairly insensitive
to changes in either the operating level, θ_i, or the gain, G, of the neurons.
A change in either of these parameters will change t_0 by at most the value
of $\sim \tau_S$.

Patterns of Correlated States   We employed formalized Hebb (1949)
learning rules to specify the strength at the synaptic connections in terms

---

[4] A model that relies on time-dependent synaptic strengths to produce rhythmic
output has been suggested by Peretto and Niez (1986). Dehaene, Changeux, and
Nadel (1987) considered a model for temporal sequences, in the context of bird song,
that uses high-order synapses. A model in which a rhythmic output is driven by
stochastic noise has been proposed by Buhmann and Schulten (1987).

[5] The period of the output is independent of λ when the response function of the
slow synapses is given by a delta function time delay, i.e., $w(t) = \delta(t - \tau_L)$; see
tables 7.2, 7.3.

of the embedded states. These rules are appropriate when the overlaps between the states in a pattern are small. However, when the states are correlated, i.e., when they have substantial overlaps, the number of states that can be embedded in the network is severely limited.

Correlations among output states are expected in biological systems. For example, some regions of the vertebrate nervous system exhibit low levels of activity, i.e., only a small fraction of the neurons fire simultaneously (Shepherd 1979). The large fraction of neurons with quiescent outputs suggests that the embedded states of these networks are substantially correlated. Correlations among the embedded states exist naturally in problems of pattern and speech recognition.

Rules that are suitable for embedding correlated states in our network are presented in Appendix 7.A. With these rules, the number of states that can be embedded scales linearly with the size of the network, independent of the correlations. The underlying mechanism for pattern generation with these new rules is the same as with the formalized Hebb (1949) rules.

Overlapping Patterns   A limitation of the model we described is its inability to generate overlapping patterns. Consider a network in which two of the patterns share the same embedded state, e.g., fig. 7.12. When the output of the network reaches the state in common to both patterns $((\mu, \nu) = (6, 1)$ in fig. 7.12), there is an ambiguity as to which state occurs next in the pattern. The reason for this ambiguity is that only transitions between consecutive states are encoded in the synaptic connections. This problem can be rectified by encoding transitions that map more "distant" states along the pattern. The delay time of these additional synaptic connections will be proportional to the "distance" between the states. For instance, the ambiguity that occurs when patterns cross (fig. 7.12) can be resolved by adding synaptic components of the form (cf. eq. 7.2)

$$T_{ij}^{L(2)} = \lambda_2 \frac{J_0}{N} \sum_{\nu=1}^{q} \sum_{\mu=1}^{r-2} (2V_i^{\mu+2,\nu} - 1)(2V_j^{\mu,\nu} - 1), \quad i \neq j, \ \lambda_2 > 0 \quad (7.29)$$

The additional contribution to the input of each neuron via the above synapses is

$$h_i^{L(2)}(t) = \sum_{j=1}^{N} T_{ij}^{L(2)} \int_0^\infty V_j(t - t') \, w^{(2)}(t') \, dt' \qquad (7.30)$$

The (normalized) synaptic response function $w^{(2)}(t)$ averages over the output histories of the neurons with an averaging time of $t \simeq 2\tau_L$. The contributions of the neural inputs $h_i^{L(2)}(t)$, together with $h_i^L(t)$, cause the transitions to depend on the previous *two* output states of the network. With reference to fig. 7.12, the network will make a transition to the state $(\mu, \nu) = (7, 1)$, and not the state $(\mu, \nu) = (7, 2)$, if the output history of the network is $(4, 1) \rightarrow (5, 1) \rightarrow (6, 1)$.

The synaptic strength and the corresponding neural inputs defined by eqs. 7.29 and 7.30 can be generalized to incorporate patterns that share several states in common (e.g., Keeler 1987). The dynamics of these generalized networks can be analyzed using the adiabatically varying energy defined in eq. 7.16, where $h^L(t)$ now represents the sum of all the time-delayed contributions. This scheme for embedding sequences in synapses with multiple time delays has been recently applied to speech recognition problems by Tank and Hopfield (1987). Their implementation used a layered neural architecture with a localized representation for both the embedded states and the patterns. The effect of adding synapses with multiple time delays on the storage capabilities of fully interconnected networks, especially those using a distributed representation, is yet to be studied.

Finally, we note that the problem of embedding correlated states as well as overlapping patterns can be circumvented by adding neurons that function as "hidden units," i.e., neurons that do not provide a direct output from the CPG. These neurons may enlarge the representation of the embedded states in a manner that reduces the overlaps between different states or patterns. This suggests that the number of motor-controlling outputs from a CPG can be much smaller than the total number of neurons in the network.

7.4.2 Biological Feasibility

Analysis of the CPG in Tritonia We used our associative network model to analyze the CPG controlling the swim rhythm in the mollusc *Tritonia*. This is a small network, yet it contains many of the basic features inherent in our model. The rhythmic output could be understood by a simplified analysis that employed threshold units as neurons and that replaced the response function of the slow synapses by a simple time delay. The simplified analysis served to emphasize the role of the connections between neurons in determining the collective output of this CPG. A more extensive analysis showed that our model accounts for the period of the observed output and for the mean operating characteristics of the individual neurons.

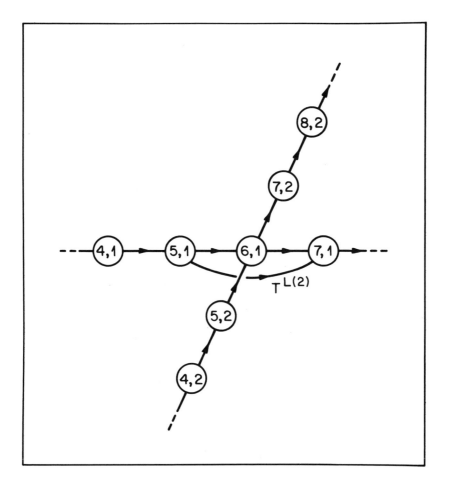

Figure 7.12
State diagram of two patterns that share a single state, i.e., $V^{6,1} = V^{6,2}$, in common. The transition labeled $\mathbf{T}^{L(2)}$ refers to a set of synaptic strengths $T_{ij}^{L(2)} \propto (2V_i^{7,1} - 1)(2V_j^{5,1} - 1)$. For a network producing the ν–1th pattern, but not for one producing the ν–2th pattern, these synaptic connections remove the ambiguity in choosing between $V^{7,1}$ and $V^{7,2}$ as the output state that should follow $V^{6,1}$.

The sign and time course of the observed synaptic strengths were in accord with the values predicted by the formalized Hebb (1949) learning rules (eqs. 7.1 and 7.2). This suggests the utility of such rules for predicting the strength of the underlying synaptic connections from the observed output states.

Our analysis demonstrates that, within the framework of our model, even a small network can function with the elimination of many of its theoretically possible connections. Many more fast synapses than slow synapses are present in *Tritonia*. The fast synaptic components stabilize the output states, and thus relatively few of these synapses can be eliminated (i.e., 25%; table 7.1). Partial elimination of the slow synaptic components can be offset by an increase in the transition strength, λ. This compensation is observed in *Tritonia*, where the relatively small fraction of slow components observed to be present (i.e., 75% of all possible connections are eliminated; table 7.1) is offset by a suitably large value for λ (i.e., $\lambda = 5$ to 10).

Our analysis also showed how the required balance between the mean operating level of each neuron and the value of its external inputs and the strength of its synaptic connections can be simply estimated. We argued (section 7.3) that the mean operating level of the VSI-A neuron in *Tritonia* is set too low. This result explained the relatively weak changes in the firing activity of VSI-A during periods of otherwise active output by the CPG (fig. 7.7). Our result further suggests that the activity of VSI-A will alternate more sharply between bursting and silence if its operating value is raised, e.g., by the injection of a small hyperpolarizing current.

Multiphasic Synapses and Synaptic Delays A variety of biophysical and biochemical mechanisms allow synaptic connections to act on more than a single time scale (for review, see Kehoe and Marty 1980). Chemically mediated synapses can show both fast and slow responses, as well as a combination of the two. For example, the synaptic connections in *Tritonia* act on time scales that differ by up to a factor of 30 (Getting 1981). Some of the chemically mediated synapses present in the network controlling the flight rhythm in the locust exhibit a delayed excitatory response (Robertson and Pearson 1985). Chemically mediated synapses in the stomatogastric ganglion of the lobster exhibit both prompt and delayed inhibitory responses (Hartline and Gassie 1979). Electrotonic connections provide a potential mechanism for the presence of both slow and fast synapses in a network. The high resistance of the electrotonic couplings between neurons in the CPG controlling feeding in the snail *Helisoma* causes their response time to be an order of magnitude slower than other synapses in the network (Kaneko, Merickel, and Kater 1978). The converse situation occurs in the circuit controlling feeding in the mollusc *Navanax*, where the electrotonic couplings act rapidly compared with the chemically mediated synaptic connections (Spray, Spira, and Bennett 1980).

Synaptic delays can result from the delays inherent in active propagation along a relatively long process. For example, the transmission delays between ganglia of neurons in the leech are much longer than the response time of individual synapses (Stent et al. 1978). Synaptic delays may also occur when the synaptic connections T_{ij}^L between pairs of neurons are mediated by interneurons. For example, the postsynaptic response observed in pyramidal cells of the olfactory cortex contains a delayed inhibitory component. The delayed component probably results from a disynaptic pathway mediated by an interneuron (Haberly and Bower 1984). It may play a role in generating the rhythmic activity of the olfactory cortex (e.g., Freeman 1975).

Neurons may contain cellular as well as synaptic delays. Cellular delays can affect the response time of a neuron to many or all of its synaptic inputs. A general theory for associative network models that contain cellular delays does not yet exist. However, when the response time of the cellular delay is short compared to the slow synaptic response time, τ_L, the separation of the time scales between τ_S and τ_L is maintained and the output properties of the network model are unaffected. Some well-characterized cellular delays can be considered in terms of an effective synaptic delay. For example, the outward potassium current I_A (Connor and Stevens 1971) is responsible for the delayed response of the VSI-B neuron in *Tritonia* (Getting 1983b, and chapter 6). This current has the effect of allowing only *slow* excitatory inputs into VSI-B, but does not affect the time scale of the inhibitory connections (see table 7.1).

Lastly, our model is capable of producing rhythmic output in large networks that contain only monophasic connections. In this case, a synapse has either a fast time response or a slow time response, but not both. The strength of each synapse is chosen according to the appropriate Hebb rule (eqs. 7.1 and 7.2). The minimum value of the transition strength, λ, depends on the relative number of fast versus slow connections (eq. 7.20). This suggests that our model may be appropriate for analyzing CPGs that do not contain multiphasic synapses.

Modulation of the Output   The output activity of many CPGs can be initiated and modulated by external inputs from command neurons

(Kennedy, Evoy, and Hanawaly 1966; Kupfermann and Weiss 1978). These neurons modulate a select fraction of neurons in the CPG. In addition, the output of CPG can be affected by the concentration of circulating neurohormones. These hormones affect the operating characteristics of neurons and possibly the strength of certain synaptic connections (e.g., Pinsker and Ayers 1983; Marder 1984; Harris-Warwick 1986).

By what mechanisms can these inputs or hormones function within the context of our model network? Large changes in the period of the output can occur if the external inputs or neurohormones affect either the time constant of the slow synaptic response, τ_L, or the transition strength, λ. For example, a neuromodulator that selectively augments the strength of the slow synaptic components, or diminishes that of the fast components, will shorten the period of the output. It will be interesting to see if neurophysiological correlates for these and related predictions are found.

It should be emphasized that we have considered so far only networks with parameters, e.g., synaptic strengths and neuron operating levels, that do not change in time. Biologically these parameters undergo slow changes, such as increases (facilitation) or decreases (fatigue) in the values of the synaptic strengths. These slow changes may modulate the overall behavior of the network. For example, a gradual *increase* in the mean operating levels will dephase the output pattern of a CPG. This will eventually terminate the oscillatory output, as observed for the CPG in *Tritonia* (fig. 7.7) (Lennard, Getting, and Hume 1980; Getting 1983b).

Networks with Only Inhibitory or Only Excitatory Connections   The connection strengths T_{ij}^S and T_{ij}^L determined by the formalized Hebb rules (eqs. 7.1 and 7.2 with uncorrelated embedded states) contain both inhibitory and excitatory components. Biological systems may contain predominantly inhibitory or excitatory connections. We thus consider whether our model network can properly function when the synaptic connections are modified so that most or all of the connections have the same sign.

The stability of the model network depends on its ability to relax to one of the embedded states. This relaxation is governed by the fast synaptic components, T_{ij}^S. The mean value of these connections is approximately zero (eq. 7.1). For the simple case in which these synaptic strengths are uniformly shifted from the values determined by eq. 7.1, the modified strengths $T_{ij}^{S'}$ can be expressed as

$$T_{ij}^{S'} = T_{ij}^S + \frac{\overline{J}}{N} \tag{7.31}$$

The mean value of the synaptic strength is now $\overline{J}/N$; $\overline{J} < 0$ if the connections are primarily inhibitory and $\overline{J} > 0$ if the connections are primarily excitatory. The components T_{ij}^S contribute to the stabilizing term in the energy function for the network (first term in eq. 7.16). The mean value $\overline{J}/N$ contributes an additional term to the energy of the form

$$-\frac{1}{2}\sum_{i=1}^{N}\sum_{j=1}^{N}(2V_i - 1)\frac{\overline{J}}{N}(2V_j - 1) = -\frac{\overline{J}}{2N}\left(\sum_{i=1}^{N}(2V_i - 1)\right)^2 \tag{7.32}$$

When the components $T_{ij}^{S'}$ are predominantly inhibitory the additional term in the energy (eq. 7.32) is positive. This contribution is at a minimum for states in which the number of neurons that are firing roughly equals the number that are quiescent. The embedded states in the network correspond to stable states of this form. Thus the additional term in the energy does not change the function of the network. Consequently, our model can describe pattern generation in networks containing fast synaptic components that are only inhibitory.

When the fast synaptic components $T_{ij}^{S'}$ are predominantly excitatory, the additional term in the energy is negative. This term is at a minimum when all of the neurons are quiescent or when all of them are firing. When the mean excitation is sufficiently large, such that $\overline{J} > J_0$ (eq. 7.1), the network will tend to generate either an output state in which most of the neurons are firing or in a state in which most neurons are quiescent. Thus the embedded states are destabilized for large values of $\overline{J}$. The above arguments also hold for Hopfield's network (Denker 1986b).

The slow synaptic components T_{ij}^L do not substantially affect the stability of the states embedded in the network when the synaptic response function $w(t)$ is a smooth function of time. Our model network will function properly if the slow synaptic components are modified, as above, to be either predominantly inhibitory or predominantly excitatory. Note that adding an offset to either the T_{ij}^S or the T_{ij}^L components requires a concomitant change in the mean operating levels of the neurons (eqs. 7.12 and 7.13).

Application to Related Biological Phenomena We have focused our study on aspects of animal behavior that involve the generation of *rhythmic* motor outputs. However, many other behaviors can be described as a fixed *linear* sequence of motor outputs, such as bird song and certain aspects of courtship (see, e.g., Lorenz 1970). The model we presented may be relevant for describing aspects of the neural circuitry that underlies this larger class of behaviors.

Another possible application of the model involves the relation between learning rules that depend on the history of a neuron's activity and the temporal associations inherent in classical conditioning (Barto and Sutton 1982; Tesauro 1986; Klopf 1987). Finally, the network models we described can be used for recognizing sequences of sensory input that correspond to a pattern of embedded states (Kleinfeld 1986; Amit 1988).

Learning and Plasticity One of the central features of the model is the simple relationship between the output patterns and the connections, i.e., the formalized Hebb (1949) learning rules (eqs. 7.1 and 7.2). These rules allow new patterns to be embedded in the network by modifying the synapses both incrementally in time and locally in space; the change to each synapse depends only on the activities of the postsynaptic and presynaptic neurons during the learning of the new pattern. Local updating of the synapses makes the present model particularly suitable for large, complex systems that are continuously updated as patterns are modified or added. Other learning rules may be used in biological systems, but they probably share many of these features (see also Appendix 7.A).

We introduced the relation between the "sequential" form of the T_{ij}^L synapses (eq. 7.2) and their slow dynamic response (eqs. 7.6 to 7.9) as an *ad hoc* assumption. These two features may, in fact, be closely related to each other. If one considers the evolution of the synaptic strengths in terms of a dynamic learning mechanism, the different final forms of the T_{ij}^S and the T_{ij}^L synaptic components may be the result of the different time scale of their dynamic response. For example, the T_{ij}^L components can relate two experiences that are separated by the characteristic response time of the slow components, while the T_{ij}^S components can only aid in recalling the presence of either experience. It would be interesting to implement this idea in a biologically plausible model for learning.

This work was supported in part by the National Science Foundation (Grant PHY82-17853). The address of David Kleinfeld is Solid State and Quantum Physics Research Department, AT&T Bell Laboratories, Murray Hill, New Jersey 07974. The address of Haim Sompolinsky is Racah Institute of Physics, Hebrew University, Jerusalem, Israel 91904. Electronic mail should be addressed to sompoli@hbunos.bitnet.

Appendix 7.A: Rules for Forming Synapses with Correlated States

In this appendix we present rules for forming the T_{ij}^S and T_{ij}^L synaptic components that are suitable for generating patterns with correlated states. These rules extend the results of a recently proposed model for incorporating correlated states into associative networks.

For mathematical convenience we define the output of the neurons in terms of a variable that ranges between -1 (quiescent) and $+1$ (maximum firing rate), i.e.,

$$S_i = 2V_i - 1 \tag{7.33}$$

The embedded states are thus given by S^1, S^2, ..., S^r, $r \leq N$, where r is the length of the pattern and N is the number of neurons. For simplicity of notation we consider networks that generate a single pattern. We assume that each component of $S^\nu = \{S_i^\nu\}_{i=1}^N$ is either $+1$ or -1, and confine our results to the high-gain limit of the network (eq. 7.14).

The model makes use of the "pseudo-inverse" method (Kohonen and Ruohonen 1973; Personnaz, Guyon, and Dreyfus 1986; Kanter and Sompolinsky 1987). This method requires that the embedded states are linearly independent, but otherwise places no restrictions on the choice of states.

We define the correlation matrix, $\mathbf{C}$, between these states by

$$\mathbf{C}_{\mu\nu} = \frac{1}{N} \sum_{i=1}^N S_i^\mu S_i^\nu, \qquad \nu, \mu = 1, \cdots, r. \tag{7.34}$$

For orthogonal states, $\mathbf{C}$ reduces to $\mathbf{C}^{\mu\nu} = \delta^{\mu\nu}$. A set of r states, O^1, O^2, ..., O^r, that are orthogonal to the S^νs can be constructed from linear combinations of the S^νs, i.e.,

$$O_i^\mu = \sum_{\nu=1}^r \mathbf{C}_{\mu\nu}^{-1} S_i^\nu \tag{7.35}$$

It is straightforward to show that

$$\frac{1}{N} \sum_{i=1}^N O_i^\mu S_i^\nu = \delta^{\mu\nu} \tag{7.36}$$

Using this property, we define the synaptic strengths T_{ij}^S to be

$$T_{ij}^S = \frac{J_0}{N} \sum_{\mu=1}^{r} S_i^\mu O_j^\mu, \quad i \neq j \tag{7.37}$$

The synaptic connections T_{ij}^S (eq. 7.37) will map the state S^μ back onto S^μ regardless of the size of the correlations between the embedded states. Thus, these connections stabilize the network in each of the embedded states.

To generate a pattern of embedded states, we define the synaptic strengths T_{ij}^L to be

$$T_{ij}^L = \lambda \frac{J_0}{N} \sum_{\mu=1}^{r-1} S_i^{\mu+1} O_j^\mu, \quad i \neq j \tag{7.38}$$

This matrix maps the state S^μ onto the state $S^{\mu+1}$ (see also Guyon, Personnaz, Nadal, and Dreyfus, 1988).

A network using the above rules (eqs. 7.37 and 7.38) generates disjoint patterns with arbitrarily selected (linearly independent) states. The maximum number of states that can be embedded is $p = r \simeq N$ (cf. eq. 7.19). The lower bound on λ is now $\lambda > (1 - a) = (1 - p/N)$, which goes to zero as the number of embedded states approaches its maximum limit. Iterative algorithms for embedding additional (correlated) states into an existing network are discussed by Denker (1986a) and Diederich and Opper (1987).

Appendix 7.B: Calculation of t_0 for a Relatively Long Pattern

In this appendix we derive an expression for the steady-state value of t_0, the time between transitions, in terms of the transition strength λ and the slow synaptic response time τ_L. This expression is calculated for a network that produces a pattern that contains a relatively large number of embedded states ($1 \ll r \leq p \ll N$) (Sompolinsky and Kanter 1986). As in Appendix 7.A, we take $S_i = 2V_i - 1$.

Let $t = 0$ be the time at which the output state of the network has just changed to S^μ. The transition to the next state, at time $t = t_0$, is initiated by those neurons whose activity changes in going from the μth to the μ+1th state, but whose activity in the μ+1th state equals that in the first through μ−1th states. For this population of neurons, $S_i^\nu = -S_i^\mu$ for $\nu < \mu$ and for $\nu = \mu + 1$. The activity of the network during the interval $t < 2t_0$ is

$$S_i(t) = \begin{cases} -S_i^\mu & \text{for } t < 0 \\ +S_i^\mu & \text{for } 0 < t < t_0 \\ -S_i^\mu & \text{for } t_0 < t < 2t_0 \end{cases}$$

where we have assumed that $\tau_S \ll \tau_L$ and that the network is operating in the high-gain limit (eq. 7.14).

The transition time is found by comparing the time-averaged inputs $h_i^L(t)$ with the stabilizing inputs $h_i^S(t)$. The inputs t_0 the neurons discussed above, for time $0 < t \leq t_0$, are given by (eq. 7.4),

$$h_i^S(t) = \sum_{j=1}^{N} T_{ij}^S S_j(t) = +S_i^\mu$$

and (eqs. 7.6 and 7.7)

$$
\begin{aligned}
h_i^L(t) &= \lambda \sum_{j=1}^{N} T_{ij}^L \int_{-(\mu-1)t_0}^{t} S_j(t')\, w(t-t')\, dt' \\
&= \lambda \left[S_i^2 \int_{-(\mu-1)t_0}^{-(\mu-2)t_0} w(t-t')\, dt' + \cdots \right. \\
&\quad + S_i^{\mu-1} \int_{-2t_0}^{-t_0} w(t-t')\, dt' + S_i^\mu \int_{-t_0}^{0} w(t-t')\, dt' \\
&\quad \left. + S_i^{\mu+1} \int_{0}^{t} w(t-t')\, dt' \right] \\
&= \lambda S_i^\mu \left[-\int_{0}^{(\mu-1)t_0+t} w(t')\, dt' + 2\int_{t}^{t+t_0} w(t')\, dt' \right]
\end{aligned}
$$

where we took $\Delta\theta_i = 0$ (eq. 7.12). A transition will occur when the inputs $h_i^L(t_0)$ and $h_i^S(t_0)$ are equal in magnitude and opposite in sign. Confining ourselves to the limit $\mu t_0 \to \infty$ (i.e., $\mu t_0 \gg \tau_L$), so that the value of the first integral is unity (eq. 7.8), we find

$$\frac{1}{2}\left(1 - \frac{1}{\lambda}\right) = \int_{t_0}^{2t_0} w(t')\, dt' \tag{7.39}$$

The above equation has a solution only for $\lambda \geq 1$.

We used eq. 7.42 to calculate the dependence of t_0 on λ for four interesting response functions (see table 7.2). These functions, normalized to unity (eq. 7.7) with a mean response time of τ_L (eq. 7.9), are: (1) A delta function, corresponding to a sharp time delay, such as that caused

Response Function		Duration of Each State[a]	
Name	w(t)	$t_o(\lambda)$	Range
Delta function delay	$\delta(t - \tau_L)$	τ_L	$1 \leqslant \lambda < \infty$
Uniform averaging with delay	$\dfrac{1}{\tau_w}$; $(\tau_L - \tau_w/2) \leqslant t \leqslant (\tau_L + \tau_w/2)$ 0 ; otherwise	$\tau_w \left[\dfrac{\tau_L}{\tau_w} + \dfrac{1}{2\lambda} \right]$	$1 \leqslant \lambda < \infty$ $\tau_L < t_o \leqslant 2\tau_L$ with $\tau_w \leqslant 2\tau_L$
Exponential averaging	$\dfrac{1}{\tau_L} e^{-t/\tau_L}$; $0 \leqslant t < \infty$ 0 ; otherwise	$\tau_L \ln\left(\dfrac{\lambda + \sqrt{\lambda(2-\lambda)}}{\lambda - 1} \right)$	$1 < \lambda < 2$[b] $0 < t_o < \infty$
Linear averaging	$\dfrac{2}{3\tau_L}\left[1 - \dfrac{t}{3\tau_L} \right]$; $0 \leqslant t \leqslant 3\tau_L$ 0 ; otherwise	$3\tau_L\left[1 - \sqrt{\dfrac{\lambda - 1}{2\lambda}} \right]$	$1 \leqslant \lambda < \infty$ $3(1-\sqrt{1/2})\tau_L \leqslant t_o \leqslant 3\tau_L$

(a) These results were derived for steady-state conditions, with $\tau_L \gg \tau_S$ and with the network operating in the high-gain limit [Eq. (2.14)]; see text for details.

(b) The network will not produce stable oscillations for values of λ in the range $\lambda \geqslant 2$.

Table 7.2
Duration of the output states for a relatively long pattern.

by active propagation along an axon. For this case, $\overline{S(t)} = S(t - \tau_L)$. (2) Uniform averaging after a delay, used for the simulations shown in figs. 7.5 and 7.6. The width of the response is τ_W and the delay is given by $(\tau_L - \tau_W/2)$. (3) Exponential averaging, corresponding to the charging relation for a capacitor or to simple low-pass filtration. (4) Linear averaging, corresponding to a linearly decreasing ramp function.

An interesting result is that stable oscillations cannot be sustained with an exponential averaging function for values of λ greater than 2. Exponential averaging heavily contributes relatively recent values of $S_i(t)$ to the time-averaged outputs $S_i\overline{(t)}$. This leads to dephasing of the transition for large values of λ.

Appendix 7.C: Calculation of t_0 for Biphasic Oscillations

In this appendix we derive an expression for the steady-state value of t_0 for a network that produces biphasic oscillations. As in Appendixes 7.A and 7.B, we take $S_i = 2V_i - 1$. Let $t = 0$ be the time at which the output state of the network has just changed to S^μ. The state of the network at all previous times, assuming $\tau_S \ll \tau_L$ and that the network is operating in the high-gain limit (eq. 7.14), is

$$S(t < 0) = \begin{cases} -S^\mu & \text{for } -(2n+1)t_0 < t < -2nt_0, \quad n = 0, 1, 2, \ldots \\ +S^\mu & \text{for } -2nt_0 < t < -(2n-1)t_0 \end{cases}$$

These states are used to determine the time-averaged output $\overline{S(t)}$. The inputs to each neuron at time t, $0 < t < t_0$, are thus (eq. 7.4)

$$h_i^S(t) = +S_i^\mu$$

and (eqs. 7.6 and 7.7)

$$h_i^L(t) = -\lambda S_i^\mu \left[\int_0^t w(t - t')\, dt' - \int_{-t_0}^0 w(t - t')\, dt' \right.$$

$$\left. + \int_{-2t_0}^{-t_0} w(t - t')\, dt' - \cdots \right]$$

where we took $\Delta\theta_i = 0$ (eq. 7.12).

At time $t = t_0$ a transition to the state S^μ occurs, implying that $h_i^S(t_0) = -h_i^L(t_0)$. This leads to

$$\frac{1}{2}\left(1 - \frac{1}{\lambda}\right) = \sum_{n=1}^{\infty} \int_{(2n-1)t_0}^{2nt_0} w(t')\, dt' \tag{7.40}$$

where use has been made of eq. 7.8. The above equation for t_0 has a solution only for $\lambda \geq 1$.

We used eq. 7.40 to calculate the dependence of t_0 on λ for the four response functions discussed in Appendix 7.B. The linear averaging function, which approximates the slow synaptic response observed in *Tritonia*, was used for the simulations shown in figs. 7.10 and 7.11. The results are shown in table 7.3. A surprising result is that stable oscillations cannot be sustained with a linear averaging function (with no missing synaptic connections) for values of λ between $(2n)$ and $(2n + 1)$,

	Response Function	Duration of Each State[a]	
Name	$w(t)$	$t_0(\lambda)$	Range
Delta function delay	$\delta(t - \tau_L)$	τ_L	$1 \leqslant \lambda < \infty$
Uniform averaging with delay	$\dfrac{1}{\tau_w}$; $(\tau_L - \tau_w/2) \leqslant t \leqslant (\tau_L + \tau_w/2)$ 0 ; otherwise	$\tau_w\left[\dfrac{\tau_L}{\tau_w} + \dfrac{1}{2\lambda}\right]$	$1 \leqslant \lambda < \infty$ $\tau_L < t_0 \leqslant 2\tau_L$ with $\tau_w \leqslant 2\tau_L$
Exponential averaging	$\dfrac{1}{\tau_L} e^{-t/\tau_L}$; $0 \leqslant t < \infty$ 0 ; otherwise	$2\tau_L \tanh^{-1}\left[\dfrac{1}{\lambda}\right]$	$1 < \lambda < \infty$ $0 < t_0 < \infty$
Linear averaging	$\dfrac{2}{3\tau_L}\left[1 - \dfrac{t}{3\tau_L}\right]$; $0 \leqslant t \leqslant 3\tau_L$ 0 ; otherwise	$\dfrac{3\tau_L}{2n-1}\left[1 - \sqrt{\dfrac{\lambda - 2n + 1}{2n\lambda}}\right]$ with $n = 1, 2, 3, \cdots$	$(2n-1) \leqslant \lambda \leqslant 2n$ [b] $\dfrac{3\tau_L}{2n} \leqslant t_0 \leqslant \dfrac{3\tau_L}{2n-1}$

(a) These results were derived for steady-state conditions, with $\tau_L \gg \tau_S$ and with the network operating in the high-gain limit [Eq. (2.14)]; see text for details.

(b) The network will not produce stable oscillations for values of λ in the range $2n < \lambda < (2n+1)$, $n=1, 2, 3, \ldots$.

Table 7.3
Duration of the output states for biphasic oscillations.

$n = 1, 2, 3, \ldots$. The network will initially oscillate for any value $\lambda \geq 1$, but if λ is in a forbidden range the oscillations will eventually decay. This phenomenon results in gaps in the allowed spectrum of $t_0(\lambda)$ (see table 7.3).

Appendix 7.D: Difference Equations for Numerical Simulations

The differential equations that describe sequence generation can be written as a set of finite difference equations. Time is quantized in terms of the discrete variable k, and the time constants τ_S and τ_L are given by the integer variables κ_S and κ_L, respectively. These equations provide a suitable representation for numerical simulation of the sequence generator. As in Appendixes 7.A through 7.C, we take $S_i = 2V_i - 1$. The discrete versions of analog dynamic equations (eqs. 7.10 and 7.12) are

$$u_i(k+1) = \left(1 - \frac{1}{\kappa_S}\right) u_i(k) + \frac{1}{\kappa_S} \sum_{j=1}^{N} \left(T_{ij}^S S_j(k) + T_{ij}^L \overline{S_j(k)}\right) \quad (7.41)$$

where $S_i(k)$ and $u_i(k)$ are related by a nonlinear gain function, e.g., $S_i(k) = \tanh[2G(u_i(k) - \theta_i)]$, and (eq. 7.7)

$$\overline{S_i(k)} = \sum_{l=0}^{\infty} S_i(k - l) \, w(l) \quad (7.42)$$

The discrete convolution for $\overline{S_i(k)}$ can be turned into a recursion relation for broad classes of $w(k)$. We present four examples.

(1) Delta function time delay, i.e.,

$$w(k) = \delta(k - \kappa_L) \quad (7.43)$$

for which

$$\overline{S_i(k)} = S_i(k - \kappa_L) \quad (7.44)$$

(2) Uniform averaging after a delay, i.e.,

$$w(k) = \begin{cases} 1/\kappa_W & (\kappa_L - \kappa_W/2) \le k \le (\kappa_L + \kappa_W/2) \\ 0 & \text{otherwise} \end{cases} \quad (7.45)$$

for which

$$\begin{aligned} \overline{S_i(k)} &= \overline{S_i(k-1)} + (1/\kappa_W)\left[S_i(k - \kappa_L + \kappa_W/2) \right. \\ &\quad \left. - S_i(k - 1 - \kappa_L - \kappa_W/2)\right] \end{aligned} \quad (7.46)$$

(3) Exponential averaging, i.e.,

$$w(k) = \begin{cases} (1/\kappa_L)e^{-k/\kappa_L} & 0 \le k \\ 0 & \text{otherwise} \end{cases} \quad (7.47)$$

for which

$$\overline{S_i(k)} = e^{-1/\kappa_L}\,\overline{S_i(k-1)} + (1/\kappa_L)S_i(k) \qquad (7.48)$$

(4) Linear averaging, i.e.,

$$w(k) = \begin{cases} (3/2\kappa_L)(1 - k/3\kappa_L) & 0 \le k \le 3k_L \\ 0 & \text{otherwise} \end{cases} \qquad (7.49)$$

for which

$$\begin{aligned}
\overline{S_i(k)} &= 2\overline{S_i(k-1)} - \overline{S_i(k-2)} + (3/2\kappa_L)\left[S_i(k) - S_i(k-1)\right] \\
&\quad -(1/2\kappa_L^2)\left[S_i(k-1) - S_i(k - 3\kappa_L - 1)\right]
\end{aligned} \qquad (7.50)$$

CHAPTER 8

Spatial and Temporal Processing in Central Auditory Networks

SHIHAB SHAMMA

8.1 Introduction

A fundamental organizational principle of the nervous system is that neurons are interconnected to form purposeful networks. This is especially relevant in higher animals where nervous function depends primarily on the patterns of interconnections among large numbers of neurons rather than on elaborate specializations of individual neurons. Thus, to understand brain function, the focus of our investigations must expand from the detailed responses and structure of single cells to include the unit response patterns in relation to the activity of other cells, and the distributions of these responses over a population of these cells, and across populations of different cell types.

Computational neurobiology plays a particularly critical role in the study of neural networks. In part, this is due to the lack of adequate experimental methods that fall in between the patch clamp, intracellular, and extracellular recordings appropriate to single cells, and the relatively coarse evoked potential recordings, EEGs, and 2-deoxyglucose labeling methods. The technology of multicellular recordings on a moderate scale is still at its infancy. Consequently, studies of neural networks have relied heavily on theoretical models to relate and explain experimental data derived from finer and coarser levels of experimentation.

Neural network models typically exhibit three distinct and equally important flavors: biological, algorithmic, and phenomenological. All styles usually serve to relate relatively peripheral measures (e.g., environmental signals and outputs of sensory organs) to higher-level functions and percepts, thus providing varied descriptions of brain function. The differences among these approaches lie mainly in the overall objectives and constraints they assume. Thus, in the biologically oriented models, the goal most often is to provide a concise mathematical description relating directly to neurophysiological and anatomical data. In the phenomenological models, abstract and "black box" models of the network components are commonly used, and the emphasis shifts to descriptions of higher functions and psychophysical percepts. Algorithmic formulations are intermediate in that computational structures replace "black boxes," but little or no attempt is made to relate them to the actual biological substrate.

In this chapter, we shall illustrate the interactions between the biological and algorithmic approaches in the study of neuronal processing in the mammalian auditory system. This system consists of several parallel pathways, beginning at the hair cells of the inner ear, passing through up to six major nuclear groups, and ending at the auditory cortex. Considerable information has been gathered over the last two decades from the peripheral levels of the cochlea and the VIII (auditory) nerve, which gives a fairly accurate picture of the patterns of neural activity at the input of the auditory system (Young and Sachs 1979). At its "output," the system derives many perceptually important measures of the sound signal such as its spectrum and pitch (primarily monaural tasks, critical for speech and music perception) and its binaural attributes (important for sound localization and signal-in-noise enhancement). However, at the intermediate neural structures responsible for these transformations, little is known about the topology and function of the neural networks that exist, despite the substantial body of anatomical and neurophysiological data available (see Irvine 1986).

Therefore, in understanding auditory function, network modeling provides the pivotal link between signal and perception. This process will be demonstrated in the context of the spectral estimation problem in monaural audition. Specifically, we shall analyze critically how three different computational algorithms are motivated and implemented as neural network models. Many general themes and conclusions will emerge that also apply to the modeling of other sensory sytems. In the following sections, we shall first review the basic organizational principles of the mammalian auditory system. Three possible strategies for the central auditory processing of sound are then discussed in relation to their performance and the details of their neural network formulations. The details and results of simulating these networks are finally illustrated in section 8.5.

8.2   The Mammalian Auditory System

An important function of the mammalian auditory system is to discriminate and recognize complex sounds based on their spectral composition. The basic underlying processing steps occur early in the auditory system at the cochlea of the inner ear (see schematic of fig. 8.1). The pressure waves of an incoming sound signal cause vibrations of the tympanic membrane (eardrum) and ossicles of the middle ear, which in turn excite mechanical vibrations in the form of waves that travel along the length of the basilar membrane of the inner ear. Because of the unique spatially distributed geometry and mechanical properties of the basilar membrane, the traveling waves acquire distinctive properties that reflect the amplitudes and frequencies of the sound stimulus.

For instance, the vibrations due to a single steady tone increase in amplitude away from the entrance (base) of the cochlea reach a maximum and then decay abruptly at a distance that is monotonically related to the frequency of the tone; the higher the frequency, the more basal is the location of the peak. Consequently, the spatial axis of the cochlea can be viewed as tonotopically ordered, with each location associated with a particular frequency, also called the characteristic frequency (CF). This tonotopic order is also reflected in the frequency-tuned responses of the auditory nerve fibers that innervate the basilar membrane, and is further preserved at all subsequent nuclei in the primary pathway of the auditory system.

Another feature of these vibrations is their finite (decreasing) velocity as they travel up the cochlea, which causes increasing arrival delays and gives rise to the impression of traveling waves. These delays become particularly noticeable near the point of maximum amplitude, where the traveling vibrations appear to slow down abruptly and become more "crowded" before collapsing. Another way to express this observation is that the spatial frequency of the traveling wave significantly increases near its apical end (or the point of resonance), compared to the basal end.

The vibrations of the basilar membrane are transduced into nervous activity on the auditory nerve fiber array via thousands of inner hair cells that are situated in the organ of corti, and are distributed along the entire length of the basilar membrane. The generator (intracellular) potential of each hair cell effectively provides a readout of the instantaneous vibrations of the membrane at a given point, but with two important modifications: (1) It is approximately half-wave rectified because of the intrinsic properties of the transducer channels; and (2) it is low-pass filtered above about 3–4 kHz because of the capacitive effects of the cell's membrane. The combined effect of these two transformations causes the higher frequency tones to produce only constant intracellular potential at their CF locations.

Figure 8.1 illustrates the intracellular potentials of an array of hair cells (128) in response to a two-tone stimulus (600, 2000 Hz), computed using detailed biophysical models of basilar membrane and hair cell function (Holmes and Cole 1984; Shamma, Chadwick, Wilbur, Rinzel, and Moorish 1986). The outputs are plotted as they would project onto the auditory nerve, i.e., they are spatially organized according to their point of origin, and thus tonotopic order is preserved. The resulting spatio-temporal response patterns display the fundamental properties of the basilar membrane traveling wave discussed earlier. In particular, note the (frequency-dependent) spatial segregation of the responses to the two tones, and the rapid changes (both in the amplitude and phase) of the response waves near the CF locations corresponding to the tones. These responses compare well with the responses recorded from a large population of cat auditory nerve fibers (Miller and Sachs 1983; Young and Sachs 1979), and reconstructed in the same format of the above figures (Shamma 1985a).

Each inner hair cell is innervated by several independent and stochas-tically firing auditory nerve fibers that encode the intracellular potential by their instantaneous firing rates. Experimentally, a poststimulus his-togram of many repetitions of a fiber's extracellular response record provides an approximate measure of the time course of the underlying hair cell potential.[1]   Central auditory neurons, receiving inputs from several converging auditory nerve fibers (of approximately equal CFs), can also reproduce the hair cell potential by integrating the independent firing patterns. Therefore, the stochastic firing of auditory nerve fibers can be viewed primarily as a means for conveying hair cell potentials to the central auditory networks, rather than as an information processing stage; and as such, modeling the synaptic transformations at the pe-ripheral and central terminals of the nerve fiber array and the stochastic nature of their firings can often be bypassed in a first-order approxima-tion. As we shall elaborate later, similar simplifications can be applied to the modeling of neuronal interactions in a network.

---

[1] There are many detailed models of various aspects of hair cell/nerve fiber trans-formations (e.g., see Deng, Geisler, and Greenberg 1987; Westerman and Smith 1984). Auditory nerve fiber responses are most often modeled as a nonstationary point pro-cess whose instantaneous rate is approximately given by the hair cell's intracellular potential (for details, see Siebert 1970).

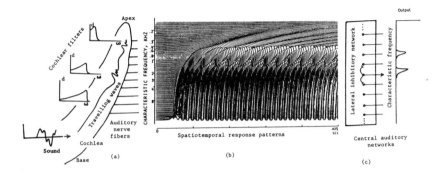

Figure 8.1

A schematic of early monaural auditory processing. (a) A two-tone stimulus (600, 2000 Hz) is analyzed by a detailed multistage biophysical model of the cochlea (Holmes and Cole 1984; Shamma et al. 1986). Each tone evokes a traveling wave along the basilar membrane that peaks at a specific location reflecting the frequency of the tone. The membrane responses are computed by a model composed of a bank of 128 filters distributed along the length of the cochlea, each representing the effective transfer function between the stimulus and the output at that location. Schematic transfer functions (d(ω)) of three such filters are shown in the figure. Note the shift in the "center frequency" of the filters from low frequencies (at the apex) to high frequencies (at the base). The filter responses at each location are further processed by a model of inner hair cell function (Shamma et al. 1986) and the output is interpreted as the instantaneous probability of firing of the auditory nerve fiber that innervates that location (corresponds experimentally to the envelope of the PST histogram of the fiber's response (Shamma 1985a). For frequencies below 3–4 kHz, the responses are phase-locked, i.e., they approximately reflect the waveform of the underlying movement of the basilar membrane. For higher frequencies, only the amplitude of the membrane's displacements (i.e., proportional to the power output of the filter) is encoded. (b) The responses thus computed are organized spatially according to their point of origin. This order is also tonotopic due to the frequency analysis of the cochlea, with apical fibers being most sensitive to low frequencies, and basal fibers to high frequencies. The characteristic frequency (CF) of each fiber is indicated on the spatial axis of the responses. The resulting total spatio-temporal pattern of responses reflects the complex nature of the stimulus, with each tone dominating and entraining the activity of a different group of fibers along the tonotopic axis. (c) The neural networks of the central auditory system (e.g., the lateral inhibitory network) generate an estimate of the spectrum of the stimulus.

8.2.1   The Spectral Estimation Problem

The composition of the frequency spectrum of an acoustic stimulus is a primary cue for its identification. A basic issue in central auditory processing has been the question of how the system makes an estimate of this spectrum from the responses of the auditory nerve. In principle, there are two sources of information in the responses that can be utilized: spatial and temporal. The spatial aspect refers to the use of the response distribution along the tonotopic axis, while the temporal aspect refers to the information available in the synchronized (or phase locked) components of the response. As we shall elaborate in sections 8.4 and 8.5, using one or both of these response properties has profound implications for the topology and characteristics of the central auditory networks that are presumed to estimate the spectrum. In the following sections we will illustrate the kind of considerations that arise in constructing different types of neural networks that implement three distinct algorithms for the spectral estimation problem: the mean-rate (purely spatial) hypothesis, the periodicity (primarily temporal) hypothesis, and the spatio-temporal hypothesis. In each case, we shall first outline the specific computational algorithm, then make the appropriate models and approximations, and finally discuss the physiological relevence of the results.

8.3   The Single-Neuron Model

The first and perhaps most critical step in modeling a neural network is the choice of its constituent neural elements. The level at which a single neuron is described mathematically (i.e., the amount of detail and the degree of abstraction) depends primarily on the nature of the application at hand. Thus, at one extreme, modeling a small circuit of morphologically and functionally different neurons may require significant detail to capture the characteristics of each neuron. At the other extreme, it may be advantageouss to bypass the single-neuron model entirely, using instead a continuum model to describe the activity of a dense and homogenous neural tissue. Both levels are useful in modeling intermediate neural networks; gravitating towards one extreme or the other would then serve to highlight different aspects of the response or, as is often the case, to facilitate analytical treatments or computer simulations.

The basic single-neuron model we shall use is shown in fig. 8.2a. It is viewed as a processor with multiple, differently weighted inputs and a single output. In many cases, such a description should be considered merely "functional" and not necessarily corresponding to specific anatomical structures (e.g., dendrites and axons). Let $x_j(t)$ represent the train of spikes arriving from the jth neuron to the ith neuron. A single spike potential at time τ_k is modeled by a delta function $(\delta(t - \tau_k))$. The influence of this spike at the soma of the postsynaptic cell (i.e., the EPSP or IPSP) is modeled by a linear time-invariant transformation with impulse response $(h_{ij}(t))$. Thus $h_{ij}(t)$ includes the efficacy, sign, and temporal properties of the synaptic response, the time constants of the cell membranes, and the effective spatial transformations due to dendritic branching and the location of the synapse relative to the cell body. Consequently, the overall intracellular potential due to N such inputs is given by :

$$y_i(t) = \sum_{j=0}^{N} \int_{-\infty}^{t} h_j(v)x_j(t - v)dv = \sum_{j=0}^{N} h_{ij}(t) * x_j(t) \qquad (8.1)$$

where $x_j(t) = \sum_k \delta(t - \tau_k)$, and $(*)$ denotes the convolution operation. Note that the above description of synaptic interactions is highly abstract and simplified, and should not be viewed at the same level of detail as that involving such physical nonlinear processes as transmitter release and conductance changes (as discussed for example in chapters 3 and 4). The impulse response $h_{ij}(t)$ is meant to embody the salient aspects of these processes at a purely phenomenological level.

We next assume that the instantaneous firing rate $(z_i(t))$ of the postsynaptic cell is approximately proportional to its intracellular potential $y_i(t)$, with possibly two important deviations: saturation and threshold. The first is due to the refractory period of axonal firing, which limits the maximum rates at which a neuron can fire (z_{max}). The second reflects the fact that the firing rate cannot be negative and that the production of an action potential requires a significant EPSP. One simple way to approximate this relation between $y_i(t)$ and $z_i(t)$ is given by the following sigmoidal function:

$$z_i(t) = g(y_i(t)) = \frac{z_{max}}{1 + e^{-b(y_i(t) - y_0)}} \qquad (8.2)$$

where b, y_0 are constants to be chosen appropriately to reflect the spontaneous firing of the cell and its maximum rate of change as a function of the input.

Finally, an important simplification often used in network models concerns the description of the stochastic firing of the cells. The output of the ith neuron is a train of spikes $x_i(t)$ similar to those impinging on it $(x_j(t))$. A particulary useful idealization is to model the stochastic

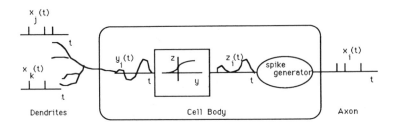

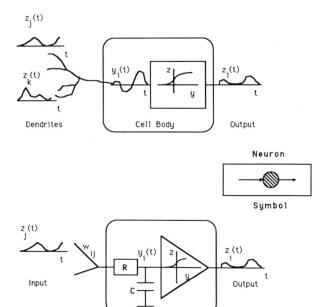

Figure 8.2
Models of a single neuron: (a) A model of a single neuron using stochastic spike
input and output descriptions. (b) A simplified version of the neuron model using
instantaneous firing rates as the input and output variables. (c) A minimal model
of the single neuron using a simple first-order description of the membrane impulse
response $(h(t) = (1/\tau)e^{-(t/\tau)})$. The "neuron symbol" indicates the input and output
ports and their directions.

behavior of the neuron $(x_i(t))$ as a nonstationary point process (see foot-note 1), with its instantaneous rate $z_i(t)$ given by $E(x_i(t))$, where $E(.)$ denotes the expectation operator (Snyder 1975). Consequently, explicit references to the stochastic firings of all cells $(x_j(t))$ can now be elim-inated if we redefine $y_i(t)$ as the ensemble mean of the instantaneous intracellular potential, i.e.,

$$y_i(t) = E\left[\sum_{j=0}^{N} h_{ij}(t) * x_j(t)\right] = \sum_{j=0}^{N} h_j(t) * E(x_j(t))$$

$$= \sum_{j=0}^{N} h_{ij}(t) * z_j(t) \tag{8.3}$$

where $h_{ij}(t)$ is assumed to be a deterministic function (see Sejonwski 1977 for more examples). The variables $y_i(t)$ and $z_i(t)$ can in principle be measured experimentally from poststimulus histograms of intracellular and extracellular records, respectively. The resulting simplified neuron model is shown in fig. 8.2b.

The choice of the exact form of $h_{ij}(t)$ depends critically on the ob-jectives of the modeling and the computational costs involved. For in-stance, if the details of the dendritic branching and function are im-portant, then $h_{ij}(t)$ may take elaborate forms that reflect the effects of the spatial spread and attenuation of the potential from the synapse to the soma (Rall 1964; Segev, Fleshman, Miller, and Bunow 1985). In other cases, such effects may be simplified to a scaling parameter that determines both the sign and efficacy of a typical synaptic "impulse re-sponse," i.e., $h_{ij}(t) = w_{ij} \cdot h_o(t)$ for all i and j, where $h_o(t)$ models the temporal characteristics of a typical postsynaptic potential, and w_{ij} is a scalar that determines its sign (excitatory or inhibitory) and the overall strength of the connection between neurons i and j. Once again, $h_o(t)$ can take many forms depending on the amount of detail required, e.g., $h_o(t) = (t/t_{peak})e^{-t/t_{peak}}$ (the so-called α function), $h_o(t) = (1/\tau)e^{-t/\tau}$ (a leaky integrator with time constant τ), or $h_o(t) = \delta(t - t_o)$ (a pure t_o time delay). In many situations, ignoring the entire temporal compo-nent of the responses $(h_o(t) = \delta(t))$ can lead to further simplifications and valuable insights into the role of the w_{ij} interconnection profiles in the network function.

We shall consider here the intermediate case of $h_o(t) = (1/\tau)e^{-t/\tau}$ as an example that can be extended or reduced to other forms. Substituting into eq. 8.3, we get:

$$
\begin{aligned}
y_i(t) &= \sum_{j=0}^{N} h_{ij}(t) * z_j(t) = \sum_{j=0}^{N} w_{ij} \int_{-\infty}^{t} h_o(t-v) z_j(v)\, dv \\
&= \sum_{j=0}^{N} w_{ij} \int_{-\infty}^{t} \frac{1}{\tau} e^{-(t-v/\tau)} z_j(v)\, dv
\end{aligned}
\tag{8.4}
$$

Taking the time derivitive (d/dt) of the above equation, a set of coupled, nonlinear, first-order differential equations results that describes the dependence of the intracellular potential of each neuron $(y_i(t))$ on the activities of all other neurons in the network (fig. 8.2c):

$$
\tau \frac{dy_i}{dt} + y_i = \sum_{j=0}^{N} w_{ij} z_j
\tag{8.5}
$$

for all i, where the explicit dependence of $y_i(t)$ and $z_i(t)$ on time has been dropped for notational convenience. Furthermore, the influences of an array of external inputs $(e_j(t))$, with synaptic weights (v_{ij}) onto neuron i, can be readily incorporated into the above equation to give:

$$
\tau \frac{dy_i}{dt} + y_i = \sum_{j=0}^{N} w_{ij} z_j + \sum_{j=0}^{M} v_{ij} e_j
\tag{8.6}
$$

This equation can be written in many equivalent forms, e.g., the vector notation in terms of $\mathbf{y}$,

$$
\tau \dot{\mathbf{y}}(t) = \mathbf{W} \cdot \mathbf{g}(\mathbf{y}(t)) + \mathbf{V} \cdot \mathbf{e}(t) - \mathbf{y} = \mathbf{F}(\mathbf{y}, \mathbf{e}; \mathbf{V}, \mathbf{W}, t)
\tag{8.7}
$$

The neuronal model of eq. 8.6 can now be used to construct a variety of neuronal networks to perform a wide range of functions. The principle task that remains is the choice of the connectivities of the network (w_{ij} and v_{ij}) so as to achieve specific goals or to describe certain topologies. This process will be illustrated in the network implementation of three algorithms. The first two (section 8.4) derive their computational properties from the temporal characteristics of the constituent neural elements, rather than from the spatial patterns of interconnections among them (as in the case of the third algorithm; section 8.5).

8.4   Neural Networks for Spectral Estimation

Two networks are illustrated in this section that perform the monaural spectral estimation task. In each case, the computational algorithm is first discussed, followed by its neural network implementation based on the single-neuron model derived above. In all cases, only the outlines of the method are presented, with more emphasis placed on the general class of computations that the resulting neural network can perform.

8.4.1   The Mean-Rate Hypothesis

According to this hypothesis the spectrum of an acoustic stimulus is encoded in the spatial profile of the mean firing rates of the auditory nerve fibers. Thus, the amplitude and frequency of a stimulus component is reflected by a relative increase in the average activity of a fiber population that is located at the appropriate CF along the tonotopic axis. Such a profile essentially reflects only the envelope of the basilar membrane vibrations (i.e., the amplitude) and ignores completely the fine structure of the traveling waves (i.e., the phase).

The computations that a central auditory network needs to perform in order to estimate this profile are rather simple. For each fiber, a running average of the firing rate is estimated over a short time interval (typically 10–20 $msec$), which is then plotted against the CF of the fiber (i.e., its location along the tonotopic axis). A simple network model to implement these computations is shown in fig. 8.3. It consists of a tonotopically organized array of neurons. Each neuron receives an excitatory input from a spatially restricted set of fibers, and integrates the activity with a membrane time constant of the order of a few milliseconds. Conceptually, there are no interconnections required in this network and hence the neuron model of fig. 8.2c and eq. 8.6 (with $v_{ij} = 0, w_{ij} = 0, i \neq j$) can readily perform this operation given the appropriate values of τ.

The simplicity of such a "network" is appealing; there are, however, several complications, most important among them being the dynamic range issue (a problem common to other sensory systems; Koch and Poggio 1987). In order for a neuron to encode the typical range of intensities seen in environmental sounds, the dynamic range of its response (between the threshold of response and its saturation) has to exceed 70–80 dB. The dynamic range of auditory nerve fiber responses rarely exceeds 30–40 dB (Sachs and Young 1979). Furthermore, experimental recordings (Sachs and Young 1979) show that at moderate sound

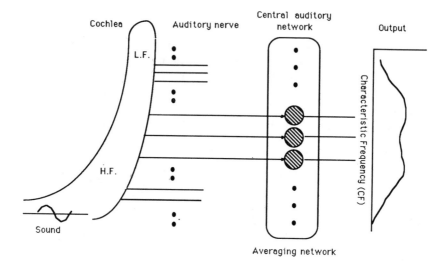

Figure 8.3
A schematic of the auditory processing stages according to the mean-rate hypothesis.
The firing rate of each auditory nerve fiber is simply averaged by the central auditory
network. The outputs are plotted as a function of space (tonotopic axis).

levels, most fibers' responses are saturated and thus are incapable of encoding the relative height of the different frequency components in the signal.[2] Consequently, for such a network to be a viable scheme for central auditory processing, additional hypotheses are needed to resolve the dynamic range problem. These include the proposition that most information at moderate and high sound levels are encoded in the firings of unsaturated high-threshold fibers (less than 20%), or that the experimental data are an inaccurate reflection of the situation in the normally behaving animal.

8.4.2   The Periodicity Hypothesis: Neural Networks for Temporal Processing

In the second view of cochlear processing, the responses of the auditory nerve are presumed to encode the stimulus spectrum primarily through the temporal modulations of their instantaneous firing rates. Consequently, in order to derive the spectral estimate, the central auditory networks would have to process the detailed temporal structure of the nerve responses, rather than the simple average measures as in the above case. It has long been observed experimentally that the firing patterns of mammalian auditory nerve fibers can phase lock to the temporal waveform of their input stimulus for frequencies up to 3–4 kHz. However, not until the series of experiments by Sachs and Young (Miller and Sachs 1983; Young and Sachs 1979) were the importance and richness of the temporal aspects of the nerve responses fully appreciated. In recordings from large populations of nerve fibers responding to speech-like stimuli, they demonstrated that the temporal structure of the responses can encode robustly the spectrum of the stimulus over large dynamic ranges and background noise levels. This work pushed to the forefront the questions of what type of computations are needed to exploit the temporal response patterns to derive the spectrum, and how they are to be implemented in the neural networks of the CNS.

Many computational algorithms have subsequently been suggested to tackle these questions (Delgutte 1984; Seneff 1984; Sinex and Geisler 1983; Young and Sachs 1979). Common to all of them is the use of some form of frequency analysis to measure the periodicities in the response waveforms, either explicitly as in Fourier transform methods, or

---

[2] Decibels (dB) are logarithmic units used often in amplitude and power comparisons of ratios r_1 and r_2 ($20log(r_1/r_2)$). A 6 dB increase in the ratio of two quantities then corresponds roughly to a doubling of the ratio of their amplitudes. Therefore an 84 dB dynamic range approximately equals a 16,000-fold change in the sound amplitude between threshold and saturation.

implicitly in the time domain by computing autocorrelation functions. Consequently, these algorithms operate on the time history of the nerve firing rate, and hence need to store and to combine in various ways the response waveform over a finite interval. In order for such computations to occur in the nervous system, neural networks need to exist that exhibit precise series of time delays that are organized in a regular topology. Such delays may arise through systematic variations in the morphological features of the network neurons, e.g., axons or dendrites with regularly changing lengths, diameters, or membrane time constants.

An Example of a Network Implementation Consider the "neural" implementation of a particularly simple example of such algorithms— called the cosinusoidal comb filter. The algorithm presented here is similar to one proposed earlier by Young and Sachs (1979) and Delgutte (1984). The basic idea behind this scheme is to estimate the spectrum by measuring the degree of phase locking exhibited by the synchronized responses of the fiber array to a bank of bandpass filters with center frequencies organized according to the CF of each fiber. The output of such a filter array would then reflect the spectrum of the input stimulus. A neural circuit that approximately achieves the bandpass transfer function of each filter is shown in fig. 8.4a. Here, the central auditory neuron receives the responses of one fiber, and in addition a delayed version through a longer axon collateral or an excitatory interneuron. The exact amount of delay (τ_c) is critical and must be consistent with the CF of the input fiber, i.e., $\tau_c = 1/(2\pi f_c)$, where f_c is the CF of the fiber. Using the neuron model of eq. 8.6, and assuming no interconnections among the central neurons ($w_{ij} = 0$) and no divergence in the inputs ($v_{ij} = 0, i \neq j$), the intracellular potential of the receiving cell is then given by:

$$\tau \frac{dy_i}{dt} + y_i = e_i + e_i(t - \tau_c) \tag{8.8}$$

for all i, where we have arbitrarily assumed unity input weights ($v_{ii} = 1$) for simplicity. The equation above is linear, and hence it is particularly convenient to use the frequency domain to illustrate the transfer characteristics of the neuron. Taking the Fourier transform on both sides and collecting the resulting terms, we obtain:

$$Y(\omega) = E(\omega) \cdot (1 + e^{-j\omega\tau_c}) \cdot \frac{1}{1 + j\omega\tau} \tag{8.9}$$

where $Y(\omega)$ and $E(\omega)$ are the transformed variables, and $\omega = 2\pi f$ is

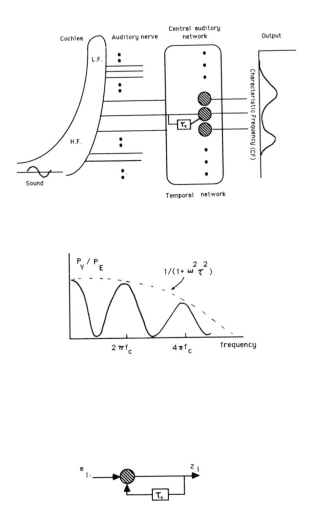

Figure 8.4
A schematic of the auditory processing stages according to the temporal processing
hypothesis: (a) A nonrecurrent network for measuring the periodicities of auditory
nerve responses. Each central neuron receives as input the instantaneous firing rate of
an auditory nerve fiber, and a second delayed version (τ_c delay). The amount of delay
varies along the network and is equal to $1/CF$, where CF = characteristic frequency
of the fiber. (b) The transfer function of each neuron in the temporal network. (c) An
alternate recurrent implementation of the temporal network elements.

angular frequency. The output power spectrum is therefore given by (fig. 8.4b):

$$P_Y(\omega) = P_E(\omega) \cdot 2(1 + cos(\omega\tau_c)) \cdot \frac{1}{1 + \omega^2\tau^2} \qquad (8.10)$$

The input spectrum P_E is therefore modified by two terms in the above transfer function. The first is due to the delayed pathway (τ_c) that emphasizes the frequency components at f_c and its harmonics relative to other frequencies (thus the name comb filter). Note also that the input DC component ($\omega = 0$) is also retained in the output. The second term is the low-pass filter due to the time constant (τ) of the cell membranes. If $\omega_c \approx 1/\tau$, the low-pass filter will attenuate further the harmonics of f_c passed through by the first (comb) filter. Thus, the remaining output signal $y(t)$ will reflect primarily the input fiber responses in the neigborhood of f_c, and a DC component that can be easily removed through such mechanisms as adaptation or self-inhibition. The final output $z_i(t)$ is a compressed version of $y_i(t)$.

In this manner, a neural circuit can approximately perform frequency measurements, a fundamental operation in a large class of temporal algorithms (Seneff 1984; Sinex and Geisler 1983; Young and Sachs 1979). Furthermore, with minor modifications on the scheme outlined above, finer control can be achieved over many of the parameters of the filters, e.g., their band widths and sharpness (Delgutte 1984). It is also possible to show that somewhat different operations and connectivities can result in essentially equivalent transfer characteristics, e.g., using multiplication (rather than addition) at the cell's input (Delgutte 1984), or substituting the delayed input with a delayed feedback from the output (fig. 8.4c) . The latter modification contrasts two basic arrangements of neural interactions that will be discussed in detail in the next section: the recurrent versus nonrecurrent topologies.

Finally, an important question that arises here concerns the biological feasibility of such neural circuits. To measure a range of frequencies f_c, a corresponding range of delays τ_c needs to exist via regular changes in axonal lengths and/or membrane time constants along the tonotopic axis. The anatomical and physiological evidence in support of such models is nonexistent at present. Furthermore, there are no examples of such arrangements from other mammalian sensory systems. This raises the real possibility that, despite the richness and robustness of the information carried in the temporal modulations of the auditory nerve responses, it may be irrelevent as far as the central auditory system is concerned. There is, therefore, a powerful incentive to formulate and

test more biologically realistic algorithms that are capable of extracting
the temporal cues.

8.5   Neural Networks for Spatial Processing: Lateral Inhibitory Networks

A simple alternative strategy for the central auditory processing of temporal cues emerges if we examine the detailed spatio-temporal structure
of the responses of the auditory nerve. Such a natural view of the response patterns on the auditory nerve (and in fact in any other neural
tissue) has been lacking primarily because of the immense technical difficulties in obtaining recordings from large populations of nerve cells.
Figure 8.1b illustrated this view of the response of the ordered array
of auditory nerve fibers to a two-tone stimulus (600 and 2000 Hz). As
mentioned earlier, each tone generates on the basilar membrane a traveling wave that synchronizes the responses of a different band of fibers
along the tonotopic (spatial) axis. The responses reflect two fundamental properties of the traveling waves—namely the abrupt decay of
the amplitude and the rapid accumulation of phase lag near the point
of resonance (Shamma 1985a). These features are in turn manifested
in the spatio-temporal response patterns as edges or sharp discontinuities between the response regions phase-locked to different frequencies
(fig. 8.1a). Since the saliency and location of these edges along the spatial tonotopic axis are dependent on the amplitude and frequency of each
stimulating tone, a spectral estimate of the underlying complex stimulus can be readily derived by detecting these edges, using algorithms
such as those performed by the lateral inhibitory networks of the retina
(Hartline 1974; Shamma 1985b).

As we shall elaborate below, the processing that an lateral inhibitory
network performs is primarily spatial in character and therefore depends on the patterns of interconnections that exist among the network elements. To illustrate this and other aspects of the network operation, we shall review the analysis of models of two possible lateral
inhibitory network topologies:[3] recurrent and nonrecurrent (fig. 8.5).
These terms refer to the presence or absence of feedback from the neural outputs. Thus in fig. 8.5a, the inputs to the nonrecursive lateral
inhibitory network $(e_i, i = 1 \ldots N)$ are combined to compute the final
outputs $(z_i(t), i = 1 \ldots N)$ without any recurrent connections, i.e., only

---

[3]See Hartline (1974) for an excellent review of the physiology and mathematics
of such networks in the retina.

feedforward computations are performed. Recurrent networks are shown in fig. 8.5b, where the output of each neuron is fed back to the input of neighboring neurons. These two types of networks can serve equivalent functions, but may also diverge considerably depending on the strength and profile of the network interconnections.

8.5.1 Analysis of the Nonrecurrent Lateral Inhibitory Network

Using the neuron model of eq. 8.6, the nonrecurrent lateral inhibitory network can be described by the following system of linear equations:

$$\tau \frac{dy_i}{dt} + y_i = \sum_{j=0}^{N} v_{ij} e_j \tag{8.11}$$

for $i = 1 \ldots N$. In order to simplify the later comparison of this network with recurrent lateral inhibitory networks, we rewrite the matrix of input weights (v_{ij}) into two parts: $v_{ii} = 1$ term that represents the weight of the excitatory input that spatially coincides with neuron i, and v_{ij} terms that represent all other inhibitory input influences (fig. 8.5a):

$$\tau \frac{dy_i}{dt} + y_i = e_i - \sum_{j=0}^{N} v_{ij} e_j \tag{8.12}$$

Note that here, unlike the neural circuit of figs. 8.3 and 8.4 earlier, each neural output y_i (or equivalently, $z_i = g(y_i)$) is influenced by inputs to other neurons in the network through the matrix of weights v_{ij}. Thus, the network output is a result of processing the spatial patterns of the input.

In order to gain better intuition of the function of these networks, we examine their input-output transfer characteristics in the frequency domain. The main simplifying assumption adopted in the remainder of this section is that the networks are either infinitely long or are circular, thus allowing us to ignore network boundary effects. The frequency domain analysis can be carried out using the network description discussed above as a system of discrete, coupled differential equations or, alternatively, using a continuum description of the network. In the following, we shall adopt the continuum formalism along the spatial axis. It should be clear, however, that the discrete analysis (corresponding to a sampled spatial axis) yields analogous formulas, the main difference being in the interpretation of the spatial variables as sampled functions, and their transforms as being periodic functions of spatial frequency.

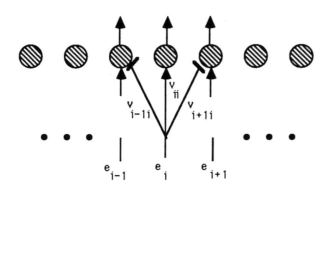

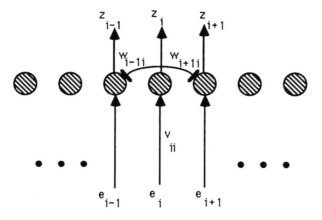

Figure 8.5
Two types of lateral inhibitory networks. (a) The nonrecurrent lateral inhibitory network. Excitatory and inhibitory "synapses" are indicated by arrows and bars, respectively. (b) The recurrent lateral inhibitory network.

To develop the continuous system equations, we assume that the number of neurons N is large and that the differences in the parameters and connectivities from one neuron (i) to another $(i+1)$ are small. A neuron therefore can be viewed as a member of a continuum—a large densely packed and homogeneous neural layer. The discrete equations (eq. 8.12) become:

$$\tau \frac{dy(s,t)}{dt} + y(s,t) = e(s,t) - v(s) *_s e(s,t) \tag{8.13}$$

where s is the spatial (or tonotopic) axis of the network, the variables $y(s,t)$ and $e(s,t)$ become continuous functions of time as well as space, and $(*_s)$ denotes the spatial convolution between the input spatial pattern at time t and the profile of inhibitory connectivities $v(s)$. We shall assume here that the network is homogeneous (i.e., that at any point s', a neuron "sees" the same weight profile $v(s - s')$) around it, and that the spatial Fourier transform of $v(s)$ exists. Taking the Fourier transforms with respect to both the spatial and temporal axes, we obtain the transfer function of the network:

$$Y(k,\omega) = E(k,\omega) \cdot (1 - V(k)) \cdot \frac{1}{1 + j\omega\tau} \tag{8.14}$$

where k and ω represent the spatial and temporal frequency variables, and E and Y represent the transformed variables.

The above equations indicate that the input is modified by two separate terms. The first $(1 - V(k))$ is purely spatial and is related to the Fourier transform of the input connectivity profile $(v(s))$. The second is purely temporal and reflects the low-pass filtering due to the cell membranes. Before discussing the properties of these networks and illustrating the outputs that result from applying the auditory nerve spatio-temporal patterns to this network, we examine and compare the processing in the recurrent version of this network.

8.5.2   Analysis of the Recurrent Lateral Inhibitory Network

In the recurrent lateral inhibitory network (fig. 8.5b), the network can be thought of as consisting of a single layer of neurons that are mutually inhibited, either directly through axon collaterals (i.e., the neurons are inhibitory), or indirectly through a second layer of inhibitory interneurons. We consider first a single-layer network of N inhibitory neurons. The dynamics can be described by the following set of equations:

$$\tau \frac{dy_i}{dt} + y_i = \sum_{j=0}^{N} v_{ij} e_j - \sum_{j=0}^{N} w_{ij} g(y_j) \tag{8.15}$$

where w_{ij} represent the inhibitory recurrent interconnections among the network elements. Due to the presence of the nonlinear function $g(.)$, the above system of equations is nonlinear and thus has the potential for considerably more complex and interesting dynamics than the linear system of the nonrecursive lateral inhibitory network above. In order to compare the two networks, we consider first the linear behavior of this lateral inhibitory network around a steady state potential y_i^* and input e_i^*, where (from eq. 8.15 above) $y_i^* = \sum_{j=0}^{N} v_{ij}e_j - \sum_{j=0}^{N} w_{ij}g(y_j^*)$. Let $y_i = y_i^* + \tilde{y}_i$ and $e_i = e_i^* + \tilde{e}_i$, where $\tilde{y}_i$ and $\tilde{e}_i$ are small-signal fluctuations around the steady states, then:

$$\tau\frac{d\tilde{y}_i}{dt} + \tilde{y}_i = \tilde{e}_i - \sum_{j=0}^{N} w_{ij}\tilde{y}_j \tag{8.16}$$

where the slope of $g(.)$ around y^* has been absorbed in w_{ij}, and we have assumed that each neuron is driven externally only by its coincident input, i.e., $v_{ij} = 0$ for $i \neq j$, and $v_{ii} = 1$.

These equations can be written in the continuum form as before:

$$\tau\frac{d\tilde{y}(s,t)}{dt} + \tilde{y}(s,t) = \tilde{e}(s,t) - w(s) *_s \tilde{y}(s,t) \tag{8.17}$$

with the same assumptions as in the nonrecurrent case applying to $w(s)$ and its Fourier transform. Taking the spatial and temporal Fourier transforms, we obtain:

$$\tilde{Y}(k,\omega) = \tilde{E}(k,\omega) \cdot \frac{1}{1 + j\omega\tau + W(k)} \tag{8.18}$$

where $\tilde{Y}, \tilde{E}$, and W are the transformed variables.

8.5.3 Spatial Processing with the lateral inhibitory network: Edge Detection and Peak Selection

Equations 8.14 and 8.18 represent the linear transfer characteristics of the two lateral inhibitory networks. We concentrate first on the spatial transformations that these networks apply to their input patterns, i.e., we assume that the temporal variations of the input are slow relative to the time constant of the network (τ). In order to compare the two networks directly, we consider identical profiles of inhibitory connectivities, i.e., $w_{ij} = v_{ij}$ (and hence $W(k) = V(k)$). Then, eqs. 8.14 and 8.18 become:

$$\tilde{Y}(k,0) = \tilde{E}(k,0) \cdot (1 - W(k))$$

for the nonrecurrent network, and

$$\tilde{Y}(k,0) = \tilde{E}(k,0) \cdot \frac{1}{1 + W(k)}$$

for the recurrent network.

For small $W(k)$, the latter equation can be expanded and approximated by the nonrecurrent equation, which suggests that the two networks can perform essentially similar functions in the spatial domain. In order to understand how the profile of connectivities $(W(k))$ is chosen, we recall that the lateral inhibitory network was initially invoked to detect the "edges" created by the rapid amplitude and phase changes of the traveling waves. These edge regions are (by definition) regions of rapid change that exhibit high spatial frequencies (k) compared to the flat (low spatial frequency) regions in between. Consequently, in order to enhance these edges and thus sharpen the input patterns, the network transfer function $(\frac{\tilde{Y}}{\tilde{E}}(k,0))$ should have spatial high-pass transfer characteristics as illustrated in fig. 8.6b. Figure 8.6a illustrates the profiles of inhibitory connections $(w(s))$ needed for both lateral inhibitory networks, and the way the strength of these connections falls off gradually with distance. For either network, the patterns of connectivity can be simply described as follows: for each neuron we require a central excitatory input and an inhibitory surround. In the recursive lateral inhibitory network the inhibition is derived from the outputs of surrounding neurons, whereas in the nonrecurrent case it is derived from the inputs to surrounding neurons. The exact shape (strength or spread) of the $w(s)$ profile determines the effectiveness of the lateral inhibitory network in sharpening the input profiles. For instance, a narrow $w(s)$ generally allows only the highest spatial frequencies to pass; similarly, a stronger $w(s)$ attenuates further the lower spatial frequencies.

A major difference between the two networks concerns their stability properties. Unlike the nonrecurrent network, which is always stable, the recurrent lateral inhibitory network may become unstable for certain $w(s)$ profiles. Specifically, when $W(k) = 1$ the denominator of eq. 8.18 is equal to zero, and the output is ill-defined. This occurs generally when the self-inhibition of each neuron of the network is small compared to the mutual inhibition.[4] The linear model of the lateral inhibitory network cannot serve a useful purpose when it becomes unstable. If, on the

---

[4] More precise statements can be made given specific profiles. For instance, for a symmetric positive profile (i.e., $w(s) \geq 0$ and hence $W(k)$ is maximum at $W(0)$), the area under the profile of inhibition ($\int_{-\infty}^{\infty} w(s)ds$) should be ≤ 1 for stability.

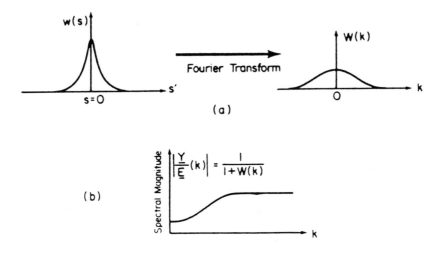

Figure 8.6
Transfer characteristics of the linear lateral inhibitory networks. (a) The profile of inhibitory connectivities and its spatial Fourier transform. (b) The spatial transfer function of the linear recurrent lateral inhibitory network.

other hand, the nonlinearities of threshold and saturation are retained in the model (eq. 8.15), then it can be shown that the instability leads to hysteresis phenomena, to the generation of spatial periodic patterns, and to other interesting and complex phenomena that may serve as models of various perceptual experiences (see Appendix 8.A; Ermentrout and Cowan 1980; Morishita and Yajima 1972).

One particularly useful function that the nonlinear lateral inhibitory network can serve is in local or global peak selection—also known as the "winner-take-all" function. In Appendix 8.A we show analytically how this behavior emerges in a simple recurrent lateral inhibitory network. It is easy to see intuitively, however, how the pattern sharpening of the linear network gives way with increasing inhibition to the all-or-none outputs of the nonlinear network. Figure 8.7 illustrates schematically the change in the inputs and outputs of the lateral inhibitory network (e.g., eq. 8.15) with varying amounts of lateral inhibition. Consider first the situation where each neuron in the network inhibits equally *all* other neurons, but not itself (i.e., in eq. 8.15, let $w_{ij} = w$ for $i \neq j$, and $w_{ii} = 0$). For small w (fig. 8.7a), the inhibition is weak enough that no neuron is shut off or saturated, and the network sharpens the input according to the linear analysis discussed above. With stronger inhibition, neurons representing the output activity due to the valleys of the input pattern become more suppressed and only neurons driven by the peaks of the input pattern continue to fire (fig. 8.7b). At the strongest inhibition (fig. 8.7c), only one neuron can survive—that representing the largest peak of the pattern—while all others are suppressed. In effect, the lateral inhibitory network has selected the largest peak in the entire input pattern (the global peak) and signaled its location by the activity of the appropriate neuron. The lateral inhibitory network can perform the same function locally if the inhibitory profile (w_{ij}) is spatially limited (e.g., $w_{ij} = w$ for $/i - j/ \leq c$, and $w_{ii} = 0$). In this case, the same peak selection (or suppression) is observed for peaks that are less than c neurons apart (Sellami 1988). Such processing is valuable in simulating the feature extraction and recognition of contaminated input patterns.

From a biological point of view, both types of lateral inhibitor networks appear feasible. Thus, the recurrent lateral inhibitory network was first found in the compound eye of *Limulus*, the horseshoe crab (Hartline 1974). Extensive elegant experiments and theoretical studies of this network have demonstrated its role in sharpening visual images by highlighting their spatial edges and peaks and by detecting and emphasizing their temporal changes. The ON-center/OFF-surround responses of the retinae of many animals can be seen as functionally equivalent to

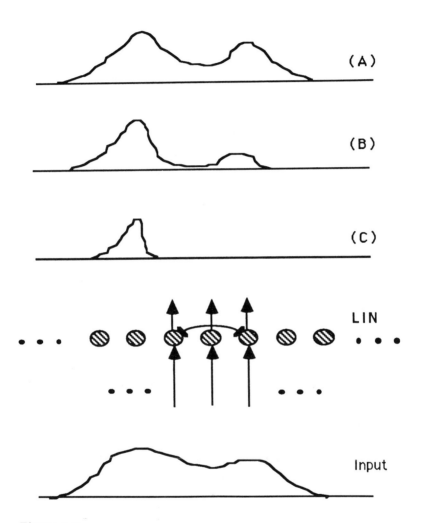

Figure 8.7
The winner-take-all function of the nonlinear lateral inhibitory networks. (a) Output
of the network with small lateral inhibition. (b) The output with medium amount
of inhibition. (c) The winner-take-all output at the highest amount of inhibition.

the lateral inhibitory network in *Limulus*, although they may exhibit additional more complex responses. Nonrecurrent lateral inhibition can be mediated via many possible anatomical arrangements, two of which are shown in fig. 8.8: inhibitory interneurons (fig. 8.8a) or dendro-dendritic synapses (fig. 8.8b). A combination of these two possibilities has indeed been found in the olfactory bulb (Rall 1970).

8.5.4 Temporal Processing with Lateral Inhibitory Network: Onset Sharpening and Oscillations

In the nonrecurrent lateral inhibitory network , the processing of the temporal fluctuations of the input pattern is decoupled from the spatial component and consists of simple low-pass filtering as seen in eq. 8.14. In the recurrent network, the processing of the spatial and temporal components is closely coupled. This becomes more apparent if we rewrite eq. 8.18 as

$$\tilde{Y}(k,\omega) = \tilde{E}(k,\omega) \cdot \frac{1}{(1 + j\omega\tau_{eff})} \cdot \frac{1}{(1 + W(k))} \tag{8.19}$$

where $\tau_{eff} = \tau/(1 + W(k))$ is now the effective time constant of the low-pass filter represented by the first term of the transfer function. τ_{eff} depends on the value of $W(k)$; thus, for higher spatial frequencies $(W(k) \rightarrow 0$; see fig. 8.6), the time constant increases and the output is attenuated at lower temporal frequencies. This can be understood intuitively by observing that for the recurrent inhibition to be effective, sufficient time is required for it to be fed back. For fast-changing inputs, the inhibition may not keep up and thus the sharpening of the instantaneous input patterns deteriorates significantly. For the processing of auditory nerve response periodicities of $\approx$1–2 kHz, the lateral inhibitory network should be relatively fast acting with time constants (τ) of the order of 0.1–0.2 *msec*. Note that although the single-layer lateral inhibitory network is first-order with respect to time, it is still capable of simulating periodic oscillatory phenomena if, for example, asymmetrical inhibitory profiles of connectivities are used.[5]

8.5.5 Processing with More Elaborate Lateral Inhibitory Network Models

The above linear analysis of the lateral inhibitory network can be extended to many more complex situations and topologies. The most com-

---

[5]Asymmetrical profiles of $w(s)$ give rise to complex forms of $W(k)$ in eq. 8.19, and hence to complex poles that result in oscillatory behavior (Morishita and Yajima 1972; Matsuoka 1985).

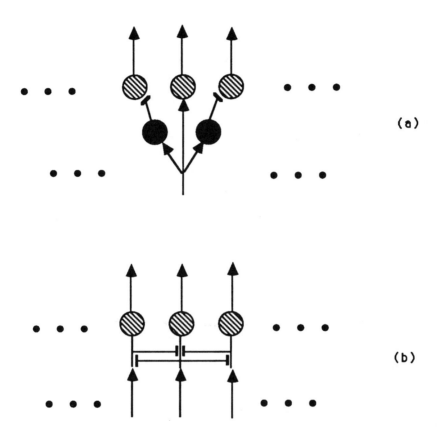

Figure 8.8
Physiological implementations of the nonrecurrent lateral inhibition. (a) Using inhibitory interneurons. (b) Using inhibitory dendro-dendritic interactions.

mon is the double-layer lateral inhibitory network where the inhibition among the excitatory cells of the first layer is mediated by inhibitory interneurons of a second layer (see Cannon, Robinson, and Shamma 1983; Cannon and Robinson 1985; Morishita and Yajima 1972). In this case, a system of second-order nonlinear differential equations results that can be used to simulate damped or periodic oscillatory responses. More elaborate single-neuron models can also be used to account for such higher-order properties as adaptation (Stein, Leung, Oguztoreli, and Williams 1974), axonal transmission delays (Oguztoreli 1979), shunting inhibition (Grossberg 1976), and dendritic processing (Poggio, Torre, and Koch 1985; Rall 1964; Segev et al. 1985). For instance, if we assume that recurrent inhibition exhibits an absolute transmission delay (τ_d) from one neuron to another, then eq. 8.17 becomes

$$\tau \frac{d\tilde{y}(s,t)}{dt} + \tilde{y}(s,t) = \tilde{e}(s,t) - w(s)*_s\tilde{y}(s, t - \tau_d) \tag{8.20}$$

with the spatial and temporal Fourier transforms given by

$$\tilde{Y}(k,\omega) = \tilde{E}(k,\omega) \cdot \frac{1}{1 + j\omega\tau - W(k)e^{-j\omega\tau_d}} \tag{8.21}$$

This lateral inhibitory network is capable of simulating considerably richer modes of temporal processing.

It should be emphasized, however, that introducing these or other details into the lateral inhibitory network models is often accompanied by heavy computational costs and stability problems. Therefore, it is best to use initially the simplest minimal model, and to modify its structure gradually when secondary details are necessary. Clearly, the choice of the minimal model is closely tied to the objectives of the problem. For instance, in the simulations discussed below, we shall sometimes forgo the computation of the temporal dynamics of the responses of the nonlinear lateral inhibitory network in order to highlight the peak selection property of the network. Including the temporal components would introduce "predictable" effects in the responses, and would also increase significantly the complexity of the simulations.

8.6   Implementations of Lateral Inhibitory Networks

We shall consider in this section the issues that arise in simulating two examples of the lateral inhibitory network models: a linear nonrecurrent and a nonlinear recurrent lateral inhibitory network. The first lateral inhibitory network (**LIN.I**) processes the auditory nerve responses directly to generate an estimate of the acoustic spectrum; the second lateral inhibitory network (**LIN.II**) selects and thus highlights the local peaks of the **LIN.I** outputs. In both cases, the discrete rather than the continuous version of the models are simulated (eqs. 8.12 and 8.15).

In general, simulations of linear networks or transfer functions are considerably faster than their nonlinear counterparts, mostly because of the availability of analytical solutions or fast algorithms to perform the forward and inverse Fourier transforms (so-called FFTs). When analytical solutions are not available, numerical methods to integrate the differential equations can be used, which are almost always computationally very expensive in a moderate system of tens of neurons. Several computational packages are available ranging from standard integration routines (e.g., the well-known DGEAR) to circuit simulation programs that compute various input-output transfer characteristics of the equivalent electrical circuit diagram of the network (e.g., SPICE; see chapter 3 for more details).

8.6.1   Simulating Nonrecurrent Lateral Inhibitory Networks

As discussed earlier in section 8.5, an estimate of the acoustic spectrum can be extracted from the responses of the auditory nerve by detecting the peaks and edges created by the travelling wave patterns due to the different components of the stimulus. To demonstrate this, the response patterns of the two tone stimulus shown in fig. 8.1 and the spoken word /magnanimous/ of fig. 8.9 were applied to the nonrecurrent lateral inhibitory network model of eq. 8.12. Although recurrent lateral inhibitory network topologies can also be used, this lateral inhibitory network was chosen both for biological and computational reasons:

1. Since the edges of the auditory nerve responses are created by phase and/or frequency mismatches between the response waveforms of neighboring fibers that are synchronized to relatively high frequencies (up to $2-3\ kHz$), it is essential that the network cells have fast inhibitory time constants (≈ 0.1–$0.2\ msec$) so as to detect and sharpen these edges. Recurrent inhibition is likely to be slow compared to nonrecurrent inhibitory dendro-dendritic synapses.

2. The nonrecurrent lateral inhibitory network can be simulated rapidly. Thus, if we assume that the time constant of the lateral inhibitory network neurons (τ) is small relative to the uppermost frequency

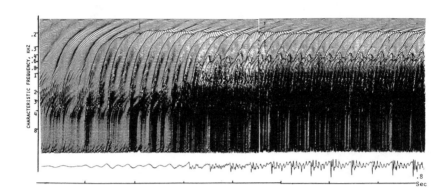

Figure 8.9
Auditory processing of cochlear outputs: spatiotemporal outputs of the spoken word
/magnanimous/ processed using the cochlear model described in fig. 8.1. Responses
to the initial part of the word /ma/ are shown, together with the input waveform fed
into the model.

of phase-locking on the auditory nerve, then eq. 8.12 simplifies
further to:

$$y_i = e_i - \sum_{j=0}^{N} v_{ij} e_j \tag{8.22}$$

where v_{ij} is the profile of inhibition around the ith neuron. The
remaining action of this lateral inhibitory network is therefore intuitively simple and computationally fast: To compute the output
trace at the ith location (y_i), subtract from the ith input trace
(e_i) a weighted sum of its neighbors.

There remain two important parameters before such a simulation can
be run: determining N and the exact inhibitory profile v_{ij}. The number of neurons in this network was determined by the prior choice of 128
as the number of auditory nerve fibers. For different applications, this
number varies depending on the desired spatial resolution of the input
patterns. Using a 128-neuron network here and in other later simulations places a high premium on using the simplest and computationally
most efficient network realizations. The choice of the inhibitory profile
v_{ij} is not critical provided that its spatial extent reflects the slopes and
the spatial resolution of the edges and peaks to be detected in the input

patterns. In the auditory system, the spatial resolution of the different, simultaneously presented frequency components is on the order of one-third of an octave, i.e., a spatial distance on the tonotopic axis of the network layer of ≈ 6 neurons. The w_{ij} profile was thus chosen to be symmetrical, five coefficients long (two on either side of the central excitatory unit input), and with values that produce zero outputs for a locally flat input (e.g., the profile used for the computations of the output in fig. 8.1c and fig. 8.10a is $+0.25, -0.75, 0, -0.75, +0.25$). Finally, the resulting trace from each neuron $(y_i(t))$ is rectified to generate the output $z_i(t)$ $(= g(y_i(t)))$. For plotting purposes, this output is averaged with a relatively long moving window (e.g., 10 $msec$, every 3 $msec$)[6] and the entire array is then displayed in one of two ways: (1) In the case of stationary signals where the location of the edges does not change with time (e.g., the two steady tones of fig. 8.1b), only one cross section is plotted; (2) for nonstationary stimuli, where the stimulus spectrum (and hence the edge and peak locations) changes with time, the entire averaged spatiotemporal output is plotted (see fig. 8.10a).

In either case, the outputs clearly mark the locations and saliency of the edges of the input auditory nerve patterns, which in turn represent the main spectral components of the acoustic stimulus. In this manner, the auditory system can easily generate an estimate of the stimulus spectrum without recourse to Fourier analysis or other temporal correlation schemes (see section 8.4.2).

8.6.2 Other Implementations of Nonrecursive Lateral Inhibitory Networks

The equations developed to describe the behavior of the nonrecurrent lateral inhibitory network suggest two other approaches for its implementation: (1) Using simulations of the equivalent electrical circuit of the network, and (2) frequency domain computations. In the first approach, an equivalent electrical circuit can be easily constructed from eq. 8.12 using such software simulation packages as SPICE (see chapter 3). There are many advantages to this approach—and some crippling limitations. On the positive side, SPICE's powerful features simplify significantly the setting up and computations of the network outputs. This is particulary true when *both* the nonlinearities and the dynamics

---

[6] In the case of the auditory system, the moving window averaging step has an important physiological interpretation based on the well-established observation that phase-locking deteriorates significantly in the responses of central auditory neurons. These neurons can only encode the averaged outputs of the **LIN.I**, i.e., such as those of fig. 8.10a.

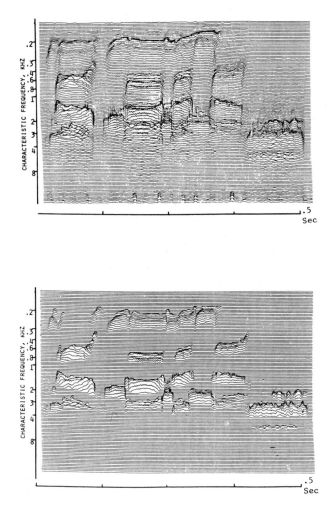

Figure 8.10
Auditory processing of cochlear outputs. (a) Output patterns generated by the **LIN.I**
nonrecurrent network. The peaks represent perceptually significant features of the
stimulus spectrum. Note the change in these features with time corresponding to the
different phonemes. (b) Further sharpening of the **LIN.I** outputs using the recurrent
LIN.II network.

of the neural responses are necessary for the description of the network function (neither of which were used in the computations above). The disadvantages of using SPICE or any similar program is the computational overhead cost required to set up and solve for the outputs of a large number of neuron models. This, coupled with the difficulties in utilizing or incorporating fast numerical methods to compute the outputs, may limit or even outweigh in some cases the benefits of simplicity (see chapter 3 for a more complete discussion).

The frequency domain approach provides significant computational advantages since it allows the use of such highly efficient algorithms as the Fast Fourier Transform (FFT) (Oppenheim and Schafer 1976). In the case of the linear network (e.g., eq. 8.14), this is the fastest method to use. Here, the input patterns are first transformed into the frequency domains, and the final output $\tilde{Y}(k, \omega)$ is inverse transformed to the spatial and temporal domains $(y(s, t))$. Simple adaptations to this approach should be used with long input sequences (e.g., a continuous stream of sound), such as the overlap-and-add or the overlap-and-save methods (Oppenheim and Schafer 1976).[7]

8.6.3   Simulating Nonlinear Recurrent Lateral Inhibitory Networks

The recurrent lateral inhibitory network model is used here to sharpen further the spectral peaks generated by the **LIN.I** (fig. 8.10a). The network performs this function by implementing a winner-take-all strategy over local regions of the input pattern. The exact behavior of the network is primarily determined by the parameters of the inhibitory profile w_{ij}. Specifically, the strength (magnitude) of the weights controls the amount of suppression the winning peak applies to the rest of the network, while the width of the profile determines the resolution of the selected peaks (or the extent of the local regions).

Since the nonlinearities of neuronal transmission play a critical role in mediating the function of this network, the simplest equations that we can use are those of eq. 8.15. A fundamental difference between these equations and those of **LIN.I** (e.g., eq. 8.12) is the fact that, in the recurrent case, the computations of all neuron outputs has to proceed in parallel since the value of $y_i(t)$ depends on the concurrent outputs $(y_j(t))$ of other neurons. In contrast, the computation of $y_i(t)$ in the feedforward **LIN.I** topology depends only on present and past inputs and not on the outputs of the other neurons $(y_j(t))$. Therefore,

---

[7] The FFT can also be used in the computations of the nonlinear equations (8.15) to evaluate the spatial convolutions between the output and connectivity profiles.

in solving eq. 8.15, the whole system has to be integrated simultaneously, which is computationally very expensive. One way to simplify the task is to ignore the settling behavior (the dynamics) of the network, and compute instead the equilibrium states achieved by the network for each input pattern, i.e., to find all the $y_i(t)$ (for $i = 0 \ldots N$) that satisfy the following equations:

$$y_i = \sum_{j=0}^{N} v_{ij} e_j - \sum_{j=0}^{N} w_{ij} g(y_j) \qquad (8.23)$$

or equivalently in terms of $z_i = g(y_i)$:

$$z_i = g(\sum_{j=0}^{N} v_{ij} e_j - \sum_{j=0}^{N} w_{ij} z_j) \qquad (8.24)$$

These equations are solved for each new input pattern e(t).

An easy way to perform these calculations is to initiate first the z vector, then compute a new value using the right side of eq. 8.24, and finally iterate until a fixed point of the mapping is achieved (z^*). The iteration can be done in one of two ways: synchronously and asynchronously. In the former, the entire vector z is updated at each iteration; in the latter, only one element of the vector is randomly chosen and updated at each iteration. In either case, the iterations are stopped when the updated vectors cease changing. This process is then repeated for each new input vector.

Two complicating factors have to be considered when performing the above computations: hysteresis and limit-cycles. Hysteresis is an inherent property of the winner-take-all function of the recurrent lateral inhibitory network (see Appendix 8.A). It is manifested in the above equation by the fact, that for a given input pattern (e), different initial states may lead to different final outputs z^*. The hysteresis property may or may not be desirable depending on the details of the task modeled. Limit cycles occur in the network iterations in rare circumstances, mostly when using the synchronous method of updating the vectors. In these situations, the updated vector usually oscillates between two states (rarely longer cycles).

An example of the recursive network output is shown in fig. 8.10b. Here, the output of **LIN.I** was applied to the network as described by eq. 8.15, with network connectivities w_{ij} given by the following symmetric inhibitory profile: 0(midpoint), 0.02, 0.05, 0.1, 0.15, 0.2, 0.25, 0.25, 0.2, 0.15, 0.1, 0.05, and its reflection; $v_{ij} = 0$ for $i \neq j$, and $v_{ii} = 1$.

There are two important regions in the inhibitory profile: the central "weakly coupled" region, and the strongly inhibitory surround. The width of the central region was chosen so as to allow the selected output peaks to be approximately equal to the typical width of the input peaks. The width and strength of the inhibitory surround were chosen such that a selected winner output peak suppresses the peaks and activity of all neighboring neurons (within $\approx$ 20 neurons). All computations were performed using the asynchronous updating method, and the output is evaluated for each input profile starting at zero output initial conditions. It should be emphasized that, in principle, the recursive network could have been applied directly to the spatio-temporal patterns of the cochlea (fig. 8.9) with similar results. However, since the **LIN.II** simulations are computationally expensive compared to those of **LIN.I**, it is much more effective to use first the **LIN.I** to process the cochlear outputs and thus reduce the sampling rate of the patterns from the 20,000 patterns/sec at the **LIN.I** input, to the 200 patterns/sec at their output. Performing the **LIN.II** computations on 20,000 patterns directly is computationally not practical.

8.6.4   Summary of the Lateral Inhibitory Network Processing of Auditory Patterns

In vision, as in the somatosensory system, the traditional role of the lateral inhibitory network has been to detect and highlight the edges and peaks in the spatial patterns defined by the mean firing rates of the sensory epithelium. This is exactly the case in the auditory system for sound stimuli where no phase-locking is present, e.g., for high-frequency stimuli ($> 4\,kHz$). For the important lower frequencies, however, the edges are primarily expressed as borders between response regions that are phase-locked to different frequencies. These edges are particularly stable with respect to sound level variations since, despite the limited dynamic range of the auditory nerve fibers and the saturation of their mean response rates at high stimulus levels, the temporal course of their instantaneous firing rates remains relatively intact (Shamma 1985b, 1986). Consequently, the overall texture of the responses, particularly the sharp discontinuities between the different response regions, is largely preserved, and thus can be exploited by the lateral inhibitory network at all sound levels (Shamma 1986).

In postulating lateral inhibitory networks as computational algorithm for monaural spectral estimation, the temporal structure of auditory nerve responses is seen to play an indirect role in encoding the sound spectrum, being only a "carrier of" the spatial features that the network detects. This view is fundamentally different from that of the purely temporal algorithms (as in section 8.4.2) that sought to derive direct temporal response measures (e.g., the absolute frequency of phase-locking), and consequently required for their implementation such neural structures as the organized time delays.

8.7   The Biological Plausibility of a Neural Network Model

A critical element in the design process of any neural network is the nature of the available constraints. Often, these constraints are formulated only as an input-output map that defines the transfer characteristics of the desired network, but not its implementation. For instance, in the case of the auditory spectral estimation problem discussed earlier, both the auditory nerve responses (input) and the hypothetical perceived spectrum (output) are known, and the objective is to design the network (algorithm) that performs the desired mapping. There are literally countless network topologies and algorithms that can perform this task, of which two classes were contrasted: the temporally based and the spatially based. Consequently, the following question arises: how is one to compare and select critically among these networks?

This question is important when the objective of the modeling is to discover the underlying biological neural substrate that performs the computations. Thus, it is relatively easy in general to come up with a network that can perform any desired task, given enough complex neuron models (systems of nonlinear differential equations) with arbitrary connectivities (arbitrary coupling). It is a different matter altogether to come up with a biologically plausible network to perform the task. Unfortunately, there are no definitive rules that lead to such network designs; rather, there are intuitive guidelines that are based on our current understanding of the function and anatomy of the central nervous system. For instance, electrophysiological studies have provided detailed results of the kind of computations and the range of speeds expected of typical mammalian neurons. Thus, a neuron cannot compute at nanosecond speeds, nor does it have access to precisely synchronized clocks. Neurons do, however, form elaborate dendritic trees and axonal arborizations, and are thus capable of establishing finely tuned connectivities with other neurons. These findings suggest that, in the absence of specific evidence to the contrary, neural networks are more likely to utilize and process input patterns that are distributed in space rather than in time.

Another important source of information for neuronal modeling concerns the representational primitives of the particular nervous system under study. Such knowledge is usually derived from psychophysical and/or neurophysiological studies. It provides valuable constraints on the type of computations that the network models perform and the output measures they seek to extract. A particularly good example of such primitives are the oriented edge and motion detectors of the mammalian visual system. The discovery of these organizational features has restricted significantly the range of plausible network models that are involved in vision processing, which in turn has led to the design of more focused and fruitful physiological and anatomical studies of the visual system. In contrast, the situation in the auditory system is considerably more vague as no comparable primitives have emerged. Consequently, only a few constraints exist in the formulation of auditory processing algorithms and network implementations, and one is forced to rely on more general plausibility arguments like those outlined above. Nevertheless, the example of the visual system remains as a powerful source of inspiration for similar networks in other sensory systems.

The address of Shihab Shamma is Department of Electrical Engineering, University of Maryland, College Park, Maryland 20742. Electronic mail should be addressed to sas@eneevax.umd.edu .

Appendix 8.A

We examine here in more detail the modes of processing in a simple nonlinear neural network, and the emergence of such phenomena as the winner-take-all and hysteresis described earlier in the chapter. The network is composed of two mutually and recursively inhibited nonlinear neurons (fig. 8.11).

The recursion of inhibition and the nonlinearity of the neuron models are essential properties of the network function.

The mathematical description of the simplified two-neuron network is derived directly from eq. 8.6 with nondivergent external inputs ($v_{ij} = 0, i \neq j; v_{ii} = 1$) and equal mutual inhibitory connections ($w_{ii} = 0$, and $w_{12} = w_{21} = -w$):

$$\tau \frac{dy_1}{dt} + y_1 = e_1 + w\, z_2 \qquad (8.25)$$

$$\tau \frac{dy_2}{dt} + y_2 = e_2 + w\, z_1 \qquad (8.26)$$

The final outputs z_1, z_2 are related to the "membrane potentials" (y_1, y_2) by a nonlinear transformation ($z_i = g(y_i)$) as shown earlier in eq. 8.2. For the purposes of the simulations shown in this appendix, the parameters of the function ($g(.)$) are chosen as follows: $z_{max} = 1$ and $a = e^{(.5b)}$. Equation 8.2 can therefore be rewritten as:

$$g(y_i) = \frac{e^{b(y_i - .5)}}{1 + e^{b(y_i - .5)}} \qquad (8.27)$$

i.e., the sigmoidal function saturates at 1, and achieves its midpoint when $y_i = .5$ (i.e., $g(.5) = .5$). The value of the parameter b affects only the steepness of the curve around the midpoint. The function $g(.)$ has its maximum slope at the midpoint ($\dot{g}_{max} = \dot{g}(.5) = .25b$). Setting $b = 4$ limits the maximum value of the slope of $g(.)$ to 1.

In the analysis of the recurrent lateral inhibitory network earlier (section 8.5), we examined and simulated the spatial processing of the network for inputs that vary slowly relative to the time constant of the network (τ), or equivalently for a fast settling network ($\tau \to 0$). Such solutions formally correspond to the so-called equilibrium or steady-state solutions of the system (see chapter 5 for a detailed discussion). In eqs. 8.25 and 8.26, these solutions correspond to the case when the variables ($y_1(t), y_2(t)$) cease changing with time (i.e., $dy_1/dt = dy_2/dt = 0$). They are given by:

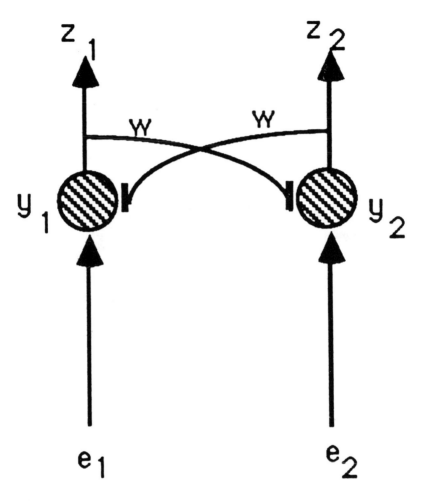

Figure 8.11
Schematic of a two-neuron recurrent lateral inhibitory network.

$$y_1 = e_1 - wg(y_2) \tag{8.28}$$

$$y_2 = e_2 - wg(y_1) \tag{8.29}$$

The equilibrium solutions therefore depend on the constant inputs (e_1, e_2) and inhibitory connections (w).

The Case of Weak Inhibitory Connections ($w < 1$)

The solutions can be obtained graphically as the intersection of the curves representing each equation. This is illustrated in fig. 8.12(top) for the case of small w ($w = 0.5$), and three different input combinations $(e_1, e_2 = (0, 1), (1, 1), (2, 1))$. In general, it can be shown that for each input combination (e_1, e_2), these equations will have only one solution when $w \leq 1$, and that the solution is stable. The stability of the equilibria can be analyzed using the methods detailed in chapter 5 (e.g., by examining the sign of the real part of the eigenvalues of the linearized equations around each equilibrium point).

The response of this network to small fluctuations in the input patterns can be directly related to the spatial sharpening observed in the linearized recurrent lateral inhibitory network (fig. 8.6b and eq. 8.18). For instance, consider the responses around the steady state ($y_1 = y_2 = y$) established by equal constant inputs ($e_1 = e_2 = e$). Any small input changes ($\tilde{e}_1$ and $\tilde{e}_2$) can now be expressed in terms of two components ($\tilde{e}_{dc}$ and $\tilde{e}_{ac}$) as follows:

$$\tilde{e}_{dc} = \frac{\tilde{e}_1 + \tilde{e}_2}{2} \tag{8.30}$$

$$\tilde{e}_{ac} = \frac{\tilde{e}_1 - \tilde{e}_2}{2} \tag{8.31}$$

where $\tilde{e}_{dc}$ represents the in-phase component corresponding to zero spatial frequency ($k = 0$), and $\tilde{e}_{ac}$ represents the out-of-phase component corresponding to the maximum spatial frequency representable by the two input elements. The corresponding outputs ($\tilde{y}_{dc}$ and $\tilde{y}_{ac}$) can be computed from the linearized versions of eqs. 8.28 and 8.29 to give:

$$\tilde{y}_{dc} = \frac{\tilde{e}_{dc}}{1 + \dot{w}} \tag{8.32}$$

$$\tilde{y}_{ac} = \frac{\tilde{e}_{ac}}{1 - \dot{w}} \tag{8.33}$$

where $\dot{w}$ represents the contribution of the inhibitory connection and the slope of the nonlinearity at the steady state ($\dot{w} = w \cdot \dot{g}(y)$). For $0 \leq w < 1$, the high-pass function (and hence the sharpening) of the network is evident by the attenaution of the $\tilde{e}_{dc}$ (eq. 8.32) and the amplification of $\tilde{e}_{ac}$ (eq. 8.33).

The Case of Strong Inhibitory Connections ($w > 1$)

An important qualitative change occurs in the behavior of the solutions for larger inhibitory connections ($w > 1$). This is illustrated in the lower part of fig. 8.12 for $w = 2$. The sigmoidal curves become so bent as to intersect at more than one point at certain input combinations. For instance, at ($e_1 = e_2 = 1$), there are three equilibrium points: $s1, s2, s3$. Only one solution exists outside an intermediate range of e_1 and e_2 values, e.g., at (e_1, e_2) = $(0, 1)$ and $(2, 1)$. An important question arises here: Where does the system relax when three equilibria exist (e.g., when $e_1 = e_2 = 1$)?

Once again, the answer to this question relates to the stability of the three different equilibria. Applying the methods of chapter 5 around each point ($s1, s2, s3$), it becomes apparent that both $s1$ and $s3$ are stable equilibria, while the inside point $s2$ is not. This means that $s1$ and $s3$ can be viewed as attractors toward which nearby output trajectories converge. The $s2$ equilibrium point, in comparison, is an unstable saddle that "repels" the output trajectories (see chapter 5 for more precise descriptions). This is illustrated in fig. 8.13 which shows an expanded view of the three equilibria and a set of trajectories starting at four different initial starting output values ($I1, I2, I3, I4$).

These outputs point to the important observation that for some inputs, e.g., $e_1 = e_2 = 1$, there are two possible final outputs ($s1$ or $s3$) depending on the initial conditions of the system. This is exactly what is understood by hysteresis. This phenomenon can be very useful in simulating a variety of nervous system functions such as the temporary storage of information and the encoding of pattern durations without resort to delay lines. The winner-take-all function of the network is also evident in these figures (lower part of fig. 8.12, and fig. 8.13) by the fact that when either output is large positive, the other is significantly suppressed and very small.

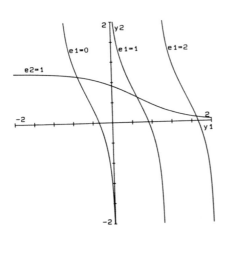

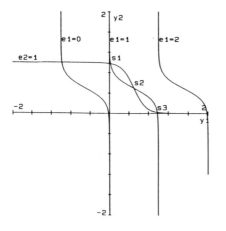

Figure 8.12
The nullclines of eqs. 8.25 and 8.26. The "vertically" oriented curves represent
eq. 8.25 for three different values of e_1. The "horizontal" curve represents eq. 8.26
with $e_2 = 1$. The intersections represent the equilibrium points of the system at the
different conditions. In the top figure, the strength of the inhibitory connections are
given by $w = 0.5$ and in the lower figure by $w = 2$.

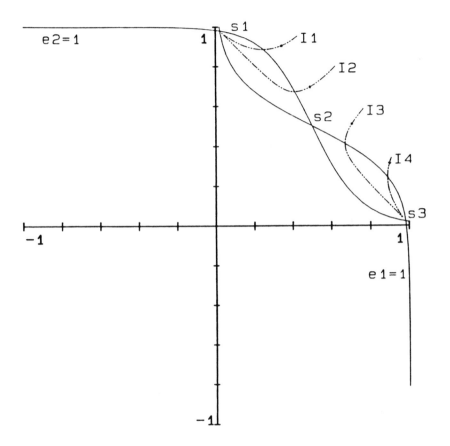

Figure 8.13
An expanded view of the equilibrium points seen in the lower part of fig. 8.12. The
trajectories (dashed) of the system outputs are shown starting at four different initial
conditions around the steady states.

CHAPTER 9

The Simulation of Large-Scale Neural Networks

MATTHEW A. WILSON and JAMES M. BOWER

9.1 Introduction

Previous chapters have described techniques used to simulate the responses of single neurons in isolation to different patterns of inputs by modeling their detailed biophysical structure. In the brain, it is the anatomical and physiological characteristics of the complex neural circuits in which single neurons are embedded that determine the actual pattern of inputs to a cell as well as the significance of the cell's output. As with single isolated cells, computer simulations can provide a means to study the complex functional relationships between neurons comprising such networks (see chapters 6, 7 and 8).

Traditionally, most models of brain circuitry have focused on simulating the macroscopic or "higher-order" functionality of systems of simplified computational or neuronal units. In fact, the prevalence of models of this type has made the modeling of neural networks, in general, synonymous with an abstracted treatment of neural processing in which the study of function takes precedence over the details of implementation. Periodic attempts have been made over the last twenty years to develop neural network models that are structurally more realistic (Pellionisz, Llinas, and Perkel 1977). However, we would argue that only recently have technical developments made simulations of realistic, large-scale neural networks truly practical. One of these technical developments is the rapid increase in affordable computational power, which allows the simulation of models with considerable complexity. Equally important for this kind of modeling is the increasing sophistication of neurophysiological and neuroanatomical techniques, which has resulted in an explosive growth in the availability of structural details on which this type of modeling relies.

In this chapter we will consider the construction and simulation of neural network models that are fundamentally based on the anatomical structure and physiological characteristics of actual biological networks. We have found, through our own modeling efforts, that this "structural" approach to modeling has several distinct advantages over strictly abstract treatments (Wilson and Bower 1988). First, biological realism allows known neuroanatomical and neurophysiological data to be used to constrain the values of many model parameters. This limits the parameter space of a model that needs to be explored to tune and characterize the behavior of complex network models. Second, biologically accurate simulations can more readily generate neuronal-like outputs comparable to data from actual physiological experiments. This increases the likelihood that predictions of the models will be relevant and testable. For example, our models generate intracellular membrane potentials, single-spike output, and extracellular field potentials (fig. 9.7; Wilson and Bower, 1980). And finally, models closely based on the structural properties of biological networks force functional hypotheses to fit within the physical constraints imposed by the actual biological system. In this way insights provided by this type of detailed modeling provide directions for more abstracted studies while at the same time assuring their relevance to actual network properties (Wilson and Bower 1988).

While structural simulations can provide a means to study the functional properties of complex networks, they are also potentially valuable to experimental neurobiology. In particular, simulations that are based on a biological system often highlight undescribed but important features of the modeled networks and thus can suggest important network or cellular parameters to characterize experimentally. This experimental/modeling interaction is especially important given the powerful experimental tools that are currently available to neurobiologists and the wide range of data that they can generate. Thus, this type of structural modeling provides a framework in which detailed experimental data can be organized and interpreted, and biologically relevant theories of brain function can be studied.

9.2   Network Modeling Considerations

Having stated the general advantages of structural neural network models, and made the claim that the revolution in computing power and neurophysiological and neuroanatomical data has made them more accessible, it is important to point out explicitly that the process of modeling still requires working within considerable limitations. In fact, even with the tremendous increases in available computing power, no existing computer can practically simulate all that is known about large neural networks, while at the same time no neural structure has yet been described in all its structural detail. Even in so-called simpler invertebrate networks, experimentalists are well aware that a vast amount of information relevant to function must still be extracted, yet modelers are still forced to simplify their networks for simulation purposes (see chapters 6 and 7). The main body of this chapter outlines our approach to these issues by describing a model of the piriform (olfactory) cortex in some detail. However, we will first consider more specifically some of the general technical factors involved in designing and implementing such a model given these limitations.

Faced with both incomplete information about the networks to be modeled and insufficient computing power to incorporate all information that is currently known, the major task in simulating large-scale, realistic networks is determining the appropriate modeling approximations. In most cases the basic test of the appropriateness of these approximations in structural models will be whether the simulated network can replicate fundamental (and measurable) behavior of the actual system. Of course, as the sophistication of the questions asked with a simulation increases so does the necessary complexity of the model. As such, the process of network modeling can be seen as a bootstrap operation that ideally goes hand in hand with experimental work. To discuss this general relationship between model complexity and simulation objectives we will consider two levels of structural organization at which approximations are often made, the cellular level and the network level.

9.2.1   Cellular Complexity

In modeling single cells, there are several types of structural details to consider. There is spatial/cellular structure, which includes characteristics such as dimension, extent, and location of cell bodies, dendrites, axons, and spines. Then there is biophysical/subcellular structure with membranes, channels, receptors, and their voltage- and time-dependent characteristics including channel conductances, membrane resistance and capacitance, the nature of receptor binding, ionic diffusion, and buffering. Previous chapters have shown that these features can be modeled in some detail if that is the primary objective. However, the network modeler must determine the relative benefit of including such details given the computational cost. Again, it is the nature of the questions asked that determines which details are most critical. For example, in our simulations of the piriform cortex the spike output of a cell is not modeled using a complete Hodgkin-Huxley model for action potentials; instead, a simple threshold criterion is applied to the membrane potential to generate discrete spike events. The occurrence of these spikes is indicated with a spike waveform "pasted" onto the actual membrane potential at the appropriate time. In this case, the details of spike generation are sacrificed for the sake of computational efficiency. As another example, if the details of dendritic interactions are significant to the question being asked in the model, then the use of an explicit multicompartmental model of individual cells and their dendritic regions is indicated (Koch, Poggio, and Torre 1982, 1983). If the nonlinearities of dendritic interaction are not of great significance to the particular response or network property of interest, then a simplified single-compartmental model of a cell might be sufficient (as in chapter 6). In other cases the type of physiological responses the simulation is expected to generate dictates the level of neuronal complexity. For example, in our model, data such as field potentials and current source density measurements require information about the spatial distribution of membrane currents in the simulated cortex to be calculated using a distributed model of the cell and its processes (see below).

9.2.2   Network Scale

At the network level a primary design consideration is one of scale. This is clearly seen in our model of piriform cortex where on the order of 10^3 cells represent a cortex that actually contains over 10^6 cells. Several basic approaches can be taken to deal with this problem. First, a modeler can reduce the scope of the model to include only a restricted portion of the actual structure. In this way a small region of the cortex can be simulated closer to its actual scale (see chapter 10). In this case the amount of cortical area simulated is restricted, but single-cell activity and local interactions are more accurately represented. Obviously, this approach is useful only if the primary aspects of the circuitry involved in the particular response being studied are preserved in this localized model, i.e., there are few relevant longer-range interactions. The second approach involves using sparse samples of single cells over a broad cortical area. This reduces the spatial resolution of simulated activity but allows the study of cortical phenomena that require nonlocal interactions. However, using cells as subsamples of a larger cortical area introduces the problem of compensation for the activity of cells not included in the simulation. This problem can be approached in several ways. For example, single modeled cells can represent the average response of a group of cells. The output of modeled "cells" in this case would consist of a continuous estimate of spatially averaged activity over a region of the ac-

tual network. This is roughly equivalent to using a rate-encoded output
as is commonly done in more abstracted network simulations (Hopfield
1984; Hinton, McClelland, and Rumelhart 1986). An alternate representation preserves the single-spike nature of actual single-cell output. In
this case the properties of single modeled cells are designed to resemble
actual single cells as closely as possible, but synaptic strengths are adjusted to compensate for missing neurons. This is the approach that we
have taken with our simulations as described in more detail below. The
use of the single-spike output representation versus the spatial-average
representation can be somewhat quantified. Appendix 9.D describes a
measure based on an estimate of the connection probability between
cells within different regions. In this case, the criterion used to select
one representation over another is the preservation of the average or expected one-to-one connection characteristics between simulated cells. A
detailed discussion of this issue with sample calculations related to the
piriform cortex model can be found in Appendix 9.D.

9.3   Piriform Cortex and Model Structure

In the remainder of this chapter we will elaborate on the general issues
outlined above by describing in detail the techniques that we have employed in carrying out structural simulations of olfactory cortex. However, because this is a structural model it will first be necessary to place
the model in context by giving a general background description of piriform cortex. A more detailed description of this cortex can be found in
Shepherd (1979) or Haberly (1985). The reader should also note that
the intention of this chapter is to describe how the cortex is simulated
and not to discuss the simulation results or conclusions themselves.

9.3.1   General Cortical Features

Piriform (olfactory) cortex is the primary olfactory cerebral cortical
structure in all mammals. This structure is the focus of our modeling efforts because of its well-defined organization, the availability of
physiological data, and its presumed capacity for memory and associative functions (Haberly 1985). The afferent sensory input to the piriform
cortex is from the olfactory bulb, which itself receives direct projections
from olfactory receptors. This cerebral cortical area is, therefore, unusually close to the sensory periphery, being just one structure removed.
Bulbar input to the cortex is delivered via a fiber bundle known as
the lateral olfactory tract (LOT). This fiber tract appears to make dis-

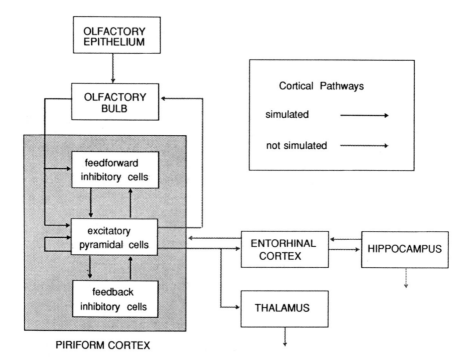

Figure 9.1
Block diagram of the olfactory system showing the basic connections between several
primary structures. Arrows show the flow of information between these structures.
The principal pathway in olfactory processing begins in the olfactory receptors, which
project to the olfactory bulb. The olfactory bulb has extensive projections to other
olfactory structures including the piriform or olfactory cortex. The piriform cortex
has feedback projections to the olfactory bulb, intracortical association projections,
as well as projections to the limbic system via entorhinal cortex.

tributed, nontopographic, excitatory connections with cortical neurons across the extent of the cortex (figs. 9.2, 9.3). This input arrives along the edge of the cortex and projects across its surface in a lateral fashion to a superficial layer (Devor 1976).

In addition to the afferent input connections from the olfactory bulb, there is also an extensive set of connections among neurons intrinsic to the cortex (figs. 9.2, 9.3). For example, the so-called association fiber system arising from the principal cortical cells, the pyramidal cells, makes sparse, distributed excitatory connections with other pyramidal cells across the cortex. There are also intrinsic inhibitory feedforward and feedback connections within the cortex mediated by two types of inhibitory interneurons with different properties. Pyramidal cell axons constitute the primary output of the piriform cortex and project to limbic structures such as entorhinal cortex (Haberly and Price 1978; Luskin and Price 1983a,b) whose neurons, in turn, project to the hippocampus. As such, piriform cortex has close ties to both the sensory periphery and to deeply buried forebrain structures of considerable current interest in neurobiology due to their postulated roles in learning and memory (Tanabe, Iino, and Takagi 1975; Devor 1977; Eichenbaum, Shedlack, and Eckmann 1980).

9.3.2   Neuronal Types

Pyramidal cells are the principal cell type in piriform cortex, and are believed to be exclusively excitatory (Haberly and Price 1978; Haberly and Bower 1984). There are also several populations of nonpyramidal cells or interneurons that can be distinguished on anatomical grounds (Haberly 1983; Haberly and Feig 1983). These neurons appear to be GABAergic and seem to mediate both feedback and feedforward inhibitory effects (see below). Our model is based on a single population of pyramidal cells plus two populations of inhibitory interneurons responsible for feedforward and feedback inhibitory influences (fig. 9.2). The model represents neurons across the full extent of the actual cortex (approximately 10 mm x 6 mm). In the simulation described here, we have modeled 1,500 cells of each type (50 cells x 30 cells) for a total of 4,500 cortical cells (fig. 9.3). The model also includes 100 cells representing the input to the cortex from the olfactory bulb.

9.3.3   Cortical Lamination

Piriform cortex, like all of the cerebral cortex, is a laminar structure that can be subdivided into layers based upon the segregation of different inputs and cell types. Piriform cortex, however, is composed of three

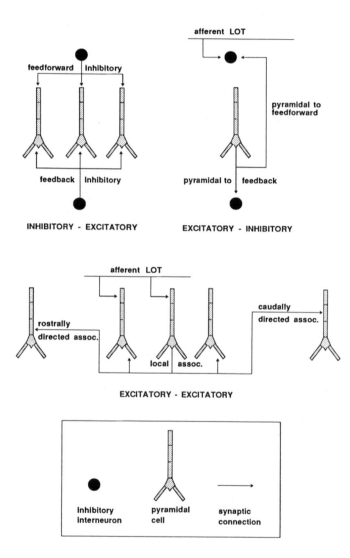

Figure 9.2
Basic interconnection patterns of cells within the model of piriform cortex as described in the text.

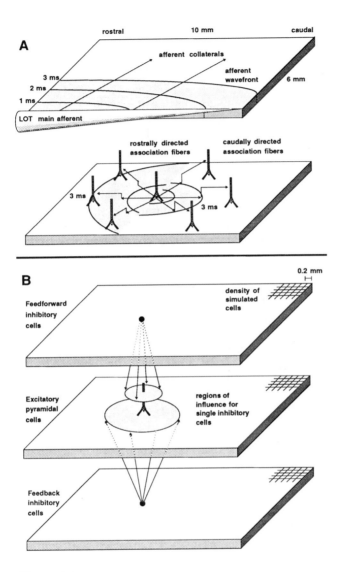

Figure 9.3
(A) The upper diagram shows characteristics of the afferent input to the cortex. The main lateral olfactory input tract (LOT) is seen at the lower edge of the diagram with bulbar input arriving from the left. The spread of activation following LOT stimulation is indicated by contours showing the location of the afferent wavefront at three successive times. The lower diagram shows the pattern of association fiber interconnection between a single pyramidal cell and pyramidal cells located rostral and caudal to it. The spread of activation is seen to be slower in the caudal than the rostral direction due to the difference in propagation velocities of the two types of association fibers. (B) A three-dimensional schematic diagram of the the three major cell types included in the model of piriform cortex—feedforward inhibitory interneurons, pyramidal cells, and inhibitory feedback interneurons. The grid in the upper right shows the scale of the model consisting of 1500 cells (50x30) of each type. Each grid site corresponds to the location of a modeled cell. The shaded regions indicate the regions of influence of the two types of inhibitory interneurons on pyramidal cells.

principal layers as compared with the six layers of neocortical structures. The most superficial layer (layer I) contains afferent axons that originate from mitral cells in the olfactory bulb as well as association axons arising from other pyramidal cells within the piriform cortex. Both fiber systems terminate on apical dendrites of pyramidal cells that extend through this layer. Based on these terminations, layer I can be further subdivided into the surface region where afferent fibers terminate (layer Ia) and the deeper regions containing terminations of the association fibers (layer Ib). There is evidence that layer Ib is further subdivided into a superficial region containing the terminations of caudally directed association fibers and a deeper region containing rostrally directed association fiber terminations (Haberly and Price 1977; Haberly and Bower 1984). Below layer I, the deeper layer II consists of densely packed cell bodies of both pyramidal cells and interneurons. Layer III contains basal dendrites of layer II pyramidal cells as well as cell bodies of deep pyramidal cells and other interneurons (fig. 9.3). Local connections between pyramidal cells terminate on basal dendrites in layer III. In the current model, only layer II pyramidal cells are simulated. The laminar pattern described serves as the basis of the compartmental model of the pyramidal cell in which distinct compartments correspond to laminar regions receiving particular types of input (see figs. 9.4, 9.5, 9.6, and Appendix 9.A).

9.3.4   Network Connections

Afferent Sensory Pathways   As mentioned above, primary afferent input enters piriform cortex via the lateral olfactory tract projection from mitral cells of the olfactory bulb (fig. 9.3). Present evidence suggests that this projection is exclusively excitatory (Biedenbach and Stevens 1969a,b; Haberly 1973a; Haberly and Bower 1984) and extremely diffuse or nontopographic. These afferent fibers make excitatory synaptic connections with pyramidal cells and feedforward interneurons in layer Ia (Haberly 1985). This afferent input to the cortex is modeled as a set of independent fibers that make sparse connections with pyramidal cells and inhibitory interneurons. The actual degree of interconnection is varied according to the experimental paradigm being simulated. For example in some simulations we seek to reproduce physiological data obtained with shock stimulation of the afferent input system. Under these conditions of massive, synchronous afferent activation, the input to the cortex is represented as a bundle of afferent fibers that make excitatory synaptic connections with all pyramidal cells and feedforward interneurons in the cortex (Appendix 9.D). In other simulations where the intention is to replicate patterns of activity seen with more natural stimuli, we treat the afferent inputs independently and connect them more sparsely (Wilson and Bower 1988).

In both the actual cortex and the model, conduction velocities along axons are finite and vary with the axonal type (Haberly 1978). Signals travel along the main input tract from rostral to caudal, and are distributed across the cortex via many small collaterals (Devor 1976). In the model, signals proceed along the main fiber tract towards caudal cortex at a speed of 7.0 m/s. Collaterals leave the main fiber tract at a 45° angle and travel across the cortex at a speed of 1.6 m/s (Haberly 1973b).

In the actual cortex there is a diminution of afferent input to pyramidal cells moving from rostral to caudal that is reflected anatomically in the number of synaptic terminals (Price 1973; Schwob and Price 1978), and physiologically in the amplitude of shock-evoked potentials mediated by the afferent system (Haberly 1973b). To simulate this effect in the model, the strength of synaptic input due to afferent signals is exponentially attenuated with increased distance from the rostral site of stimulation (see w_{static} in eq. 9.5).

Association Circuitry   In addition to the input connections from the olfactory bulb, there is also an extensive set of connections between the neurons intrinsic to the cortex (figs. 9.2, 9.3, 9.4). A principal component in these connections is the association fiber system that arises from pyramidal cells and makes sparse, distributed excitatory connections with other pyramidal cells all across the cortex (Biedenbach and Stevens 1969; Haberly and Bower 1984; Bower and Haberly 1986). The fibers appear to spread out radially from the originating cell and travel rostrally at a speed of 1.0 m/s, and caudally at a speed of 0.5 m/s (Haberly 1973b; Haberly 1978) making local connections on basal dendrites of other pyramidal cells and distant connections on apical dendrites. In the model, fibers originating from pyramidal cells follow the same pattern of interconnectivity and signals are propagated along each fiber with the corresponding delays (eq. 9.2). In the model, as a consequence of simulation scaling considerations (see section 9.2.2 and Appendix 9.D), association fiber interconnectivity is greatly increased as compared to that of the actual cortex.

The effect of monosynaptic association fiber input to a simulated cell is strictly excitatory. In the model, there is an attenuation over distance of the strength of synaptic input to other pyramidal cells reflecting a presumed decrease in a particular cell's influence with distance. The attenuation is consistent with the fall off in numbers of axon terminals

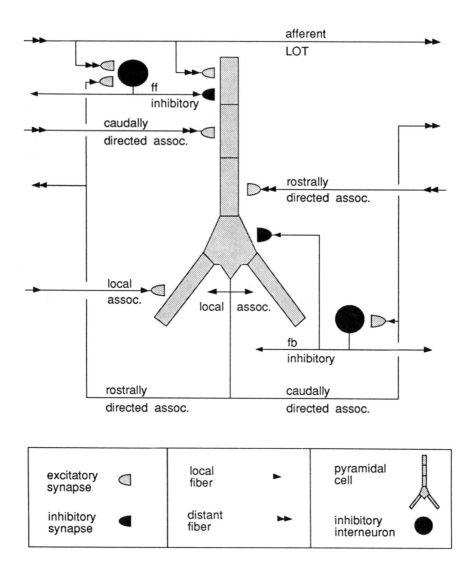

Figure 9.4
Simplified diagram of the local circuitry contained in the model of piriform cortex.
The cell in the center represents a pyramidal cell, which is the primary excitatory
cell type in the piriform cortex. Two other inhibitory cell types are shown as darkened circles adjacent to the pyramidal cell. The small semi-ellipses that appear next
to the pyramidal and inhibitory cells indicate the location of synaptic connections.
Darkened connections are inhibitory while lightened connections are excitatory. Arrows indicate the direction of propagation of signals originating from the various cell
types, as well as the distance these fibers travel.

in local axon collaterals at greater distances from the originating neuron (Haberly and Bower 1982; Haberly and Presto 1986) and is modeled with an exponential function (see eq. 9.7). Rostrally and caudally directed association fibers have unique spatial attenuation constants. The level of attenuation asymptotically approaches a minimum value for each direction, consistent with physiological studies of association fiber systems in deafferented piriform cortex (L. Haberly, unpublished). In the model, the local region of excitation surrounding the cell, which terminates on the basal dendrites of its neighbors, has a radius of 2 mm. This value is an approximation since the actual value is not precisely known. Beyond this radius, connections are made onto apical dendrites. In the model, a pyramidal cell has no excitatory connection to itself (autapse), consistent with anatomical data (Haberly and Presto 1986).

Inhibitory Circuitry   There is good evidence for two types of inhibition in piriform cortex, both of which are incorporated into the model. A well-documented Cl^- mediated feedback inhibition is thought to be generated by local interneurons that receive input primarily from local pyramidal cell association fibers as well as some afferent fibers (Biedenbach and Stevens 1969a,b; Haberly 1973a; Satou, Mori, Tazawa, and Takagi 1982; Haberly and Bower 1984; Tseng and Haberly 1986). The outputs of these inhibitory interneurons feed back to nearby pyramidal cells where significant conductance increases suggest a current shunting inhibitory mechanism (Scholfield 1978; Satou et al. 1982; Haberly and Bower 1984; Tseng and Haberly 1986). In the model these interneurons make inhibitory connections with the group of nearby pyramidal cells that lie within a 2 mm radius (again an estimate) where they activate a significant conductance increase to Cl^- at the level of the cell body (see below).

In addition to this shunting type inhibition, in the actual cortex a K^+ mediated inhibition appears to be generated by local inhibitory interneurons receiving primarily direct afferent input from the LOT as well as some associational input from pyramidal cells (Satou et al. 1982; Tseng and Haberly 1986). The outputs of these interneurons generate a long-latency, long-duration hyperpolarizing inhibitory potential in nearby pyramidal cells. Available evidence (Galvan, Grafe, and Bruggencate 1982; Satou et al. 1982; Tseng and Haberly 1986) suggests that this potential has a modest associated conductance increase and therefore may exert its inhibitory effect primarily via membrane hyperpolarization. In the model this hyperpolarizing inhibition is activated on the apical dendrites of pyramidal cells by inhibitory neurons with both feedforward and feedback input.

9.3.5 Membrane Properties of Neurons and Synaptic Inputs

Channel Types   In the model each population of neurons consists of single cells whose modeled membranes include synaptically activated ionic channels obeying simple channel kinetics and having a membrane capacitance and resistance (figs. 9.5, 9.6). The parameters that describe these properties have all been adjusted to replicate the temporal characteristics of transmembrane potentials found with intracellular recording using both *in vivo* (Haberly and Bower 1984) and *in vitro* (Haberly and Bower 1984) experimental preparations.

The membranes of modeled neurons include three types of ionic channels (table 9.1). The first type of channel is a modest-conductance sodium ion channel ($G_{peak} = 50\ nS$). This channel is activated by excitatory afferent and association fiber synapses, with an equilibrium potential of $100\ mV$ above the average firing threshold of the cell ($E_{Na} = 55\ mV$). In this channel the time to onset of the conductance change following the arrival of a presynaptic action potential is $800\ \mu sec$, or a single synaptic delay. The duration of the change is $10\ msec$.

The second type of synaptically activated channel is a high-conductance, Cl^- mediated type. This channel is activated by inhibitory synapses from feedback interneurons and exerts a powerful current-shunting effect ($G_{peak} = 200\ nS$) on the membrane that drives it to a potential $20\ mV$ below the average firing threshold ($E_{Cl} = -65\ mV$). In this channel the time to onset of the conductance change following the arrival of a presynaptic action potential is again a single synaptic delay. The duration of the change is 20–$60\ msec$.

The third type of synaptically activated channel is a modest-conductance ($G_{peak} = 5\ nS$), K^+ mediated type. This channel is activated by the inhibitory synapses of feedforward interneurons, with an equilibrium potential $45\ mV$ below the average firing threshold ($E_K = -90\ mV$). The time course of the conductance change induced in this channel is characterized by a long latency to activation following the arrival of a presynaptic action potential (30–$50\ msec$) and a long duration (100–$600\ msec$).

Cellular Structure   The two types of inhibitory neurons are each modeled as single compartments, while two models of the excitatory pyramidal cells are used alternately during simulations. A simplified single-compartment pyramidal cell model (fig. 9.5) is used during large-

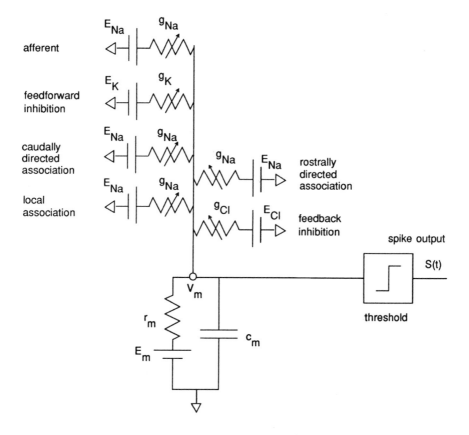

Figure 9.5
The circuit representation of a single-compartment pyramidal cell used in the model.
Synaptic inputs arrive at channels containing a variable conductance g, and an ionic
equilibrium potential E. The cell body is represented by a membrane resistance and
a membrane capacitance. Spike events are generated when the potential across the
membrane exceeds the threshold of the cell. These spike events are then propagated
to other cells along delay line axons.

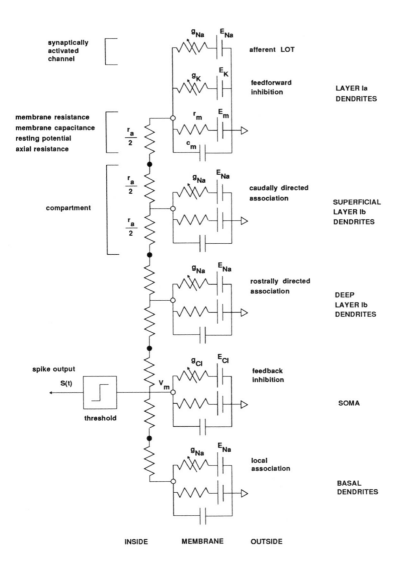

Figure 9.6
The circuit representation of a multicompartmental pyramidal cell used in the model.
There are five compartments, each containing a membrane resistance, membrane
capacitance, and resting potential, as well as one or more synaptically activated
conductances.

scale simulations to establish the macroscopic cortical behavior. A more detailed five-compartment model (fig. 9.6) is then used to generate the spatial distributions of current flow within a single neuron using patterns of inputs generated by the large-scale model. These current distributions are needed for the calculation of extracellular field potentials (see Appendix 9.B).

As discussed in general above, this approach reflects a compromise between the number versus complexity of the neuronal elements simulated. In using the single-compartment model during network simulations it is assumed that the spatial interactions of current flow within the dendritic tree of the neurons are not significant to the responses being modeled. While this assumption must be made with caution, comparison of somatic membrane potentials generated by both the single- and multicompartmental approaches show good agreement with real experiments. Therefore, this simplification may be appropriate as an initial approximation, in order to study basic cortical phenomena. However, synaptic events occurring in the dendritic tree can impose significant nonlinearities on the integration of currents at the somatic level (Koch et al. 1983). Network simulations that include explicit dendritic structure will allow more detailed study of the effects of patterned dendritic activation on cellular activity. This is particularly important in exploring the more complex questions concerning computation within the network.

9.4   Specific Network Implementation

We will now consider the mathematical details of the implementation of the model of piriform cortex. While the network being considered represents a specific region of cerebral cortex, the general mathematical formulation is actually quite generic. In fact, it has served as the basis for the development of a general-purpose network simulation software package, which is capable of simulating a wide range of cortical as well as noncortical network structures. This software is described briefly in the last section of this chapter. This simulation has also served as a model for studying the general question of how neural network simulations can be implemented on parallel computers as discussed in chapter 12.

9.4.1   Neuronal Output and Transmission Delays

The output of each modeled cell i consists of an all-or-none action potential S_i with unit amplitude that is generated when the membrane potential V_i of the cell crosses a threshold T_i and the cell has not fired for a refractory period t_r. The thresholds for each cell have a normal distribution with a mean of -45 mV and a variance of 5 mV. The resting membrane potentials are set uniformly at -70 mV.

$$S_i(t) = \begin{cases} 1 & V_i(t) \geq T_i, \text{ and } S_i(\lambda) = 0 \quad \text{for} \lambda \in [t - t_r, t] \\ 0 & \text{otherwise} \end{cases} \tag{9.1}$$

This output S_i propagates along fiber q to neurons j with a delay $t_{p(ijq)}$. The propagation delay from cell i to cell j along fiber q is

$$t_{p(ijq)} = \frac{L_{ij}}{\nu_q} \tag{9.2}$$

where L_{ij} is the the radial distance from the originating neuron i to the target neuron j, and ν_q is the velocity along the fiber type q that connects them.

There is an additional latency term $t_{\epsilon(ijq)}$ that represents the delay incurred at the synaptic junction. This corresponds to the time lag between the arrival of the presynaptic event and the generation of a postsynaptic response, nominally 800 μsec. Therefore the total time delay between generation of an action potential in the source cell and the generation of a postsynaptic event in the destination cell is

$$t_{t(ijq)} = t_{p(ijq)} + t_{\epsilon(ijq)} \tag{9.3}$$

9.4.2 Channel Conductance

When an action potential arrives at a destination cell it triggers a conductance change in a particular ionic channel described by the characteristic function $G(t)$ (see Appendix 9.C for the forms of this function). As already discussed, each class of ionic channel has a distinct set of parameters governing the time course, amplitude, and waveform of the conductance function (table 9.1). Therefore, the net channel conductance due to a single synaptic input $\hat{g}(t)$ is a function of presynaptic activation described by the function $S(t)$, and postsynaptic activation described by $G(t)$.

Since the characteristic postsynaptic conductance waveform $G(t)$ can have a time course longer than that of the presynaptic action potential, the influence of the discrete action potential event must be extended over the equivalent postsynaptic period. This effect can be described as the convolution of presynaptic events $S(t)$ with the postsynaptic conductance waveform $G(t)$. The net conductance in channel k of cell j due to input from cell i along fiber q is

$$\hat{g}(t)_{ijkq} = \int_0^{t-t_{t(ijq)}} G_{jk}(\lambda)S_i(t - \lambda - t_{t(ijq)})d\lambda \tag{9.4}$$

where $t_{t(ijq)}$ is the total delay time for presynaptic events $S_i(t)$ to reach cell j along fiber q. This function describes the synaptic transformation for spike activity across a single connection. The implementation of this synaptic transformation is discussed in Appendix 9.C and in section 9.7.3.

9.4.3   Synaptic Connections

In many simulations, especially those exploring possible learning mechanisms (Wilson and Bower 1988), it is important to be able to change the strengths of individual synaptic connections as a consequence of network activity. These synaptic strengths are specified by a weight term $\hat{w}_{ijq}$ in the basic synaptic transformation function, which describes the strength of connection between cell i and cell j along fiber q.

Physiological experiments in piriform cortex suggest that synaptic effects on postsynaptic cells vary in an activity-dependent manner both in the short term (Bower and Haberly 1985) and in the long term (Bower and Rao 1986). In the model the effects of variable synaptic efficacy are simulated using a synaptic weight term of the form

$$\hat{w}_{ijq}(t) = w_{ijq}^{static} w_{ijq}^{variable}(t) \tag{9.5}$$

where w^{static} does not vary during a simulation and corresponds to the static distribution of synaptic terminals, and $w^{variable}$ is, in general, a function of presynaptic activation S, postsynaptic state V, and time t. Since these weights modulate the amplitude of the postsynaptic conductance they must be non-negative.

The resulting conductance change induced by the activation of a single synapse is given by

$$\hat{g}(t)_{ijkq} = \int_0^{t-t_{t(ijq)}} G_{jk}(\lambda)S_i(t - \lambda - t_{t(ijq)})\hat{w}_{ijq}(t)d\lambda \tag{9.6}$$

This results in the weight applied in a "postsynaptic" fashion with the peak amplitude of the conductance continually varying at each time step.

A slightly modified form results in a "presynaptic" weighting in which the peak amplitude of the conductance is set at the time of arrival of the presynaptic signal S and remains at that value for its duration.

$$\hat{g}_{ijkq}(t) = \int_0^{t-t_{t(ijq)}} G_{jk}(\lambda)S_i(t - \lambda - t_{t(ijq)})\hat{w}_{ijq}(t - \lambda - t_{t(ijq)})d\lambda \tag{9.7}$$

9.4.4   Single-Cell Integration

The total conductance change induced in channel k of cell j is calculated by summing over all synaptic inputs to that channel.

$$g_{jk}(t) = \sum_{i=1}^{n_{cells}} \sum_{q=1}^{n_{fibers}(i)} \hat{g}_{ijkq} \qquad (9.8)$$

The membrane potential V for a single compartment (cell) j with n_c channels is computed by integrating

$$\frac{dV_j}{dt} = \frac{1}{c_m} \sum_{k=0}^{n_c} [E_k - V_j(t)]g_{jk}(t) + I_{inject} \qquad (9.9)$$

where I_{inject} takes into account any explicit current injection into the compartment and E_k is the equilibrium potential for channel type k. (See Appendix 9.A for the multicompartmental formulation.)

9.5   Setting Model Parameters

The majority of parameters in the model, such as axonal conduction velocities, time delays, the general properties of neuronal integration, and the major intrinsic neuronal connections, are estimated from anatomical and physiological measurements made within the actual cortex as described above (table 9.1). The weight term associated with each synapse is one of the primary variables subject to adjustment in the model. Determining actual values for synaptic weights in a cortical network as complex as piriform is an extremely difficult task. However, given that these weights modify conductance amplitude, modifying weights affects both the amplitude and time constants of membrane potentials. Therefore, actual experimental measurements of these factors can serve to constrain the operational range of weights. The second significant model variable not strongly constrained by experimental data is the pattern of specific cell-to-cell connections. In this case, experimentalists may never know the full matrix of interconnectivity for large-scale neural networks like piriform cortex. In the model, we constrain connectivity based on general connectivity patterns seen using anatomical and physiological techniques. However, it is an implicit assumption in this work that specific replication of actual connection patterns will not be necessary to derive functional information from these models.

9.6   Generation of Physiological Responses

Overall, our modeling of piriform cortex has proceeded in two stages. Our first objective was to replicate known cortical responses to various stimulation conditions (figs. 9.7, 9.8; Wilson and Bower 1988). Once this was accomplished we then proceeded to explore the possible functional capacities of this model (Wilson and Bower 1988). In both stages, to allow evaluation of simulated results, two neuronal output forms are generated by the simulation. First, time-varying values of membrane potential in modeled neurons are generated and directly compared with *in vivo* and *in vitro* intracellular recordings (fig. 9.7). Note again that the actual spike waveforms were not explicitly calculated but were "pasted" onto the actual membrane potential at the times corresponding to simulated spike output. Second, the simulations generate extracellular field potentials taken at discrete locations within the simulated cortex (fig. 9.7). This data is important for piriform cortex because of the wealth of field potential results available in both anesthetized and unanesthetized behaving animals (Freeman 1968, 1979a,b; Gault 1963, 1965). Field potential responses (evoked potentials, EEGs) are calculated by using a compartmental model of a pyramidal cell to establish the depth distribution of membrane currents given the pattern of input conductance changes generated by network simulation (see fig. 9.8 and Appendix 9.B). As mentioned above, further discussion of these results is beyond the scope of this chapter. The model has also allowed us to look at the spatial distribution of network activity (fig. 9.8).

9.7   Technical Implementation Issues

While the above discussion details the mathematical structure of the piriform cortex model, the computer simulation of this type of model raises specific technical implementation . In this section we will address several of these.

9.7.1   Integration Technique

Simulation of these models requires the numerical solution of systems of differential equations that describe the state of neurons as a function of time and space. These numerical techniques describe how one advances the state variables of the simulation (e.g., membrane potential) from time i to time $i+1$ through integration of the differential equations that describe the system. As discussed in Chapter 13, the primary factors

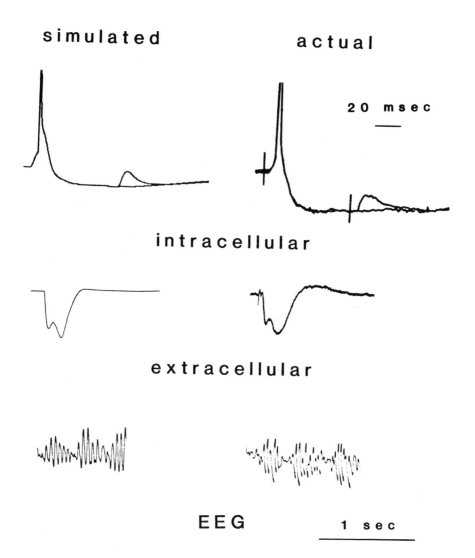

Figure 9.7
Upper right: Actual intracellular response recorded *invitro* (Bower and Haberly 1985) in response to paired shock stimuli applied to the LOT. The membrane potential of the cell was artificially depolarized to enhance the inhibitory hyperpolarization. Upper left: Simulated response under similar conditions. Middle right: Actual evoked potential response recorded *invivo* (Haberly and Bower 1984) in response to a single shock of the afferent LOT. Middle left: The simulated evoked potential contains the basic components of the actual data. Lower right: Actual EEG recorded from piriform cortex (Freeman 1960) consisting of a fast oscillatory component (30–80 Hz) modulated by a slower (3–8 Hz) component. Lower left: Simulated EEG with fast oscillations produced by alternating activation of excitatory and feedback inhibitory processes. The slow component coincides with the activation of the long-duration feedforward inhibitory process.

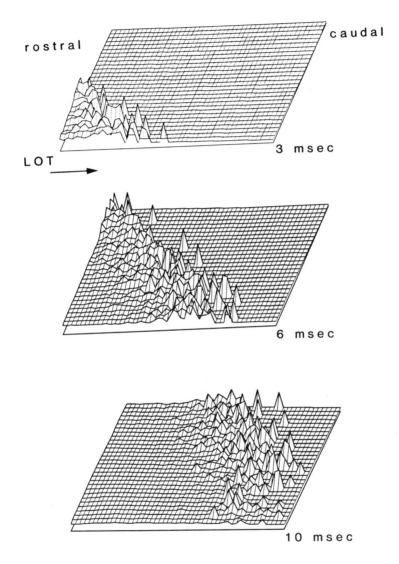

rostral

caudal

LOT

3 msec

6 msec

10 msec

Figure 9.8
Three successive snapshots taken of the membrane potential of all simulated pyramidal cells following a shock stimulus applied to the afferent LOT. LOT input enters in
the lower left corner of each frame. Activity is seen to propagate from rostral cortex
to caudal cortex in a wave-like fashion. In frame 1 the activity is carried primarily
along the fast, principal afferent fibers. By frame 3 the principal direction of the
wavefront has changed as afferent input weakens and pyramidal cell spike activity
begins propagating along the slower association fibers. (See fig. 9.3.)

that must be considered in selecting a particular technique are efficiency, accuracy, and stability. Efficiency refers to the amount of computation required to perform the integration. Accuracy reflects the degree to which solutions obtained match actual solutions. Stability is the behavior of the solution as time progresses. A system is convergently stable if it converges to a finite solution. However, methods that are stable are not necessarily accurate. Because the proper use of integration techniques is extremely important in these types of simulations, we have included a brief discussion of our results using several different techniques. For a thorough treatment of these methods refer to Chapter 13 as well as Press, Flannery, Teukolsky, and Vetterling (1986) or Smith (1985).

Large-scale networks can generally be treated as loosely coupled systems of ordinary differential equations that do not need to be solved simultaneously. In other words, evaluation of the state of any neuron in the system requires only past state information from other neurons and therefore can be solved independently for each neuron at every time step. These types of equations can typically be solved using simple numerical integration techniques. Two general categories of integration techniques will be discussed—explicit and implicit. In the following equations Δt refers to integration step size, y_i refers to the state variable at time i, and dy_i/dt is the time derivative of y evaluated at time i. For our purposes the state variable will typically be the membrane potential.

Explicit Techniques Explicit techniques solve for the state at discrete time $i + 1$ using derivatives evaluated at or before i. They are referred to as explicit because the new state is based on the known history of the system. Explicit techniques include forward Euler and Adams/Bashforth multi-step.

Forward Euler:

$$y_{i+1} = y_i + \Delta t \frac{dy_i}{dt} \tag{9.10}$$

Euler is the least accurate with marginal stability.

Adams-Bashforth: the following is the two-step Adams-Bashforth algorithm.

$$y_{i+1} = y_i + \frac{\Delta t}{2}(3\frac{dy_i}{dt} - \frac{dy_{i-1}}{dt}) \tag{9.11}$$

The Adams-Bashforth methods are more accurate but are also somewhat unstable.

Exponential: assuming a first-order form for the state equations with constant coefficients A and B over the interval Δt

$$\frac{dy}{dt} = -By + A \tag{9.12}$$

we can directly integrate the differential equation and obtain the solution. Through experimentation with our model, we have found that this technique has good stability and accuracy characteristics when used to solve membrane equations (MacGregor 1987).

$$y_{i+1} = y_i e^{-B\Delta t} + \frac{A}{B}(1 - e^{-B\Delta t}) \tag{9.13}$$

For example, given the membrane equation 9.9

$$\frac{dV}{dt} = \frac{1}{c_m}\left[\sum_{k=0}^{n_{channels}} (E_k - V)G_k + I \right] \tag{9.14}$$

$$A = \frac{1}{c_m} \sum E_k G_k + I \tag{9.15}$$

$$B = \frac{1}{c_m} \sum G_k \tag{9.16}$$

Implicit Techniques   Another class of numerical integration schemes are the implicit techniques that solve for the state at time $i + 1$ using the derivative evaluated at $i + 1$. Common implicit techniques include Gear second-order and trapezoidal integration.

Gear:

$$y_{i+1} = \frac{4}{3}y_i - \frac{1}{3}y_{i-1} + \frac{2}{3}\Delta t \frac{dy_{i+1}}{dt} \tag{9.17}$$

Trapezoidal:

$$y_{i+1} = y_i + \frac{\Delta t}{2}\left(\frac{dy_{i+1}}{dt} + \frac{dy_i}{dt}\right) \tag{9.18}$$

Implicit techniques are stable and are typically used in systems of stiff equations where the presence of widely differing time constants can result in instability using more conventional explicit techniques.

Comparison Overall, the explicit exponential and the implicit trape-zoidal technique were found to be the best integration algorithms for solving neuronal membrane equations in terms of efficiency, stability, and accuracy.

9.7.2 Step Size

Several factors are involved in selecting the simulation step size Δt. One consideration is the maximum integration step size that can be used to update the neuronal state variables. This can be affected by the nu-merical algorithm used as well as the conditions being simulated. As a general rule the integration time step should be less than 1/5 of the fastest time constant of interest to minimize integration errors. In prac-tice, lower-order integration techniques such as forward Euler require substantially smaller time steps.

The characteristics of the conductance waveform $G(t)$ will have a strong influence on the errors introduced during integration and there-fore on the step size selected. Sudden or high amplitude conductance changes can result in rapid changes in the transmembrane current (eq. 9.9), which must be integrated with small step sizes to minimize errors. Another consideration in step size selection is the minimum propagation delay between elements. The step size chosen should not be made larger than this quantity if accurate intercell propagation tim-ings are to be preserved. In general the maximum error in intercell propagation times will be equivalent to one-half the step size selected, and therefore the maximal timing error between events arriving at a cell from different sources will be equivalent to the step size. In cases where there is a large discrepancy between the step size dictated by integration and by intercell delay an approach involving multiple step sizes may be appropriate.

9.7.3 Implementation of the Synaptic Transformation

The transformation of neuronal output (spikes) to dendritic input (con-ductance) can be described as a convolution of the incoming spike signal with a characteristic conductance waveform. Two basic techniques can be used to perform this operation.

Explicit Convolution Two approaches can be taken to directly im-plement the convolution described in eq. 9.4. In both cases a history of spike signals $S(t)$ must be maintained for each cell. To reduce com-putation time, we restrict the interval over which incoming spikes are convolved with the channel conductance waveforms $G(t)$ to t_d. The

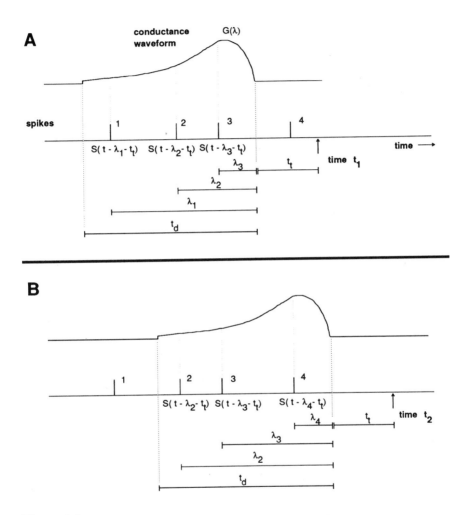

Figure 9.9
A schematic representation of the convolution operation used to transform spike output $S(t)$ into synaptic conductance change $\hat{g}(t)$ (eq. 9.4). (A) shows the spike history of a single cell being mapped onto a synaptic target at time t_1 using the conductance waveform $G(t)$. The total conductance change induced by the source cell is computed as $\hat{g}(t_1) = G(\lambda_1)S(t_1 - \lambda_1 - t_t) + G(\lambda_2 - t_t)S(t_1 - \lambda_2 - t_t) + G(\lambda_3 - t_t)S(t_1 - \lambda_3 - t_t)$. (B) shows the same mapping at a later time t_2. The time between the leading edge of the conductance waveform G and the current time t_2 remains constant (total delay t_t, eq. 9.3) while the spikes contained within the convolution interval t_d change. The total conductance change induced by the source cell at the new time t_2 is computed as $\hat{g}(t_2) = G(\lambda_2)S(t_2 - \lambda_2 - t_t) + G(\lambda_3 - t_t)S(t_2 - \lambda_3 - t_t) + G(\lambda_4 - t_t)S(t_2 - \lambda_4 - t_t)$.

length of time over which history must be maintained is given by $t_t + t_d$. The t_t factor is required to implement propagation delay. This results in a modified expression for the conductance

$$\hat{g}_{ijkq}(t) = \int_0^{t_{d(k)}} G_{jk}(\lambda) S_i(t - \lambda - t_{t(ijq)}) d\lambda \qquad (9.19)$$

Assuming that the conductance waveform function $G(t)$ is only a function of time, the convolution with the discrete signal $S(t)$ can be precalculated over the interval $[0, t_d]$ and stored at the destination site. Since the time spent communicating information between cells is a significant computational overhead, this approach can potentially reduce the amount of computation at the cost of storage proportional to $t_d / \Delta t$ per synaptic target.

An alternate approach involves evaluating eq. 9.17 at each point within the interval t_d in step with the simulation. This requires no additional storage but adds additional communication proportional to $t_d / \Delta t$ since the term $S(t)$ (the signal sent between neurons) must be accessed at each step.

Second-Order System   A second approach uses a time differential representation of the conductance waveform. The conductance is modeled as a damped oscillator that has an impulse response of the form shown in eqs. 9.33 and 9.36. The impulse is provided by the spike input $S(t)$. In this case the value of the conductance is computed using current state information and explicit convolution is not necessary. This reduces the amount of history that must be maintained from $t_t + t_d$ to t_t. See Appendix 9.C for the implementation details.

Comparison   The advantage of explicit convolution is that arbitrary conductance waveforms are easily implemented. The disadvantage is that there is either a storage or computational overhead that is on the order of the number of synaptic connections. The second-order or differential representation typically requires less computation and storage but implementation of arbitrary conductance functions is not straightforward. See Appendix 9.C for detailed comparisons.

9.7.4   Computational Requirements

The simulations of piriform cortex described were carried out on a Sun Microsystems 3/260 model microcomputer equipped with 32 *Mbytes* of memory and a floating point accelerator. These simulations of 4,500 cells (1,500 of each type) ran at a nominal rate of approximately 10 *cpu sec* per step. With a step size of 0.1 *msec* the average time for a 200 *msec* simulation was 300 *cpu min*. Using explicit convolution to compute the conductance, over 90% of the computation involved the distribution of information between elements, with the remaining time spent updating the states of individual elements. The overall computation time was very sensitive to fluctuations in activity level. Using the second-order representation, the computation was more evenly balanced between spike distribution (60%) and state update (40%) with less sensitivity to fluctuations in activity. The memory required for these simulations exceeded 24 *Mbytes* primarily due to storage of synaptic connections. This scale of simulation was operating at the upper limits of the computing resources available. As would be expected, simulations that are on the scale of hundreds of elements operate at a considerably faster rate and utilize more modest amounts of memory. For example, equivalent simulations using 300 cells (100 of each type) ran at a rate of 0.05 *cpu sec* per step. The average time for a 200 *msec* simulation was 1.5 *cpu min* and the memory required for this scale of simulation was approximately 2 *Mbytes*. Thus implementation of this type of simulation on the scale of hundreds of cells is quite feasible even on currently available PC class machines.

9.7.5 Storage Considerations

A problem in using individually specified synaptic weights and delays is that their number can expand as the square of the number of neurons in the simulation. This overhead in storage can limit the size of the network. An alternative representation for synaptic connections can be used if uniqueness of individual synapses is not critical. This representation takes the form of connection rules that describe how a representative cell connects with other cells using coordinates relative to the representative cell. The information stored in this source-relative connection scheme is both a delay and synaptic weight term. In this way a representative connection pattern takes up an amount of space proportional to that required by connections from a single cell.

9.8   The Simulator

Instructed by the model of piriform cortex just described, we have been developing a general-purpose simulation tool that allows the construction of arbitrary neuronal simulations. This effort was motivated by several factors. First, we believe that powerful but flexible simulation software will increase the likelihood that neurobiologists will build structural models of their systems. Second, we hope that the availability of a standard for simulations of this type would provide a means for exchange of modeling data and results and therefore accelerate progress in understanding these exceedingly complex neuronal structures. Third, we believe that a critical issue for the acceptance of simulations as a tool in neurobiology is the degree to which simulation results can be replicated. The availability of standard simulation software makes this much easier to accomplish. Fourth, while any neural network simulation designed with a particular network in mind can be optimized for maximum efficiency, a tremendous time investment is required to build such a system. In the process of designing the simulator we have found that the principal features of most neuronal networks are common enough that a general network simulator is not only possible but also remarkably efficient.

9.8.1 Overall Simulator Structure—in Brief

Within the network simulator GENESIS, components are constructed out of basic building blocks called elements. In the most general sense, an element is a structure that receives inputs, performs transformations on these inputs, and generates outputs. Thus, an element can represent a membrane compartment, a simple cell, or a complex dendritic structure. This is the principal source of the simulator's generality. Once constructed, these components can then be combined into networks that have varied classes of interconnectivity, from graded signals sent with no delay, to discrete signals that propagate with finite velocity. Single elements maintain lists of input and output transformation modules. The simulator maintains a library of these modules that can be extended by the user. This extendible modularity allows multiple classes of transformations within an element. Since each element is a distinct functional unit, homogeneous structure within a network is also not a limitation. Elements are maintained in a hierarchical form allowing the simulation of models at various levels of complexity and detail. Figure 9.10 shows a block diagram of the simulator implementation of the model of piriform cortex.

The simulator shell environment allows interactive access to user-expandable network specification functions and allows interactive run-time specification and manipulation of model structures and parameters. The graphical specification and display tools provide the means to construct custom graphics interface environments for individual simulations.

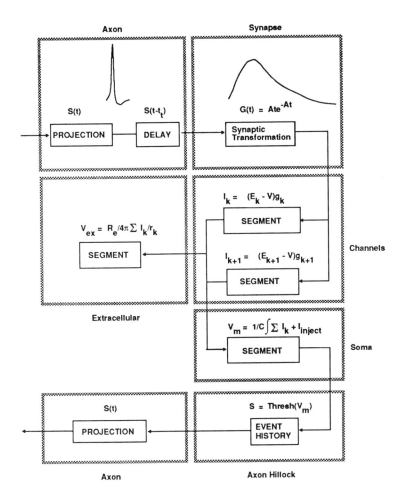

Figure 9.10
Schematic diagram showing the primary components of the single-cell model used in
the simulations of piriform cortex and their mathematical correlates. The structure
reflects the implementation of the model in the network simulator GENESIS.

9.8.2   Parallel Implementation

The object-oriented nature of the simulator design allows the basic simulator components to be easily broken up into functional pieces. The way in which these pieces can then be distributed across a parallel architecture is discussed in chapter 12. An important point is that since information is constrained to flow through simulator communication facilities, support for parallel architectures can be provided in a transparent, controlled fashion while still allowing the flexibility of user-defined functionality. The ability for the user to easily add varied functionality to the basic simulator framework is a critical factor in the simulator design.

9.8.3   Simulator Requirements

The simulator itself requires 300 *Kbytes* of memory. The optional graphics module adds an additional 300 *Kbytes*. A moderately complex cell requires from 500–1000 *bytes* with an additional 16 *bytes* for each connection. Thus, a small fully connected network on the scale of 100 cells uses approximately 200 *Kbytes*. The simulator runs under the Unix operating system. The graphical specification and display facilities have been written using the X windowing system for maximum portability. The simulator runs on a number Unix-based systems including SUN3, SUN4, SUN386i, and Masscomp computers. It is designed to be easily portable to other Unix-based systems.

The address of Matthew Wilson and James Bower is Division of Biology 216-76, California Institute of Technology, Pasadena, California 91125. Readers interested in further information on the simulator should send requests via electronic mail to genesis@aurel.caltech.edu .

Appendix 9.A: Multicompartmental Model

In the multicompartment implementation of the pyramidal cells, each compartment consists of one or more synaptic input channels, a membrane resistance r_m, and a membrane capacitance c_m (fig. 9.6).

$$r_m = \frac{R_m}{\pi l d} \tag{9.20}$$

$$c_m = C_m \pi l d \tag{9.21}$$

where l is the length of the dendritic segment, and d is its diameter. R_m is the membrane resistivity and C_m is the capacitance per unit area.

As in the case of single-compartment neurons, each channel k consists of a time-varying conductance $g_k(t)$ in series with a voltage source E_k representing the equilibrium potential of the ion associated with the channel. However, in this case, each compartment is also coupled to its adjacent compartment(s) with an axial resistance r_a. This axial resistance is divided in two and placed on either side of the lumped membrane representation for a symmetric compartment.

$$r_a = \frac{1}{2} \left[\frac{4 R_a l}{\pi d^2} \right] \tag{9.22}$$

where R_a is the axial resistivity. Therefore, the input to each compartment has two primary components, an axial and a transmembrane current.

If we select a compartment and designate its two axial ends with $+$ and $-$ then the total axial current into the compartment is given by

$$I_a = I_a^- + I_a^+ \tag{9.23}$$

where the individual axial components from the two adjoining compartments are calculated by

$$I_a^- = \frac{V^- - V}{r_a^- + r_a} \quad , \quad I_a^+ = \frac{V^+ - V}{r_a^+ + r_a} \tag{9.24}$$

V is the membrane potential of the compartment. V^{+-} is the membrane potential of the compartment on the $+$ and $-$ side of the compartment respectively and r_a^{+-} is the axial resistance of that compartment. I_a^{+-} is the current entering the compartment from the $+-$ side. To simplify notation the time-dependent variables $V(t)$ and $I(t)$ are written as V and I.

The boundary conditions assume sealed ends with $I_a^{+-} = 0$. This can be extended to a branching structure using

$$I_a^{+-} = \left[\sum_{j=1}^{N^{+-}} \frac{(V^{j+-} - V)}{r_a^{j+-}} \right] \left[1 + r_a \sum_{j=1}^{N^{+-}} \frac{1}{r_a^{j+-}} \right]^{-1} \tag{9.25}$$

where N^{+-} is the number of compartments adjoining the $+$ and $-$ side of the compartment respectively.[1] With $N^{+-} = 1$ this simplifies to eq. 9.20, which applies a dendritic cable.

The ohmic portion of the transmembrane current is given by

$$I_m = \frac{E_{rest} - V}{r_m} + \sum_{k=0}^{n_{channels}} (E_k - V) g_k(t) \tag{9.26}$$

The first term represents the passive leakage component with resting potential E_{rest} and leakage resistance r_m. The summation term gives the input through synaptically activated conductances $g_k(t)$. These conductances are activated by the arrival of presynaptic signals.

The membrane potential V of each compartment is calculated by integrating the current across the membrane capacitance. The differential change in membrane potential with time is given by

$$\frac{dV}{dt} = \frac{1}{c_m}(I_a + I_m) \tag{9.27}$$

Appendix 9.B: Field Potentials

Field potentials are generated when membrane currents generated by neurons pass through the extracellular space. These currents can be set up both by active output processes such as action potentials, as well as by input processes such as synaptic currents. The field potential at any point will be composed of the linear superposition of fields generated by current sources (current from the intracellular space to the extracellular space) and sinks (current from the extracellular space into the intracellular space) distributed along multiple cells. In the following discussion the term "current source" will be used to refer to both sources and sinks.

The value of the field potential depends on the extracellular resistivity, the location and amplitude of the current sources, and the location of the

---

[1] Note that this formulation is identical to that for asymmetric compartments with the addition of the right-hand denominator term. Thus the symmetric compartment requires slightly more computation than its asymmetric counterpart but is a more accurate representation of neurons consisting of smaller numbers of compartments.

recording electrode relative to the current sources. For example, when the recording electrode is approximately equidistant from a large number of current sources it will measure the spatially averaged field produced by these sources. This corresponds to an electrode placed on the cortical surface measuring the fields generated by a sheet of neurons beneath it (as in the EEG). As a separate example, an electrode placed very close to a smaller number of current sources would preferentially record the fields generated by those sources. This corresponds to a microelectrode placed close to the spike-generating mechanism of a single cell to measure its isolated spike output (as in extracellular single-unit recording).

The exact contributions to the field potential by neuronal activity depend largely on the geometry of single cells and network circuitry, as well as the spatial and temporal patterns of activity both within a cell (e.g., sequence of dendritic activation), and among groups of cells (e.g., synchrony of firing).

Consider the multicompartmental model used to generate the spatial distributions of membrane currents. The model computes a single transmembrane current I_m intended to represent the "lumped" current across a section of membrane. If we assign each compartment an x, y, z coordinate, we can treat each lumped transmembrane current I_m as a point current source located at those coordinates.

For point current sources distributed in a linear noncapacitive medium we have (Nunez 1981)

$$V_f(t) = \frac{R_e}{4\pi} \sum_{j=1}^{n_{cells}} \sum_{k=1}^{n_{compartments}} \frac{I_{m(jk)}(t)}{r_{jk}} \qquad (9.28)$$

where

$$r_{jk} = \left[(x' - x_{jk})^2 + (y' - y_{jk})^2 + (z' - z_{jk})^2 \right]^{\frac{1}{2}} \qquad (9.29)$$

The coordinates (x', y', z') give the location of the recording site. The coordinates (x^{jk}, y^{jk}, z^{jk}) give the coordinates of the compartment k in cell j. r_{jk} is the distance from compartment k in cell j to the recording site. $I_{m(jk)}$ is the transmembrane current in compartment k of cell j. R_e gives the extracellular resistivity per unit distance assuming a homogeneous extracellular medium (constant resistivity). V_f is an estimate of the extracellular field potential at (x', y', z').

Thus, in order to compute an estimate of the field potential the total transmembrane current for each compartment in each cell is summed according to the inverse distance of the current source (compartment) from the simulated recording site.

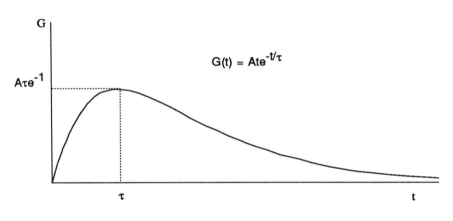

Figure 9.11
Waveform of the alpha function (eq. 9.33).

Appendix 9.C: Synaptic Transformation

Synaptic Convolution Operation

Truncating the conductance function $G(t)$ after time t_d as in eq. 9.19 can introduce rapid changes in transmembrane current. These fast transients can induce numerical instability in the integration of the membrane potential. Several methods can be used to avoid this problem. One technique is to extend the integration interval t_d such that it is many time constants τ in duration. This approach minimizes the discontinuities at the expense of increased computation. Another approach involves modifying the conductance function to eliminate discontinuities. One modification of the conductance function uses a quarter-period of a cosine function applied after the peak of $G(t)$ to force it smoothly to zero after the desired duration t_d. In this way the peak amplitude, peak latency, and rise time of the original conductance function $G(t)$ are preserved while discontinuities at time t_d are eliminated.

$$\hat{G}(t) = G(t)\left[(1 - U(t - t_{peak})) + U(t - t_{peak})cos\left[\frac{\pi}{2}\frac{(t - t_{peak})}{(t_d - t_{peak})}\right]\right] \quad (9.30)$$

where t_{peak} is the time to peak of the conductance function and $U(t)$ is the unit step function.

Second-order Synaptic Transformation

The general second-order form of the differential transformation equation is

$$\ddot{G} + \alpha\dot{G} + \beta G = x(t) \tag{9.31}$$

$$\alpha = \frac{\tau_1 + \tau_2}{\tau_1 \tau_2}, \beta = \frac{1}{\tau_1 \tau_2} \tag{9.32}$$

The impulse response of this system $(x(t) = \delta(t))$ with initial conditions of $G(0) = 0$ has two basic forms.

Alpha function   Under the condition where $\tau_1 = \tau_2 = \tau$,

$$G(t) = te^{-t/\tau} \tag{9.33}$$

The time to peak of this form is

$$t_{peak} = \tau \tag{9.34}$$

and the peak value at that time is

$$G_{peak} = \tau e^{-1} \tag{9.35}$$

Dual exponential   For $\tau_1 \neq \tau_2$,

$$G(t) = \frac{\tau_1 \tau_2}{\tau_1 - \tau_2}(e^{-t/\tau_1} - e^{-t/\tau_2}) \tag{9.36}$$

The time to peak is given by

$$t_{peak} = \frac{\tau_1 \tau_2}{\tau_1 - \tau_2}\ln(\frac{\tau_1}{\tau_2}) \tag{9.37}$$

and the peak value at that time is

$$G_{peak} = \frac{\tau_1 \tau_2}{\tau_1 - \tau_2}(e^{-t_{peak}/\tau_1} - e^{-t_{peak}/\tau_2}) \tag{9.38}$$

Practical implementation   The objective is to solve the second-order equation for $G(t)$ at each time step t and then solve for the net conductance change $\hat{g}(t)$. The second-order system can be described by two first-order equations.

$$\dot{z} = \frac{-1}{\tau_1}z + x(t) \tag{9.39}$$

$$\dot{G} = \frac{-1}{\tau_2}G + z \tag{9.40}$$

In our case $x(t) = S(t - t_t)$. If "presynaptic" weighting is included this becomes $x(t) = S(t - t_t)w(t)$.

These equations can be numerically integrated to yield $G(t)$ using the techniques mentioned in section 9.7.1. The net conductance is then calculated by

$$\hat{g}(t) = \frac{g_{peak}}{G_{peak}}G(t) \tag{9.41}$$

or with "postsynaptic" weighting

$$\hat{g}(t) = \frac{g_{peak}}{G_{peak}}G(t)w(t) \tag{9.42}$$

where g_{peak} is the desired peak conductance value.

The following equations describe one method for advancing the solution to $G(t)$ from time t to time $t + \Delta t$. If spikes are considered to take the form of impulse functions then $x(t) = S(t - t_t)/\Delta t$, where $S(t - t_t)$ is the amplitude of a spike that occurred at time $t - t_t$. The variable z can then be evaluated as

$$z_{t+\Delta t} = z_t e^{\Delta t/\tau_1} + \frac{S(t - t_t)}{\Delta t}\tau_1(1 - e^{\Delta t/\tau_1}) \tag{9.43}$$

and the conductance G is given by

$$G_{t+\Delta t} = G_t e^{\Delta t/\tau_2} + z_t\tau_2(1 - e^{\Delta t/\tau_2}) \tag{9.44}$$

The net conductance is then obtained as in eqs. 9.41 or 9.42.

Comparisons

We can compare the computational overhead associated with various implementations of the synaptic transformation by calculating estimated simulation time.

N_{sp} = the number of spikes in the interval t (total simulation time)
N_{syn} = number of synaptic connections
N_{st} = number of time steps in the interval t_d (convolution interval)

N_t = number of time steps in the interval t
N_{ch} = number of channels or synaptic targets
T_c = computation per step for communication (spike propagation)
T_s = computation per step for second-order conductance calculation
T_g = computation per step for convolution conductance calculation
$N_{st} = t_d/\Delta t$
$N_t = t/\Delta t$

In the main text, three methods for performing the synaptic transformation are described. The first is explicit convolution using precalculation of the conductance waveform with storage. The second is explicit convolution involving no storage. The third is the differential or second-order method.

The method of convolution with precalculation requires an amount of computation proportional to

$$T_{computation} = N_{syn}N_{sp}T_c + N_{syn}N_{sp}N_{st}T_g \qquad (9.45)$$

with additional storage proportional to $N_{syn}N_{st}$.

For explicit convolution without storage we have

$$T_{computation} = N_{syn}N_{sp}N_{st}T_c + N_{syn}N_{sp}N_{st}T_g \qquad (9.46)$$

We can see that there is an additional factor of N_{st} in the first term (communication) while the second terms (calculation) are equivalent.

For the differential representation we have

$$T_{computation} = N_{syn}N_{sp}T_c + N_{ch}N_tT_s \qquad (9.47)$$

In this formulation we see that the first term is as efficient as the convolution with precalculation without the storage overhead. The second term can be compared with the explicit convolution methods by looking at the factors N_{ch} versus N_{syn} and N_t versus $N_{st}N_{sp}$. Typically the number of synaptic targets or channels will be much less than the number of synapses N_{syn}. Additionally, factor N_t will be smaller than $N_{st}N_{sp}$ if there is overlap of the conductance intervals. Therefore, in general, the differential representation will be more computationally efficient than either of the explicit convolution methods.

As a sample calculation, we will examine a simulation of 100 cells each containing 5 synaptically activated channels. The simulation duration is 200 $msec$ with $\Delta t = 1$ $msec$. All synaptic conductances have duration of 10 $msec$.

N_{syn}	10000 synapses	N_{ch}	500 channels
N_{st}	10 steps	N_t	200 steps
T_c	0.02 msec/synapse	T_s	0.1 msec/channel
T_g	0.005 msec/synapse		

for $N_{sp} = 20$

	communication	calculation	total
T_1	4 sec	10 sec	14 sec
T_2	40 sec	10 sec	50 sec
T_3	4 sec	10 sec	14 sec

for $N_{sp} = 100$

	communication	calculation	total
T_1	20 sec	50 sec	70 sec
T_2	200 sec	50 sec	250 sec
T_3	20 sec	10 sec	30 sec

for $N_{sp} = 100$ and $\Delta t = 0.1$, which gives $N_{st} = 100$, and $N_t = 2000$.

	communication	calculation	total
T_1	20 sec	500 sec	520 sec
T_2	2000 sec	500 sec	2500 sec
T_3	20 sec	100 sec	120 sec

where T_1 is the computation time required for convolution with pre-calculation, T_2 is for explicit convolution, and T_3 is for the differential representation.

Appendix 9.D: Sample Calculation for Evaluation of Output Representation

In the following discussion the term "source" will refer to cells which are generating output while "target" will refer to cells receiving input.

N_s^s = the number of simulated cells in the source region
N_s^a = the actual number of cells in the source region to be simulated
N_t^a = the actual number of cells in the target region to be simulated
N_c = the number of connections on a target cell from cells in the source region of the actual network

What we wish to obtain is a simple measure of the appropriateness of the single-spike representation versus the spatially averaged output representation as discussed in the main text. This measure is based on an estimation of the number of connections between a cell in the target region and cells within the representative source region.

The total number of connections made in the target region is given by

$$T_c = \sum_{\lambda}^{N_t^a} N_c(\lambda) \tag{9.48}$$

In the case of uniformly distributed connections $T_c = N_c N_t^a$.

The number of connections made per source cell is

$$C_s = \frac{N_c N_t^a}{N_s^a} \tag{9.49}$$

The number of cells in the representative source region is

$$N_r = \frac{N_s^a}{N_s^s} \tag{9.50}$$

The estimated number of cells in the source region that project to a single target cell is given by

$$N_p = \frac{C_s N_r}{N_t^a} = \frac{N_c}{N_s^s} \tag{9.51}$$

The measure of output representation can be summarized as

$N_p > 1$ spatial average approximation with N_p discrete levels
$N_p \leq 1$ single-cell approximation with connection sparsity equal to N_p

Therefore, for valid single-spike approximation of cell output

$$N_s^s \geq N_c \tag{9.52}$$

For example, in the simulations of piriform cortex, looking at connectivity between cells within the cortex we have $N_s^s = N_c = 10^3$, giving $N_p = 1$ Thus the scale of the piriform cortex simulations lies at the transition point between fully connected single-cell output and discrete-level spatial average output.

For small N_s the spatial average technique provides an estimate that is more sensitive, in a relative sense, to variability in output levels given variability in input levels. The continuous approximation for the output level will be a function of N_p. As N_p increases the resolution or number of discrete levels that the averaged output can take increases, making a continuous or at least a higher resolution output desirable. Single-cell input and output parameters must take into account the continuous nature of the output. We will assume that the effect of the averaged output will be to activate a synaptic conductance change in the target cell consistent with the single-spike effect. The instantaneous value of conductance should reflect the expected value of the conductance given input from multiple sources. If the components of the input are assumed to be independent in time, then the expected value is simply the sum of the mean value of the individual conductance waveforms. This allows the conductance to be represented as a function of input amplitude alone. The assumption of independence is clearly a major simplification. The presence of local excitatory and inhibitory connectivity would indicate that cells in a region are not independent but are influenced by the structure of local circuitry. Yet both the single-spike and spatial-average approaches make implicit assumptions concerning the significance of local variability in the output of a region of cells. Unfortunately this issue cannot be resolved without increases in simulation size or complexity of local transformations, both of which require a deeper understanding of the structure and function of local circuitry.

Synchronous coactivation of cells within a source region reduces the independence of output activity. This has the effect of reducing the number of independent connections N_c on the target cells, thereby reducing the single-spike criterion N_p. In the extreme case of complete coactivation, which is the approximate effect of commonly used shock stimulation, $N_c = 1$ and the input can be safely reduced to a single fiber that has single-valued spike output.

Table 9.1: Model parameters for piriform cortex

t_r	absolute refractory period	10 $msec$
t_ϵ	synaptic delay	0.8 msec
$t_{\epsilon(ff)}$	feedforward inhibitory delay	50 $msec$
τ_{Na}	excitatory conductance time constant	3 $msec$
τ_{Cl}	feedback inhibitory conductance time constant	10 $msec$
τ_K	feedforward inhibitory conductance time constant	50 $msec$
$G_{peak(Na)}$	peak excitatory conductance	50 nS
$G_{peak(Cl)}$	peak feedback inhibitory conductance	200 nS
$G_{peak(K)}$	peak feedforward inhibitory conductance	5 nS
r_m	membrane leakage resistance	100 $M\Omega$
c_m	membrane capacitance	100 pF
E_{Na}	excitatory equilibrium potential	55 mV
E_{Cl}	feedback inhibitory equilibrium potential	−65 mV
E_K	feedforward inhibitory equilibrium potential	−90 mV
E_m	resting membrane potential	−90 mV
ν_{LOT}	main afferent LOT velocity	7 m/s
ν_{col}	afferent collateral velocity	1.6 m/s
ν_{ros}	rostrally directed velocity	1.0 m/s
ν_{cau}	caudally directed velocity	0.5 m/s
ν_{inh}	inhibitory velocity	1.0 m/s

Multicompartmental pyramidal cell parameters

C_m	membrane capacitance	1 $\mu F/cm^2$
R_m	membrane resistance	2000 Ωcm^2
R_e	extracellular resistance	50 Ω/cm
R_a	intracellular resistance	50 Ωcm

Cellular dimensions

segment	length (μm)	diameter (μm)
apical Ia dendrites	100	1.5
superficial Ib dendrites	100	1.5
deep Ib dendrites	100	1.5
soma	30	30
basal dendrites	200	1.5

CHAPTER 10

Modeling the Mammalian Visual System

UDO WEHMEIER, DAWEI DONG, CHRISTOF KOCH, and
DAVID VAN ESSEN

10.1 Introduction

The previous chapter dealt extensively with the problem of simulating
the electrical activity of a large number of neurons based on the anatomical and physiological constraints imposed by experimental data. These
simulations included an explicit representation of time, for instance by
accounting for axonal propagation times, and were applied to modeling
the mammalian olfactory cortex. However, given the widespread interest in the mammalian visual system from both the neuroscience and the
computer vision community, we felt that it would be useful to have one
chapter exclusively devoted to this particular system. Accordingly, we
will describe detailed computer simulations of the early visual system in
the cat, extending from the retina to the cortex. We will mainly discuss
those aspects of the model that differ from the previous chapter.

The principal aim of the work discussed here is to understand the
neuronal circuitry underlying one of the most elementary properties of
cells in the visual cortex of mammals, namely their preference to maximally respond to elongated bars of a certain orientation (for a review
see Ferster and Koch 1987). Cells can be so selective to this particular
feature that a mere $10°$ angle displacement off the optimal orientation
can reduce the maximal neuronal response by a factor of 2. The major question that any model of this phenomenon must address is how
the response of cortical neurons is so critically dependent on the orientation, even though their input fibers, arising from cells in the lateral
geniculate nucleus (LGN), are largely insensitive to orientation. The
first—and most influential—model for orientation selectivity was proposed over twenty-five years ago (Hubel and Wiesel 1962). It postulated that orientation selectivity arises from an appropriate alignment
of synaptic input, such that cells whose receptive fields fall along a row
excite the cortical cell (see fig. 10.1).

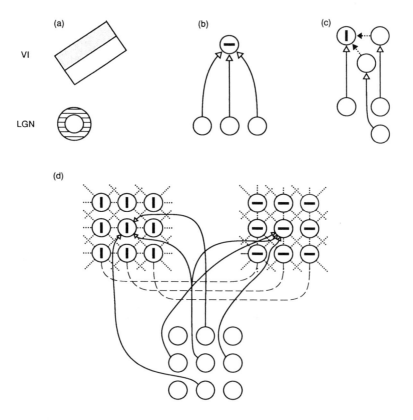

Figure 10.1
Wiring underlying orientation selectivity. (a) The concentric center-surround receptive field of geniculate cells contrasts with the elongated receptive fields of their
cortical target cells. (b) The excitatory-only model put forth by Hubel and Wiesel
(1962). A number of geniculate cells whose receptive fields are located along a given
axis monosynaptically excite the cortical cell (open arrows). Here and in the following, only the excitatory centers of the geniculate cells are drawn. (c) One instance of
an inhibitory-only model. Nonoriented cortical inhibitory (filled arrows) interneurons
shape the orientation tuning of their target cell by suppressing its response at nonoptimal orientations. In the example shown, a horizontal bar will lead to activation of
the interneuron, which will inhibit the vertically oriented cortical cell. (d) Eclectic
model combining features of all models (Koch 1987; Ferster and Koch 1987). An
excitatory Hubel and Wiesel type of presynaptic arrangement is superimposed upon
two inhibitory ones: reciprocal inhibition among similarly oriented cortical cells with
spatially nonoverlapping receptive fields (dotted lines) and cross-orientation inhibition among orthogonal oriented cells (dashed lines). Due to the massive feedback
among the participating cortical neurons, each cell acquires orientation selectivity
via a collective computation.

Alternative models have invoked the use of inhibition to shape orientation tuning (Benevento, Creutzfeldt, and Kuhnt 1972; Bishop, Coombs, and Henry 1971; Braitenberg and Braitenberg 1979; Morrone, Burr, and Maffei 1982; Sillito 1975; Sillito, Kemp, Milson, and Berardi 1980; Heggelund 1981, 1986; Orban 1984): the cell is prevented from firing at nonoptimal orientations by the action of inhibitory cortical interneurons. Current electrophysiological evidence is ambiguous, since support can be found for both classes of models.

These models are all instances of what Sejnowski, Koch, and Churchland (1988) term simplifying brain model, in that they show how orientation can be computed by invoking some of the principal structural features of the visual system, for instance center-surround receptive fields or the columnar organization of cortex. In other words, these models demonstrate that—given some general anatomical and physiological constraints—orientation can be computed in the manner postulated. However, in order to answer the question of which of these models is compatible with all of the relevant anatomical and physiological data, for instance with the large amount of divergence between the lateral geniculate nucleus and visual cortex or with the massive feedback within cortex, much more detailed simulations have to be attempted.

Since our detailed model of orientation selectivity incorporates a novel idea—that massive inhibitory cortical feedback can establish orientation selectivity without the need for nonoriented interneurons—we first evaluated its ability to correctly compute orientation using a very simplified model of neurons, based on Hopfield's elegant (1984) formalism (see chapter 7). Given the great simplicity of this model—compared to our detailed simulations—it allows us to understand quickly some of the key aspects of the model without a heavy programming burden. For instance, massive inhibition among cortical cells (fig. 10.1d) establishes orientation selectivity for all cortical cells and enables the system to work over a large range of stimuli contrast values (Ferster and Koch 1987). Questions such as the dynamic behavior of the system (for instance, the convergence time) cannot be tested on the other hand, since the Hopfield model does not account for dendritic and axonal propagation times. Moreover, detailed biophysical modeling directly mimics electrophysiological results and can thus lead to new and very specific predictions, a crucial requirement of any successful theory. The price one pays for the added realism is a substantial increase in effort on the part of the programmer and the requirement of more powerful computers. The distinction between these two types of models is strongly reminiscent of Chomsky's (1965) distinction between competence and performance models in language understanding. A competence model mimics the behavior of the system, i.e., in producing oriented cells. The performance model does the same but in a manner commensurate with the internal properties of the system, i.e., in agreement with the anatomy and physiology.

Thus, to reiterate, the aim of the kind of very detailed model discussed in this chapter is not to demonstrate that any particular circuitry could lead to cortical orientation selectivity, but to study and gain an intuitive understanding—based on numerical simulations—of how the existent circuitry is responsible for establishing orientation tuning.

10.2   The Structure of the Model

Instead of modeling the visual system in a generic mammal, we chose to simulate the early visual pathway of the adult cat in view of the considerable amount of anatomical and physiological cat data available in the literature. Thus, unless otherwise mentioned, all experimental data will refer to the cat. Although the organization of the visual system of most mammals is similar, compared to say the visual system of birds, there do exist sufficient differences within mammals (for instance, all cells in area 17 in cat are orientation-selective while cells in layer IVc in monkey visual cortex are still of the center-surround type) to make it difficult to generate specific electrophysiological predictions for a given animal in such a generic model. In keeping with this approach, we chose to model only a small monocular patch of the visual system of the cat, instead of attempting to simulate the entire system. Given the limitation on computing time, we feel that for our type of model a detailed, finely-grained model of part of the system is superior to a coarser description of the entire system. Accordingly, we simulate a small monocular patch of the X pathway comprising 2° by 2° of visual angle at approximately 4° eccentricity. This permits modeling a field of view adequate for the presentation of an effective visual stimulus without representing the high cone density within the *area centralis*. Rather than sparsely modeling the complete field of view, we are thus able to represent the neural circuitry with realistic cell densities, and at the appropriate scale, to specify individual connections. This 2° by 2° patch of the visual scene is subsequently traced through each of the anatomical structures of the early visual system, from retina to the lateral geniculate nucleus, and subsequently to layer IV of area 17visual cortex in visual cortex.

Neurons in the early visual system of mammals have been classified according to a host of different electrophysiological properties (for a thorough review see Rodieck 1979; Sherman 1985; Stone 1983). The principal classification is in terms of X and Y cells and is based on the capacity of cells to integrate input linearly throughout their receptive field (Enroth-Cugell and Robson 1966). Retinal ganglion cells of the X type respond in a linear fashion to a sine-grating, have a sustained response when stimulated in the center of the receptive field, and respond to higher spatial and lower temporal frequencies as compared to Y cells, which are not capable of linear summation. The response of Y cells is also much more transient than the response of X cells, and their receptive field is significantly larger than that of X cells at the same eccentricity. Finally, the conduction velocity of X cell axons is roughly half that of Y cells. A popular but overly simplistic view associates the X system with high-acuity form vision while the Y system is generally linked with the system relaying temporal information, such as motion, to the cortex. A third, very inhomogeneous class of cells, called W or non-X, non-Y, contains cells with large receptive fields, sluggish responses, and a number of nonlinear properties, such as direction selectivity (Cleland and Levick 1974). In the retina, X, Y, and W cells correspond to very distinct anatomical classes (Boycott and Wässle 1974). Using the physiological classification combined with intracellular dye injection, X cells have been identified with β cells, Y with α cells, and W cells with γ and δ cells (Peichl and Wässle 1979; Wässle, Boycott, and Illing 1981; Wässle, Peichl, and Boycott 1983). In the present model, we constrain our model in that we only implement the X pathway. Furthermore, for reasons of computational efficiency, we have limited the retinal population under consideration to only those β cells belonging to the physiological on-center classification, which corresponds to half of the β ganglion cells in the retinal patch. In other words, all retinal neurons described here are excited if a stimulus falls within their center and are inhibited if the stimulus falls on the surround. This system then provides input to the lateral geniculate nucleus, acting as simple relay in our present model, and subsequently to the input layer IV in striate cortex. While our cortical model is currently restricted to this single cortical layer, we are engaged in a long-term effort to model subsequent transformations of the retinal signals, both within the striate and between striate and extrastriate cortex.

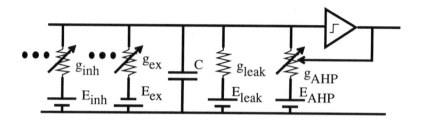

Figure 10.2
Electrical equivalent circuit of a single geniculate or cortical neuron (see eq. 10.1).
Each neuron consists of a single lumped soma with a number of excitatory and
inhibitory synapses in series with a capacity (C) and a leakage pathway (g_{leak} in
series with the battery E_{leak}). In the absence of any synaptic input, the intracellular
potential will be stabilized at $E_{leak} = -71 \ mV$. Each synapse is modeled by a time
varying conductance g_{ex} or g_{inh} in series with the synaptic reversal potential E_{ex}
or E_{inh}. For silent or shunting inhibition, $E_{inh} = E_{leak}$, while for hyperpolarizing
synaptic inputs, $E_{inh} < E_{leak}$. An action potential is assumed to be initiated if the
potential exceeds the threshold V_{thresh}. Subsequent to this event, a time-varying
inhibitory synaptic input g_{AHP}, corresponding to the potassium conductance seen
during the afterhyperpolarization, is activated (with $E_{AHP} < E_{leak}$). This will lead
to a period during which initiation of action potentials is more difficult (refractory
period).

10.3   Single-cell Model

As the purpose of this simulation is to model the time-varying behavior
of real cells, our simulated neurons exhibit realistic responses very similar to the properties of cells in chapter 9 or in chapter 6. Each cell has a
set of features that includes its membrane potential, spiking threshold,
level of spontaneous activity, and its set of synaptic connections. The
dynamic behavior of each neuron is described by the simple electrical circuit in fig. 10.2, and is determined by a first-order, nonlinear differential
equation.   Each cell is modeled by a single compartment with a passive, leak conductance (g_{leak}) in parallel with a membrane capacity C.
The passive time constant of the cell is $\tau = C/g_{leak}$. The contribution
of an activated synapse is given by the time-varying conductance change
$g(t)$, in series with the synaptic battery E. In contrast with the computation of continuous valued membrane potentials and conductances,
action potentials are modeled as discrete, binary events. If $V(t)$ exceeds
a fixed threshold, V_{thresh}, at any time, an action potential is generated
(that is, a binary variable is set) and relayed, with the appropriate delay

times, to all postsynaptic target cells. Following each action potential, the neuron experiences an afterhyperpolarization and is inhibited from spiking for a specified interval by increasing a membrane conductance (g_{AHP}) with a reversal potential negative to the cell's resting potential ($E_{AHP} = -90\ mV$). Functionally, this mimics the activation of the fast potassium currents (I_C and/or I_K) seen following action potential generation (see chapter 4). The action potential has no other direct effect on the cell's voltage trajectory. The equation of motion for the subthreshold voltage response is thus given by:

$$C\frac{dV_m(t)}{dt} = \sum_{j=1}^{k} g_{ex}(t - t_j)(V_m(t) - E_{ex})$$

$$+ \sum_{j=1}^{l} g_{inh}(t - t_j)(V_m(t) - E_{inh}) + g_{leak}(V_m(t) - E_{leak})$$

$$+ g_{AHP}(t - t_{spike})(V_m(t) - E_{AHP}) \tag{10.1}$$

where k and l are the total number of excitatory and inhibitory synapses for this particular cell, t_j the arrival time of its presynaptic action potential to the associated synapse, $g_{ex}(t)$ and $g_{inh}(t)$ the induced conductance changes (given by the α function $te^{-t/t_{peak}}$; if $t < 0$ then $g(t) = 0$; see Appendix 9.C in Chapter 9 for details regarding the efficient implementation of this function for large neuronal networks), E_e and E_i the associated synaptic batteries, and t_{spike} the time at which the neuron generated an action potential, that is $V_{thresh} < V_m(t)$. Shunting or silent inhibition is modeled by setting E_inh to the resting potential of the cell, given by E_{leak} in our model (see table 10.1), while for hyperpolarizing inhibition the battery is set to the reversal potential of potassium, $-90\ mV$. All cellular parameters are constant within any given neuronal population with the exception of the voltage threshold V_{thresh}, which was randomly chosen from a uniform distribution of values falling between -45 and $-35\ mV$. This introduced sufficient stochastic elements into our simulation to prevent phase-locking among neurons. With the exception of a low spontaneous activity introduced in the retinal β ganglion cells, additional noise is not incorporated into our cells, although this may be easily accomplished. It can be seen that our model, similar to the one described in the previous chapter, represents an elaboration of the simpler integrate-and-fire model, but stops short of a full Hodgkin and Huxley-type description as in chapter 4. This results in a physiological realistic behavior of individual neurons without requir-

ing a computationally expensive implementation of specific channels and
dendritic geometries. Once again, the selection of appropriate scale at
which to implement our model determines the computational feasibility
of the simulation.

Table 10.1: Parameters for geniculate and cortical cells

Symbol	Parameter	LGN	Cortex
C	membrane capacitance	$1nF$	$2nF$
g^*_{leak}	leakage conductance	$0.1\mu S$	$0.1\mu S$
E_{leak}	leakage reversal potential	$-71mV$	$-71.0mV$
g^*_{ex}	peak excitatory conductance	$0.15\mu S$	$0.011\mu S$
E_{ex}	excitatory synaptic reversal potential	$20mV$	$20.0mV$
g^*_{inh}	peak inhibitory conductance	-	$0.055\mu S$
E_{inh}	inhibitory synaptic reversal potential	-	$-71.0mV$
g^*_{AHP}	peak afterhyperpolarization conductance	$0.59\mu S$	$0.59\mu S$
t_{peak}	time to peak for all conductance changes	$1.0ms$	$1.0ms$
V_{thresh}	spiking threshold	$-40\pm 5mV$	$-40\pm 5mV$

* $g_{peak} = g(t = t_{peak})$

10.4   Retina

As previously described, our simulated retina comprises a two-dimensional distribution of on-center β ganglion cells with circular receptive fields.
Wässle et al. (1981) showed that upon injecting HRP into the lateral
geniculate nucleus, all retinal β cells were labeled. In this way they could
show that all β on-center and off-center cells are located on two independent lattices. The amount of spatial jitter in the exact positions of the
ganglion cells did not allow Wässle and colleagues to distinguish between
a rectangular and a hexagonal lattice. In the absence of more precise
information, we located all of our retinal ganglion cells on a noisy hexagonal grid. Instead of modeling a patch of retinal cells around the *area
centralis* with its β on-center cell density of 3250 *cells/mm²*, we located
our patch at 1 *mm* away from the *area centralis*, where the on-center β
density drops to 900 *cells/mm²* (Peichl and Wässle 1979). Since 1° is
equivalent to 0.226 *mm* in the cat retina (Bishop, Kozak, and Vakkur
1962), 1 *mm* eccentricity corresponds to about 4.5°. The associated in-

tercellular distance of a hexagonal array is $(2/(\sqrt{3}\rho))^{1/2} = 36\ \mu m \approx 9.5'$, where ρ is the cell density and $\sqrt{3} \cdot 9.5' = 16.5'$ is the distance between the cells on the hexagonal grid (Peichl and Wässle 1979). Using this spacing, we are modeling a 1 mm by 1 mm patch of cells, corresponding to about 900 cells. Thus, our model retina subtends about 4.5° by 4.5° of visual angle (see fig. 10.3 for the retinal layout).

The response of individual ganglion cells is based on extensive physiological evidence that their receptive fields can be readily described by Gaussian sensitivity profiles for both center and surround (Rodieck 1965; Enroth-Cugell and Robson 1966; Linsenmeier, Frishman, Jakiela, and Enroth-Cugell 1982). The spatial receptive field is then obtained by subtracting the surround response from the center. Thus the name of this filter, "difference of a gaussian" or DOG for short. The center response is described by

$$G_c(x,y) = \frac{K_c}{2\pi\sigma_c^2}\, e^{-\frac{x^2+y^2}{2\sigma_c^2}} \tag{10.2}$$

and the surround response by

$$G_s(x,y) = \frac{K_s}{2\pi\sigma_s^2}\, e^{-\frac{x^2+y^2}{2\sigma_s^2}} \tag{10.3}$$

Using measurements of contrast sensitivity of ganglion cells in response to drifting gratings, Linsenmeier et al. (1982) obtained four parameters that characterize the sizes (σ_c, σ_s) and peak sensitivities (K_s, K_c) of the center and surround fields. A typical X cell receptive field profile is described using $\sigma_s/\sigma_c = 3$ and $K_c/K_s = 17$ (fig. 10.3). Peichl and Wässle (1979), measuring the receptive field center size of X cells using three different methods, found sizes between 20' and 40'. We choose a value of $30' = 0.5°$, which corresponds to a σ_c of 10.6'. Since we only assigned a value to the ratio of the sensitivities, we have one free parameter in our model, which allows us to scale the total response of our simulated ganglion cells. We can now compute the physiological coverage factor, which is given by the area of the excitatory receptive field (diameter of 30') divided by the area per cell. For the above values, we find a coverage factor of 9, in good agreement with data (Peichl and Wässle 1979).

The ratio of the center to the surround signal in response to full-field light stimulation is given by $K_c\sigma_c^2/(K_s\sigma_s^2) = 0.53$. In a perfectly balanced cell, this ratio will be 1 and no response will be elicited for a full-field stimulus. However, while most retinal neurons still respond weakly

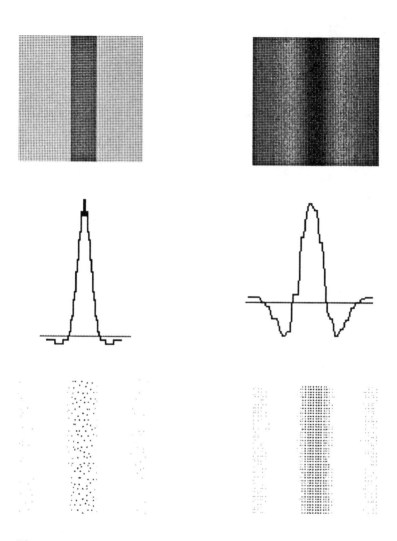

Figure 10.3
The retinal layout. The upper left panel shows our standard stimulus, a bar of variable contrast, orientation and width. This pattern is now convolved with the spatio-temporal kernel of the X ganglion cells (eqs. 10.6 and 10.7). The result is displayed in the upper right corner. The spatial part of the receptive field is shown on the same spatial scale in the left middle panel. The middle right plot shows a horizontal cross section of the convolved image. This convolved image is then subsampled on a noisy hexagonal grid, corresponding to the location of the 900 simulated on-center β ganglion cells (lower left-hand corner) and thresholded. The only difference between the retina and the LGN (lower right-hand corner) is the four times increased geniculate cell density.

to a full-field stimulus, this number is most likely an underestimate. $\sigma_s/\sigma_c = 4$ should yield a more physiological result (Linsenmeier et al. 1982). A perfectly balanced receptive field, such as the Laplacian of a Gaussian filter proposed by Marr and Hildreth (1980), would give a zero response to such a diffuse light stimulus. However, in order to approximate the Laplacian of a Gaussian filter by a DOG, the ratio of σ_s/σ_c should be equal to 1.6 (Marr and Hildreth 1980), which is clearly not the case.

The temporal response of both the center and the surround response are modeled by low-pass filters

$$L_c = \frac{1}{\tau_c} e^{\frac{-t}{\tau_c}} \tag{10.4}$$

and

$$L_s = \frac{1}{\tau_s} e^{\frac{-t}{\tau_s}} \tag{10.5}$$

with $\tau_c = 10 \; msec$ and $\tau_s = 20 \; msec$. Richter and Ullman (1982) compared the temporal response of sustained X-like ganglion cells in the primate retina against this model and found good qualitative agreement. Equations 10.4 and 10.5 are simplifications, however. Victor (1987) studied the dynamics of the center of X type cat retinal ganglion cells and derived a complete—but substantially more complex—description of their temporal behavior. We introduced a delay $\delta t = 3 \; msec$ between the center and surround response, in agreement with the theoretical prediction of Richter and Ullman (1982) as well as with the experimental evidence of Enroth-Cugell, Robson, Schweizer-Tong, and Watson (1983).

Under the assumption that the spatio-temporal receptive field is separable into a purely spatial and a purely temporal component,[1] we can now compute the response of the center and surround to a light stimulus $I(x, y, t)$ by the following convolution integrals

---

[1] Dawis, Shapley, Kaplan, and Tranchina (1984) examined this assumption in cat retinal X cells and found that separability holds for the center response but that the spatial extent of the surround depends on the temporal frequency of the stimulus and thus separability does not hold for the surround. However, for our purposes eq. 10.7 seems more than sufficient to account for cortical properties like orientation selectivity.

$$C(x, y, t) = \int_0^t \int_{-\infty}^{+\infty} \int_{-\infty}^{+\infty} G_c(x', y') L_c(t') I(x - x', y - y', t - t') dx' dy' dt'$$

(10.6)

and

$$S(x, y, t) = \int_0^t \int_{-\infty}^{+\infty} \int_{-\infty}^{+\infty} G_s(x', y') L_s(t') I(x - x', y - y', t - t') dx' dy' dt'$$

(10.7)

with the total response of the ganglion cells given by

$$F(x, y, t) = C(x, y, t) - S(x, y, t - \delta t) \tag{10.8}$$

For reasons of computational economy, the Gaussian kernel $G(x, y)$ is only being integrated within $2\sigma_s$. For any particular ganglion cell located at x, y, we can then compute its response $F(x, y, t) = F_{x,y}(t)$. Since the output of the retinal ganglion cells $F_{x,y}(t)$ represents a sort of neuronal excitability, it can never be negative. Thus, if $F_{x,y}(t) < 0$, $F_{x,y}(t)$ is set to zero. If we were to model off-center ganglion cells, their response would be given by $S(x, y, t) - C(x, y, t - \delta t)$.

This continuous neuronal excitability function $F_{x,y}(t)$ needs to be converted into discrete, stochastic, all-or-none events corresponding to action potentials. Assuming that the action potentials have a Poisson distribution, the probability that the ganglion cell fires an action potential in the small interval between t and $t + \Delta t$ (with $\Delta t << 1$) is given by

$$p_{x,y}(t) = p_0 \cdot \Delta t \cdot F_{x,y}(t) \tag{10.9}$$

where p_0 is an appropriate normalization constant. This neglects the the small probability of two or more action potentials occuring within t and $t + \Delta t$ (an event with a probability of the order of $(p_0 \cdot \Delta t)^2$). We are superimposing onto the neuronal spiking rate in response to the visual stimulus $I(x, y, t)$ a low, spontaneous spiking activity of 10 Hz (Bullier and Norton 1979). Figure 10.4 illustrates the firing rate of one retinal ganglion cell in response to a vertical bar. We simulate the effect of varying the contrast of the stimulus $I(x, y, t)$ by modulating the probability of action potential generation via variation of p_0. Equivalently, we could pass the light intensity distribution falling onto the retina through a compressive nonlinearity, such as $log(I)$ or $I/(I + I_c)$, to mimic the

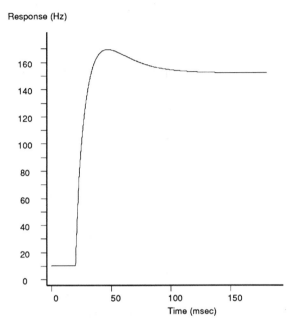

Figure 10.4

Poststimulus time histogram of a single β ganglion cell in response to a vertical, high-contrast bar as computed via eq. 10.8. At 20 $msec$ the bar (of 0.5° width) is superimposed onto the middle of the receptive field. Following the initial burst of activity, the response decays to a sustained level as a result of the delayed activation of the inhibitory surround. This continuous function is then converted into discrete action potentials used as geniculate inputs via eq. 10.9. The spontaneous firing frequency of the retinal cell is 10 Hz.

gain control properties of the rod and cone pathways in the retina (for a review see Shapley and Enroth-Cugell 1984), prior to evaluating the convolution integrals in eqs. 10.6 and 10.7. However, we can essentially achieve the same result using the simple trick of varying p_0 in eq. 10.9. This technique has the added advantage that the convolution integrals need only be evaluated once.

It should be noted that a realistic approximation of retinal activity is all that is needed to investigate the geniculate and cortical activity patterns, and selecting the correct precision and scale with which to simulate the retina results in considerable computational savings. Thus, for our purposes, it appears to be sufficient to model the retina as a linear system without explicitly modeling photoreceptors, horizontal, bipolar, and amacrine cells (for an example of this type of approach, see Gremillion, Mandell, and Travis 1987).

10.5   Lateral Geniculate Nucleus

All retinal ganglion cells project heavily to the lateral geniculate nucleus, or LGN. With few exceptions, each geniculate cell seems to receive its innervation from a single or a few retinal ganglion cells of the same class and the response properties of these geniculate neurons are essentially the same as those of their retinal counterparts with closely overlapping receptive fields (Hubel and Wiesel 1961; Singer and Creutzfeldt 1970; Cleland, Dubin, and Levick 1971). Thus, there is no significant receptive field transformation in the relay of retinal information on its way to cortex, although the massive corticofugal pathway from layer VI is most likely involved in controlling the transmission of visual information via its action on geniculate cells (Crick 1984; Sherman and Koch 1986). Retinal X ganglion cells project mainly into the A layers of the LGN, lamina A receiving input from the contralateral and lamina A1 from the ipsilateral eye. Of the approximately 450,000 cells in the LGN (Sanderson 1971), two-thirds are located in the A and A1 laminae and about two-thirds of these are of the X type. Thus, on the average each retinal X on-center ganglion cell from one eye innervates three to four geniculate relay cells. In our current model, we neglect the small degree of convergence seen among LGN cells and assume that each retinal cell projects onto four neighboring geniculate cells. Thus, the coverage factor increases to 36.

This projection from 900 retinal ganglion cells to 2,304 geniculate relay cells[2] is strictly topographic and thus preserves the spatial ordering of the original input image. The axonal propagation delay between retinal X ganglion cells and their geniculate target cells varies between 3 and 4 $msec$ (Cleland et al. 1971). The passive time constant τ for the geniculate X cells is 10 $msec$ (based on intracellular current injections; Bloomfield, Hamos, and Sherman 1987); hence the LGN introduces an integrating component into the early visual stream. For the other cellular parameters see table 10.1.

Since our model geniculate cells derive their input exclusively from a single retinal ganglion cell, they share its nonoriented, circular symmetric receptive field. This assumption neglects the somewhat stronger in-

---

[2]Not every retinal cell from our retina projects to exactly four geniculate cells.

hibitory surround effects reported for geniculate cells (Hubel and Wiesel 1961; Cleland et al. 1971; Shapley and Lennie 1985) as well as the orientation bias seen by Vidyasagar and Heide (1984) in response to moving sine wave grating of high spatial frequency. Such effects could easily be incorporated into our model by explicitly including inhibitory geniculate interneurons. These interneurons, staining positive for γ-aminobutyric acid (GABA), the principal inhibitory neurotransmitter used in subcortical and cortical structures, comprise perhaps 20–30% of the neurons in the A and A1 laminae (Fitzpatrick, Penny, and Schmechel 1984).

10.6   Visual Cortex

The primary target for geniculate relay cells is the primary visual cortex (also called area 17 or V1). While X cells from the geniculate A layers appear to project only to area 17, geniculate Y cells project to a number of areas in extrastriate cortex (reviewed in Sherman 1985). Both X and Y cells project mainly into layer IV and to a lesser extent into the upper part of layer VI. The question of whether the projection from these two cell populations (X and Y) is segregated into a lower and an upper part of layer IV (confusingly termed layers IVa and IVb by one school and layers IVab and IVc by another) is still controversial. In the current model, we are assuming that the X on-center cells in the LGN project to the lower part of layer IV. This layer, which is devoid of the large neurons seen in the upper part of layer IV, is approximately 250 μm thick (as compared to the total cortical thickness of $\approx 1,600$ μm; Beaulieu and Colonnier 1983) and contains on the order of 14,000 neurons per mm^2 (as compared to 80,000 neurons per mm^2 for all layers combined; Beaulieu and Colonnier 1983).

The projection of the visual image onto the surface of cortex is topographic, such that adjacent points in the visual field map onto adjacent points in the visual cortex. However, there is a certain degree of scatter superimposed onto this orderly representation such that nearby cells (during tangential, i.e., within the cortical plane, electrode penetrations) have receptive fields whose centers are not adjacent in visual space. For cells separated by less than 200 μm cortical distance the fluctuation in receptive field center appears to be random (Albus 1975). In other words, the projection is topographic on a macroscopic but random on a microscopic scale (for a fact-filled treatise on the physiology of cat visual cortex see Orban 1984). Finally, the visual field is distorted in a systematic manner when projected onto the cortex, such that much more area is devoted to representing the *area centralis* than the visual periphery. In fact, this projection can be roughly approximated by a logarithmic mapping (Fischer 1973; Tusa, Palmer, and Rosenquist 1978; Schwartz 1980). The cortical magnification factor M specifies how many mm of cortical distance correspond to one degree of visual angle (Albus 1975; Orban 1984). For our chosen eccentricity of $4.5°$, M is approximately 0.6 mm per $1°$ (Albus 1975). Thus, our $2°$ by $2°$ visual field projects onto a 1.2 by 1.2 mm^2 area of visual cortex, comprising roughly 20,000 cells, of which half are primarily driven by input from one eye.

We will not attempt to model all of these cells but, in accordance with the model of orientation selectivity postulated by Koch (1987), only the subclass of inhibitory interneurons. The presence in the mammalian cerebral cortex of the classical inhibitory neurotransmitter GABA and its synthesizing enzyme, glutamic acid decarboxylase (GAD), has been known for a long time (for more information on the form, function, and distribution of inhibitory interneurons see the "Cerebral Cortex" series by Peters and Jones 1984). Quantitative assessments in monkey cortex indicate that approximately 25% of the neuronal population in any cortical area is GABA- or GAD-immunoreactive (Hendry, Schwark, Jones, and Yan 1987). Morphologically, these neurons are nonpyramidal, their dendrites lack significant populations of dendritic spines, and their axons seem to be intrinsic to the cortex. In the visual cortex of the cat, these cell types included basket cells, clutch cells, and chandelier, cells or axo-axonic cells (Martin, Somogyi, and Whitteridge 1983; Kisvarday, Martin, Whitteridge, and Somogyi 1985; Jones, Hendry, and DeFelipe 1987). Electron microscopic studies of the visual cortex of the cat (Tömböl 1974; Winfield, Gatter, and Powell 1980) indicate that about 30% of all cells are small stellate cells, presumably using GABA as neurotransmitter. All of these inhibitory cells receive direct excitatory synapses from the cells in the lateral geniculate nucleus (Freund, Martin, Somogyi, and Whitteridge 1985a,b; LeVay 1987) and make extensive contacts among each other as well as onto excitatory pyramidal cells. Based on these numbers, we assumed that 25% of cortical cells are inhibitory, which brings our total cell count down to 2,300 cells in a 1.44 mm^2 patch of layer IV in area 17 (see Plate 3). We do not identify these cells with any particular subpopulation of inhibitory interneurons.

What is the divergence and the convergence associated with the geniculo-cortical pathway? When HRP was injected intracellularly into physiologically identified geniculate X cells, their axons terminate within a single continuous clump of surface area between 0.6 and 0.9 mm^2, with an average of 0.72 mm^2 (Humphrey, Sur, Uhlrich, and Sherman 1985), with anywhere between 300 and 3,000 synaptic boutons. In other words, since the cell population in a 0.72 mm^2 patch of layer IVb is about 10,000, the potential coverage factor is very large. Using a sophisticated double staining method, Freund et al. (1985a, b) revealed that the maximum number of synapses made between one geniculate axon and a single postsynaptic cell in cortex was 8, although in many cases it was only 1. Thus, with an average of 4 synaptic contacts per cell, an X cell afferent could in principle contact anywhere between 70 and 700 cells. Since we are only concerned with the 25% inhibitory interneurons, the divergence in our model, that is the number of cortical cells postsynaptic for a single geniculate cell, is roughly 220. This can be easily seen in Plate 3a.[3] The axonal propagation delay of the geniculate-cortex pathway is set to 2 $msec$ with some small random variations from cell to cell (Lee, Cleland, and Creutzfeldt 1977; Hoffman, Stone, and Sherman 1972).

The most dramatic difference between geniculate and cortical receptive fields is their organization and shape. One population of cortical cells, the simple cells, is distinguished by the discrete subregions that can be found in their receptive fields (see fig. 10.1a). These cells, which are found throughout layer IV and the upper part of layer VI, have regions that resemble the centers of the receptive fields of on-center and off-center neurons in the LGN in that light increment in an ON region or light decrement in an OFF region excites the cell. In contrast to geniculate cells, however, cortical cells have elongated receptive fields, their width being similar to the diameter of the receptive field centers of neurons in the LGN (Stone and Dreher 1973; Shermann 1985). Simple receptive fields vary in the number of subregions observed, in the elongation of each subunit, and in the overall elongation of the field. The aspect ratio of these subfields, i.e. the ratio of width to length, varies with the type and the layer of the neuron. Observed values for simple cells range from 0.2 (1:5 elongation) to 0.92 (nearly round), although cells in layer IV tend to have aspect ratios between 0.5 and 0.66 (Watkins and Berkley 1974; Gilbert 1977; Jones, Stepnoski, and Palmer 1987). Note that the aspect ratio directly determines the amount of orientation tuning in the feedforward Hubel and Wiesel type model (a smaller aspect ratio increases the tuning), while it is one among many factors shaping orientation tuning in the mixed models.

---

[3]Given this large divergence over a relatively large area (relative to the size of our cortex), only the central 2° by 2° patch of geniculate cells projects completely to the cortex. This subfield is outlined in Plates 3 and 4 by a small white rectangle superimposed onto the LGN.

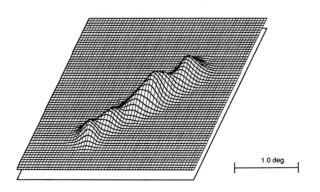

Figure 10.5
Shape of the full, two-dimensional receptive field profile of a simulated cortical cell
with a diagonal preferred orientation, similar to the one shown in Plate 3c. The
receptive field is computed by superimposing the receptive fields of all geniculate
cells projecting to this particular cell. Only the ON subfield is shown.

For our current simulations, we wired simple cells with an aspect ratio varying between 1:2.5 and 1:4. The appropriate receptive fields can
be visualized by retracing all the geniculate afferents to any particular
cortical cells. The result is illustrated in Plates 3b and 3c. Note that
these cells currently do not contain any OFF subunits. The convergence of the geniculo-cortical pathway can be visualized by retracing
all geniculate afferents to these cells (marked in red in Plates 3b and
3c). On the average, simple cells receive input from 20 to 30 cells whose
centers are aligned along a row in visual space, as postulated by Hubel
and Wiesel's original model (1962). These numbers are in rough agreement with the convergence ratio obtained from cross-correlation studies
(Tanaka 1983). The profile of the full, two-dimensional receptive field
structure is visualized in fig. 10.5.

The receptive fields are too flat across their elongated dimension, missing the pronounced peak in response seen experimentally at the center
of the ON and OFF subunits. Using a very detailed reverse correlation
technique, Jones and Palmer (1987), concluded that a two-dimensional
Gabor filter function (Daugman 1985) provides a reasonably accurate
description of simple receptive fields. We are currently including OFF
type excitatory subunits in our receptive field structure.

The mean width of the orientation tuning curve at half height for layer IV simple cells varies between 14° and 20° (Orban 1984). Although cells with elongated subfields tend to be more orientation-tuned than cells with less asymmetric receptive fields, the correlation between the aspect ratio and orientation tuning is only moderate ($r = 0.70$; Watkins and Berkley 1974), implicating other, presumably inhibitory mechanisms for the generation of orientation tuning. Cells in visual cortex are organized into orientation columns, such that nearby cells with similar orientation preferences are grouped together (Hubel and Wiesel 1962, 1963). One complete set of orientation columns, spanning all orientations, and including input from both eyes, makes up one hypercolumn. Simple cells have a number of other salient properties, such as direction selectivity and disparity tuning (for a review see Orban 1984), none of which we will consider any further. Our cortex currently does not include complex cells.

Since we do not attempt to trace the detailed development of the visual system from the young kitten to the adult cat, we construct the receptive fields of our simple cells as follows. For a cell within a given orientation column we first decide where the receptive field should be located. To do this, we backproject the cell into the LGN (e.g., a cell in the upper left corner is projected back into the upper left corner of the LGN). A rectangle of a given size is centered (for instance, 3° by 4°) around this geniculate cell and divided into a number of vertical strips (eight 3° by 0.5° strips). The size of this rectangle depends on the extent of the geniculo-cortical arborization (in our case 0.72 mm^2). Each of the geniculate cells within this rectangle could then, in principle, make a synapse with the simple cell under consideration. We then randomly choose one of these strips. In a final step, we again choose randomly from all cells within this strip (assuming a uniform probability distribution) those cells that actually project to the simple cell. This procedure (1) leads to jitter in the exact receptive field position but preserves the overall topography, and (2) generates oriented simple cells using the scheme proposed by Hubel and Wiesel (1962). Note that this scheme explicitly computes the afferent projection into cortex (Plates 3b and 3c) but only implicitly the efferent projection from the LGN (Plate 3a).

In our current version of the model, two separate inhibitory, intracortical pathways are implemented. One system corresponds to long-range inhibition among cells with approximately overlapping receptive fields but different preferred orientations. This pathway represents an anatomical substrate of cross-orientation inhibition, for which both physiological and pharmacological evidence exists (Bishop et al. 1971; Sillito 1975; Morrone et al. 1982; Ramoa, Shadlen, Skottun, and Freeman 1986; however, see also Ferster 1986, 1988). In our model, each cell projects into the three neighboring orientation columns and has a given and fixed probability of forming inhibitory synapses onto these cells. Both pre- and postsynaptic cells have spatially overlapping receptive fields but different preferred orientations (Plate 3d). We usually assume that each cortical neuron inhibits 40 cells out of a 12 by 12 patch of cells in the orientation column orthogonal to its own orientation and a somewhat smaller number of neurons in the two directly adjacent orientation columns (see Plate 3d). A second inhibitory projection is assumed to exist between neurons with similar preferred orientations but spatially offset receptive fields. Intracellular recordings support the existence of such a system (Ferster 1986). The pattern of this local inhibition varies and depends on the preferred orientation of the column. Given the spatial jitter in the receptive field locations of neighboring cells, this inhibition can, in principle, suppress firing activity among cells with identical receptive fields (in terms of their orientation and location) and could therefore act to dampen the response of the entire population. It is possible that such inhibitory synapses could be selectively removed and pruned away during development.

Both inhibitory pathways take account of the propagation times of action potentials, which are computed on the basis of the distance between the pre- and postsynaptic cell and the conduction velocity of the particular axonal process (usually assumed to vary between 1–2 m/sec). The high degree of divergence witnessed in the inhibitory projections leads to a very large number of intracortical synapses (2,300 cells each of which makes about 100 synapses or a total of 250,000 synapses) and to dramatically enhanced simulation times. In fact, as discussed more fully in chapter 12, the most time-intensive portion of the computer simulation of these networks (up to 90%) involves propagating action potentials among cortical cells. Updating the state of the individual neurons (i.e., evaluating eq. 10.1) requires a far smaller fraction of computing resources. Thus, everything possible should be done to keep the number of intracortical connections to a minimum, while the complexity of single neurons can be significantly increased, for instance by adding dendrites, without incurring significantly slower simulation times.

10.7   Simulation Results

The model was implemented on SUN workstations in C using the techniques described in the previous chapter. Some results are illustrated in color in Plate 4, for the case of a cortex where all inhibitory cortical interactions have been blocked and only a Hubel and Wiesel (1962) type of geniculo-cortical arrangement is assumed (see fig. 10.1b). The selectivity of the system can be monitored by the action potential count displayed above each orientation column. This is simply the total number of spikes occuring in any cell within that particular orientation column.

Stimulus conditions were as follows. Initially, the "cat" sees a blank screen. Under these conditions, the spontaneous spiking activity (10 Hz) in the optic nerve can be seen to activate geniculate cells and depolarize cortical cells (Plate 4a). At 20 $msec$ a vertical, 0.5° wide and elongated light bar is projected onto the retina (figs. 10.3 and 10.4). The response in the LGN reflects this stimulus (Plate 4b). The nonexcited regions in the LGN correspond to the perceptual phenomena of Mach bands, caused by inhibitory interactions mediated by the inhibitory surround mechanism of retinal ganglion cells. Spontaneous activity is actually suppressed, as can be seen by comparison with the outside regions next to the geniculate boundary. In cortex, neurons in the vertical orientation column respond vigorously to the vertical bar, while simple cells in the neighboring orientation columns fail to generate action potentials; they are, however, nonetheless depolarized to some degree (between 5 and 20 mV from rest as can be seen in the intracellular potential plots of two cortical cells; Plate 4). This is a natural consequence of the finite aspect ratio of the receptive fields. If we had used aspect ratios of 1:1.5 to 1:2.5, which is more in tune with experimentally observed values (Watkins and Berkely 1974; Gilbert 1977; Jones et al. 1987; Jones and Palmer 1987), the selectivity of the model would degrade. Since such excitatory postsynaptic potentials at nonoptimal orientations are not observed during intracellular recordings (Ferster 1986, 1988), inhibitory mechanisms must be introduced in order to block or shunt these EPSPs. At 150 $msec$ the bar is rotated into the horizontal position and cells in the geniculate start responding to this new stimulus (Plate 4c). Note that, different from most conventional neural networks where a new stimulus requires the reinitialization of the network (usually resetting the activity state of all neurons to zero or some other median value), traces of the old stimulus are still visible, in form of the intracellular potential, at the cellular level in both the LGN and in cortex. Cells in the horizontal orientation column now respond to the horizontal bar (Plate 4d). The

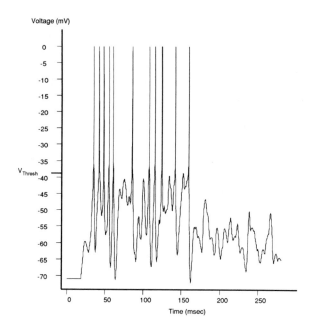

Figure 10.6
Intracellular potential of a vertically oriented simple cell during the same stimulus
sequence as in Plate 4. At 20 *msec* a vertical bar is projected onto the retina,
switching to a horizontal bar at 150 *msec*. However, unlike before, intracortical
shunting inhibition among cells with different preferred orientations suppresses the
EPSPs evoked at the nonoptimal orientation. This record should be compared against
the intracellular plot in Plate 4.

nonexcited neurons at the top and bottom in the horizontal column are
an artifact caused by the small size of the LGN.

A detailed plot of the intracellular potential of a cell in the vertical
orientation column in response to a similar stimulus sequence is shown in
fig. 10.6.   However, unlike before, intracortical inhibition among cells
with different orientations is now included in the simulation, as specified
in Plate 3d. While the cell is as responsive to a properly aligned stimulus as before, its response to nonoptimal stimuli is significantly reduced.
Individual EPSPs, caused by the geniculate afferents, are still visible, as
well as fast steep reductions in the intracellular potential caused by the
action of intracortical inhibition, which is assumed to reverse around the
resting potential of the cell (silent or shunting inhibition). Under these

conditions, IPSPs should never be visible, except when the cell is depolarized by current injections (e.g., Ferster 1986, 1988). The intracellular potential will have a smoother time course if a larger divergence is used for the intracortical inhibition.

While the color graphic display of the intracellular potential of all cortical neurons greatly facilitates understanding the working of the model, detailed quantitative measures must be used to assess the validity of the different models of orientation selectivity. Here, the modeler is in a somewhat similar situation to the experimentalist using multielectrode recordings, facing an embarrasing wealth of data. The main quantitative measure we use is spike counts for individual cells or for large cell populations. Other measures, such as simulating the total current flow in the three-dimensional extracellular cortical matrix (something akin to an electroencephalogram) as in the previous chapter, can be used.

If the contrast of the visual stimulus is decreased, retinal and geniculate cells will be less excited. Ultimately, in the straightforward excitation-only Hubel and Wiesel model, cortical cells will stop responding to the bar, since not enough geniculate-induced EPSPs will be present to carry the somatic voltage in the cortical cell above threshold (fig. 10.7). In other words, this model lacks gain control properties. If, however, cortical inhibition is superimposed onto a Hubel and Wiesel type of synaptic arrangement, a smaller contrast stimulus results in less geniculo-cortical excitation, but consequently also in less intracortical inhibition. Thus, the range of contrast values for which the eclectic model still responds is significantly higher, as borne out in fig. 10.8. Experimentally, the orientation tuning of area 17 simple cells changes little when varying the contrast between 2% and 80% (Skottun, Bradley, Sclar, Ohzawa, and Freeman 1987).

Finally, what are the limitations of this class of detailed models? Considering that area 17 contains on the order of 18 million cells (Beaulieu and Colonnier 1983), we simulate a mere 0.014% of this population, one area among many. In terms of simulation time, the principal constraint is the number of synapses to update and keep in memory (on the order of cn, for n cortical neurons with a divergence or fan-out of c). Thus, using today's technology, it is clearly not feasible to simulate anything more than a few mm^2 of cortical tissue (across all layers). However, in order to understand such relatively local computations as orientation selectivity, direction selectivity, or disparity tuning, it may not be necessary to simulate larger areas of cortex. It is in this respect somewhat disconcerting that excitatory interactions among cortical cells of the same orientation are know to occur over horizontal distances of several millimeters (Ts'o,

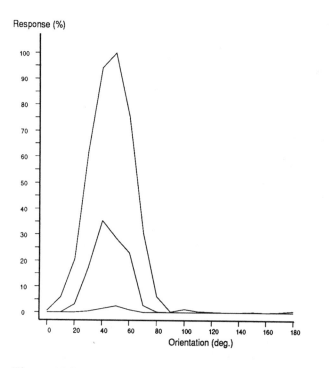

Figure 10.7
Sensitivity of the Hubel and Wiesel model to visual contrast. The total number
of action potentials within one orientation column during a 500 $msec$ presentation
of a bar of varying orientation (at 10° increments) is shown (normalized to peak
response) at three different contrast values. The retinal activity in the three curves
is multiplied by 1.0, 0.75, and 0.5, via variation of p_0 in eq. 10.9. At the lowest
contrast value, cortical cells are barely excited, reflecting the lack of gain control of
the straightforward Hubel and Wiesel wiring scheme.

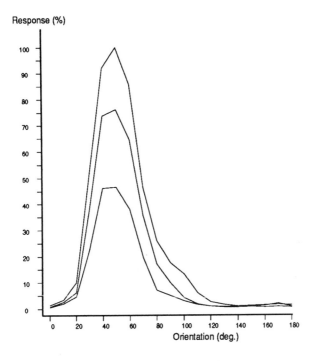

Figure 10.8
Sensitivity of a mixed excitation and inhibition model to visual contrast. The presence of cross-orientation inhibition superimposed onto a Hubel and Wiesel synaptic arrangement leads to a much improved gain control. While the response of the cortex decreases with decreasing stimulus contrast, the bandwidth remains virtually unchanged, in agreement with experimental data (Skottun et al. 1987). For details see fig. 10.7.

Gilbert, and Wiesel 1986) and that the response of cat striate cortex cells can be modified over an area considerably larger than the classical receptive field (Orban, Gulyas, and Vogels 1987). An alternative strategy is to model only a few percent of all existing cells within a given area, instead of attempting to model all cells.

The address of Udo Wehmeier, Dawei Dong, Christof Koch, and David Van Essen is Division of Biology 216-76, California Institute of Technology, Pasadena, California 91125. Electronic mail should be addressed to koch@hamlet.caltech.edu or koch@caltech.bitnet.

CHAPTER 11

Simplifying Network Models of Binocular Rivalry and Shape-from-Shading

SIDNEY R. LEHKY and TERRENCE J. SEJNOWSKI

11.1 Introduction

In this chapter we will review two neural network models of visual processing. These simplifying brain models are at a level of organization in the nervous system between the single cell and the cortical column, and at a level of analysis between the computational and the implementational (Marr 1980; Churchland, Koch, and Sejnowski 1989). The goal of these models is to provide explanations for perceptual phenomena based on the representation and processing of visual information in neural populations.

As experimental data accumulate at the level of single neurons, more and more detailed models become possible that mimic more closely the processing of particular circuits. This approach, which might be called realistic brain models, is most useful when the function of the circuit is already known and the knowledge about the circuit is almost complete down to the biophysical level. The model of central pattern generation in chapters 6 and 7 is a good example of this approach. One of the lessons learned from modeling invertebrate circuits is that a wiring diagram is not nearly enough to specify a circuit—specific biophysical membrane properties are also crucial (Selverston 1985). Unfortunately, in most parts of the vertebrate central nervous system we have only a vague notion about the function of circuits, and information about the biophysical level is at best incomplete. Even the patterns of connectivity are uncertain in cerebral cortex.

Another approach to the network level is to start with a function such as a perceptual ability and design simplified neural circuits that can perform the function within the constraints of the state of knowledge. One example of this "simplifying" approach was the Marr and Poggio (1976) cooperative model of binocular depth perception, which demonstrated that a network of simplified neurons could fuse random-dot stereograms

(Julesz 1971). These models can be simulated on a digital computer and their properties compared with human performance. However, these models are often too general to compare directly with physiological experiments, and at best they serve as a demonstration of one way that a problem can be solved.

Neither the top-down nor the bottom-up approach is ideal—what is needed is some approach that combines the strengths of both strategies. The value of a model is that it can incorporate both the existing knowledge at the biological level and the performance of the system from psychophysical measurements. The two examples given here illustrate the usefulness of such a combined style of network modeling, taking advantage of both the realistic and simplifying approaches. They are at a level that is beyond that of modeling the details of identified neurons, but not so general that essential features such as response properties of single neurons can no longer be identified.

11.2   Binocular Rivalry

The first model presented here is concerned with interactions between visual processing in the two eyes. Binocular rivalry occurs when incompatible images are presented to the two eyes, such as vertical stripes to one eye and horizontal stripes to the other. In such a situation the visual system is thrown into oscillation, so that first the image from one eye is visible, and then the other, typically for a period of about one second. In general, the entire visual field does not oscillate in unison unless the rival stimuli are sufficiently small (less than 1° in diameter), but rather it breaks up into a constantly changing mosaic of the two images.

In choosing this topic, the desire was to study an aspect of binocular vision that has received less theoretical attention than stereopsis, not only because of its intrinsic interest, but also because its study may provide clues and constraints in constructing a biological model of stereopsis. Rivalry appears to be a problem of intermediate complexity in the sense that the issues can be formulated in terms relevant to the biological concerns of the experimental neurophysiologist as well as the global concerns of the psychophysicist.

11.2.1   Experimental Data

A large body of psychophysical data related to rivalry has accumulated over the past century (O'Shea 1983). The durations of alternating left and right dominance show statistical variation, and the mean durations depend on the stimuli. The nature of this dependence is unusual. When the stimulus strength (contrast, for example) is increased to one eye, the duration of time for which the opposite eye is dominant decreases. It is therefore possible to independently vary the duration for which each eye is dominant. Also, the oscillations follow a rectangular waveform. This is indicated by the observation that a spot of light flashed to the suppressed eye has its detectability reduced by a constant amount over the entire duration of the suppressed phase, interpreted as showing that the strength of suppression remains constant until being abruptly cut off.

Neurophysiological data on the matter is more sparse. John Allman (unpublished data) has observed in the superficial layers of primary visual cortex in an alert owl monkey some neurons whose neural activity switched on and off in synchrony with behavioral indications that an eye had undergone a transition from suppressed to dominant states. A significant proportion of the cells in the middle temporal area (MT) show similar behavior (Nicos Logothetis, personal communication). This is the only neurophysiological report of oscillations associated with binocular rivalry. Varela and Singer (1987) have recorded from relay cells in the lateral geniculate nucleus (LGN) of anesthetized cats exposed to rival stimuli. They found that strong inhibition occurred when stimuli to the two eyes were unmatched. This inhibition had a latency of hundreds of milliseconds, and was abolished by disruption of corticofugal inputs through ablation of the cortex. Although no oscillations were observed (possibly because of the anesthesia), these data suggest a binocular inhibitory process at an early stage of the visual system whose activity is related to the degree of correlation between images to the two eyes. Together with the results of J. Allman and N. Logothetis, these studies indicate that although rivalry has been chiefly a concern of psychophysics, it is feasible to approach the phenomenon with neurophysiological techniques. This may be one of the simplest experimental paradigms that could link conscious awareness of sensory stimuli with neural activity.

11.2.2   Neural Network Model

By its very nature, binocular rivalry suggests some sort of reciprocal inhibitory linkage between signals from the left and right eyes prior to the site of binocular convergence. Reciprocal inhibition is common at all levels of the nervous system, from peripheral processing in the retina to visual cortex. The simplest neural network implementation of such a system is illustrated in fig. 11.1, which shows the responses of the network under different stimulus conditions, as discussed below (see also

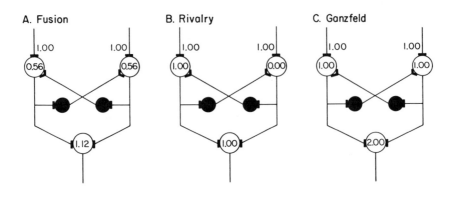

Figure 11.1
Activities in the neural network for three patterns of binocular input. (A) correlated contours (fusion), (B) uncorrelated contours (rivalry), and (C) no contours
(*Ganzfeld*). Numbers indicate relative levels of activity when inputs are arbitrarily
set to 1.0. Differences in activities are explained by postulating that binocular spatial correlation affects the strength of inhibitory coupling between the left and right
sides.

Lehky 1988). The open circles represent excitatory neurons and the filled
circles inhibitory neurons. There are two excitatory neurons, one from
the left side and one from the right, which converge upon a binocular
neuron. These two neurons receive sensory information along inputs
from the periphery, indicated by the lines originating from the top of
the diagram. Finally, there are two inhibitory neurons, each inhibiting
the other side in feedback fashion. This circuit is intended to model
binocular processing for only a small, isolated patch of visual field, and
is incomplete in the sense that it does not include lateral interactions.

The point of the network is to model in as simple a way as possible the
essential neural interactions that may underlie the oscillation of binocular rivalry, without considering many of the biophysical details of actual
neurons. Oscillations of course imply a system whose state is changing
as a function of time, or a dynamical system. The qualitative behavior
of a dynamical system can be found using the mathematical methods of
stability theory, as developed in chapter 5. Stability analysis gives the
general conditions under which the system will fall into different behavioral states (oscillating or nonoscillating) without providing quantitative
information about those states. When a stability analysis is performed
on a reciprocal inhibition network, it can be shown that two conditions

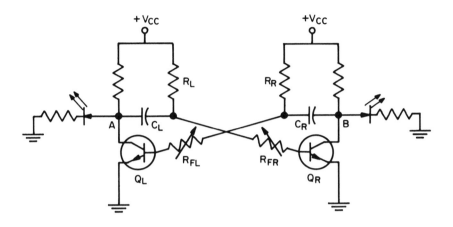

Figure 11.2
Circuit diagram of an astable multivibrator. This circuit is meant to be a physical
analog of the neural networks shown in fig. 11.1, in which the two transistors Q_L
and Q_R represent the two monocular excitatory units in that figure (open circles),
resistors R_{FL} and R_{FR} control strength of inhibitory coupling in the reciprocal
feedback inhibition pathway, and capacitors C_L and C_R control the adaptation time
constant of the inhibition. The subscripts L and R refer to the left and right sides
respectively.

are required for it to go into oscillations (Matsuoka 1984, 1985): (1) the
inhibitory coupling must be sufficiently strong, and (2) adaptation of
inhibition must also be sufficiently strong.

11.2.3   Analog Electrical Circuit

In order to go beyond a simple qualitative analysis and look at some
of the actual properties of the oscillations produced by the network,
it is necessary to simulate the behavior of the system. The dynamics
of the system are governed by coupled nonlinear differential equations
that are not analytically soluble. Therefore one must either solve them
numerically on a computer or find an equivalent physical system that is
subject to the same equations but can be more easily studied.

Following the second approach, the system that was chosen as an
analog to the neural network for rivalry was the electronic circuit shown
in fig. 11.2 (analog in the sense that its behavior shared the dynamical
features of interest with the neural network).   The circuit is called
an astable multivibrator and is essentially an oscillating flip-flop, whose

behavior is described in many electronic textbooks and which is easily built.

The analogy between this circuit and the neural network can be seen as we step through the operation of the circuit. The two transistors Q_L and Q_R represent the left and right excitatory neurons. The points labeled A and B in the circuit are equivalent to the outputs of those two neurons, and LEDs were placed at those points to allow visual monitoring of the output voltages at those points. Nothing in the electronic circuit corresponds to the binocular neuron. It would have been straightforward to model a binocular neuron by including circuitry that linearly summed the voltages from points A and B, but that would not have added to our conceptual understanding of what was going on, and would have cluttered and complicated the circuit. The left and right transistors are connected in a manner that may be described as reciprocal inhibition. The "inhibitory" pathway from Q_L to Q_R runs through C_L and R_{FR} to the base of Q_R, and analogously from point B to the base Q_L on the other side. If the voltage at point A is high, that forces the voltage at point B to be close to zero, and vice versa. As the circuit oscillates, the voltages at points A and B alternately go high and low.

The slow charging of the capacitors C_L and C_R along the circuit path connecting the two transistors can be thought of as "adaptation" of inhibition, and this adaptation is necessary for the system to go into oscillation. When the voltage of capacitor C_L on one side gradually charges up to the threshold of transistor Q_r on the other side, the system flips state. At this point the whole process starts over with the other capacitor and transistor, and so on back and forth indefinitely as the system oscillates (the transistors here effectively act as switches; that is to say, their transfer function between "input" base voltage and "output" collector voltage can be approximated by a very steep sigmoid).

Finally, the values of the variable resistors R_{FL} and R_{FR} in the feedback pathway can be thought of as determining the strength of "inhibitory coupling" between the right and left sides. Small resistances correspond to strong inhibitory coupling and large resistances to weak coupling. As we said before, the strength of inhibitory coupling is one of the factors that determine whether a system with reciprocal feedback inhibition will oscillate or not. This can easily be demonstrated in this circuit, for as one increases the values of the feedback resistance (decreases inhibitory coupling) by turning the knob of a potentiometer, a particular point is reached at which the oscillations suddenly stop. Instead of each LED being alternately fully lit or completely dark, both are now on simultaneously, but at some intermediate level of brightness.

In the language of dynamical systems theory this is called a bifurcation point, a point at which a discontinuous change in the behavior of the system (from oscillating to nonoscillating) occurs as one of the system variables (feedback resistance) is continuously changed.

Now we can compare the behavior of this astable multivibrator circuit with that of binocular rivalry. One similarity is that the astable multivibrator produces rectangular oscillations. In addition, the duration of time that the left or right side is "dominant" can be varied independently by changing the value of a parameter (time constant for charging the capacitor) on the opposite side. This is analogous to the behavior of rivalry, if one substitutes "change contrast" for "change capacitor (adaptation) time constant." Although it will not be discussed in detail here, the statistical distribution of the durations of dominance and suppression can also be replicated by the system under consideration here by adding random noise to the model (Lehky 1988). Finally, the electronic circuit passes from an oscillating to nonoscillating state as the value of the feedback resistances (strength of inhibitory coupling) is varied. In the binocular visual system, we know that the behavior goes from oscillating (rivalry) to nonoscillating (fusion) as the correlation of images presented to the two eyes is varied.

This last point brings up an important physiological prediction of the astable multivibrator model, which is that not only is there reciprocal feedback inhibition prior to the site of binocular convergence, but this inhibition involves synapses whose strength is affected by the degree of correlation between the left and right images. High correlation would lead to weak inhibitory coupling across the synapses, and low correlation would lead to strong inhibitory coupling. Furthermore, it has already been mentioned that changing stimulus strength (contrast) in rivalry and changing the adaptation time constant in the astable multivibrator circuit have analogous effects. Therefore, a second prediction would be that the binocular reciprocal inhibition postulated here shows adaptation whose time constant depends on contrast. In other words, adaptation occurs at a faster rate when contrast is increased.

Going back to fig. 11.1, the activities within the neural network as postulated by the model are shown for binocular fusion and rivalry (the values for fusion are in fact taken from an earlier model (Lehky 1983) that considered psychophysical results about how various luminances presented to the two eyes combine to form the perception of binocular brightness). The last diagram in the figure shows some psychophysical data from Bolanowski (1987) that show that when no contours are present (uniform field or *Ganzfeld* conditions) the binocular reciprocal inhibition disappears, so that luminances presented to the two eyes add up linearly to form the percept of binocular brightness. This is included here in support of a central point of the modeling, that the strength of inhibitory coupling in binocular vision is a function of the spatial patterns presented to the two eyes. The strength of inhibitory coupling for the three conditions can be ordered as follows: uncorrelated contour (rivalry) > correlated contour (fusion) > no contour (*Ganzfeld*).

It is important to point out that the model as presented here is incomplete, since it just says that the degree of correlation between the left and right spatial patterns affects the strength of inhibitory coupling, but does not give any mechanism by which this may occur. This postulated effect of spatial correlation on binocular inhibition is presumably mediated by various lateral interactions not considered in the model.

A functional model such as the one presented here cannot define anatomical location. However, the physiological data of J. Allman and N. Logothetis (personal communication) and of Varela and Singer (1987) suggest that the processes under consideration here are already occurring at an early stage (primary visual cortex and area MT). Varela and Singer further propose that the correlation between the left and right images computed at the cortical level controls, through known feedback connections, inhibitory circuits in the LGN or perigeniculate nucleus that gate the signals passing through the LGN to the cortex. Certainly the precise binocular alignment of layers in the lateral geniculate nucleus points to an important role in binocular vision beyond the inadequate notion of the LGN as the recipient of a rather amorphous set of modulatory influences from the brainstem, or the simple notion of the LGN as a "relay center" (Sherman and Koch 1986; Koch 1987).

In conclusion, although the model presented here was at a much simplified level, it both fits the available data well and suggests new lines of experimental investigation that might not have been otherwise considered.

11.3   Computing Surface Curvature from Shaded Images

In the previous example, intuition was coupled with knowledge of anatomy and physiology of the visual system to arrive at a plausible network model of binocular rivalry. The network is a small but important part of a larger, more complex system. As processing is traced into the visual cortex, it becomes more difficult to find plausible network models based on intuition.

Recently, new "learning" algorithms have been devised as constructive techniques for designing networks that can perform specified transformations between input and output. In this section we describe the application of one of these algorithms, called "error back-propagation," to a problem in visual processing (see Appendix 11.A). Specifically, the algorithm is used to construct a network that can extract certain shape parameters from shading information contained in continuous images of simple surfaces (Lehky and Sejnowski 1988).

Our interest here is in the properties of the receptive fields in such a network, and how they compare to receptive fields actually found in visual cortex. The general finding is that the receptive fields developed by the network are surprisingly similar those found in primary visual cortex. We conclude that neurons that can extract surface curvature can have receptive fields similar to those previously interpreted as bar or edge detectors (Hubel and Wiesel 1962). The receptive field of a sensory neuron is necessary but not sufficient to determine its function within a network. We emphasize the importance as well of the "projective field" of a neuron in determining its function, where the projective field is the output pattern of connections that the neuron makes with other cells.

The approach taken here to the "shape from shading" problem differs fundamentally from that which has been used by researchers in machine vision (Ikeuchi and Horn 1981; Pentland 1984). In that work, explicit rules for extracting the parameter of interest from the image are given in the form of mathematical equations. In this network model, the rules are implicitly contained within the thousands of "synaptic weights" between the units of the network, and do not lend themselves to a more compact description.

It may be useful to compare the machine vision and network models in terms of the three levels of analysis set forth by Marr (1980): the computational level, the algorithmic level, and the hardware or implementation level. They differ most obviously, and perhaps most importantly, in the last level, that of implementation. The reason this may be the most important difference is that the properties and limitations of the hardware influence the choice of algorithm. When constrained to deal with the problem using a network architecture similar to that occurring in the brain, the resulting solution is quite different from what was conceived when the computational problem had been considered in isolation. The machine vision algorithms are local, dealing with the relation between adjacent pixels. Whatever globality they achieve is done serially, by pasting together a sequence of local analyses. In contrast, the algorithm that the network implements appears to be intrinsically global and parallel, reflecting its architecture. The network seems to handle shape-from-shading as a problem in pattern recognition, looking for particular configuration of light and dark over a fairly large patch of surface (large relative to a pixel). For more difficult problems it may be necessary to have feedback connections, such as those used in the binocular rivalry network, which would give the network a more complex temporal dynamics.

11.3.1   The Task of the Network

The local curvature is an important descriptor of the shape of a surface. The network model described here is intended to extract surface curvature from shaded images. Curvature is defined as the rate of change in the orientation of the surface normal vector as a function of arc length as one moves along a curve lying on the surface. It was selected as the parameter of interest for the network because it is a relatively robust indicator of shape. The magnitude of surface curvature is independent of rotations or translations of the surface (which is not true for shape described in terms of surface normals).

In general, the curvature at a point on a surface depends upon the direction one travels along the surface. The directions for which curvature assumes maximum and minimum values are called the principal directions, and the maximum and minimum curvatures themselves are called the principal curvatures. There is a theorem in differential geometry that states that the two principal curvatures always lie along orthogonal directions on a surface.

Knowing the principal curvatures at a point provides useful information about the local properties of the surface. If both principal curvatures are positive, the surface is convex; if both are negative, it is concave, and if they have opposite signs, the surface is saddle-shaped. If one principal curvature is zero, the surface is cylindrical, and if both are zero the surface is planar. Aside from curvature sign, the magnitudes of the principal curvatures themselves are an indication of the spatial scale of features on the surface. Hence it would be helpful to have a way of estimating principal curvatures and their orientations directly from the shading information in an image. Of course, the shading of an object depends on the direction of illumination. To be interesting and useful, the network should be capable of determining surface curvature independently of illumination direction (i.e., the network should find some aspect of the image related to curvature that remains invariant as illumination direction is changed). Furthermore, the parameters extracted by the network should not depend on the image being precisely aligned at any particular position in the overall receptive field of the network.

To summarize, the task of the network is to find the magnitudes and orientations of the principal curvatures at the center of a simple geometrical surface patch, independently of illumination direction and the position of the surface.

11.3.2   Designing the Network Model

As in the binocular rivalry model, the network to be presented here is meant to correspond to a small circuit receiving input from only a very limited region of the visual field, perhaps a region subserved by a single cortical column. The network therefore determines curvatures for a small patch of a large, complex image. To generate descriptions of images, we believe that the network here would have to be replicated at different spatial locations to cover the entire visual field, and also replicated at different spatial scales, which would all feed into higher-level networks that integrated local curvatures into more general shape descriptions (see Pentland 1986 for discussions of synthesizing descriptions of complex shapes from simple shape primitives).

The network is constructed to extract principal curvatures from a set of simple geometrical surfaces (elliptic paraboloids). The eventual relevance of this to more complex images is contained in the assumption that any surface patch can be locally approximated by such a simple geometrical surface. Since curvature is proportional to the second derivative of surface position, an arbitrary surface having the same curvature as the actual surface forms a second-order approximation to that surface. This is probably sufficiently accurate, given that the psychophysical evidence indicates that the human visual system does not generate very good estimates of surface shape from shading information alone (Mingolla and Todd 1986).

As stated before, the input images to the network were of elliptic paraboloids (parabolic cross section in depth and elliptical cross section in the fronto-parallel plane). This surface was selected because, unlike ellipsoids for example, it has no edges (occluding contours) other than edges caused by the limits of the network receptive field itself. We were interested in studying network responses to shading, without the confounding presence of edges in the images.

Reflection from the surface was assumed to be matte, so that scattering of light from the surface is independent of the location of the viewer. Illumination was also assumed to have a diffuse or Lambertian

component, so that although light came predominantly from a particular direction, there were components from all directions arising from
light reflected and scattered about by the general environment of the
surface (see Appendix 11.B for details). This diffuse illumination was
used in order to eliminate hard shadow edges from the image, again in
keeping with our desire to study network responses purely to shading.
In any case, illumination in reality almost always has a diffuse component. Specular reflections, which are also common in nature, were not
included.

Another concern in constructing the network was ambiguity in the
sign of the curvature. Without knowing the direction of illumination, it
is impossible to distinguish a positively curved surface from a negatively
curved one. The appearance of a convex surface with light coming with
a tilt of 30°, for example, is physically indistinguishable from a concave
surface illuminated at a tilt of −30°, and a saddle-shaped surface can be
found that is also indistinguishable. The inherent ambiguity in curvature sign is well illustrated by the picture of the inside-out mask face in
Gregory (1966, p. 127), in which surface curvatures are perceived as the
opposite of what they actually are. Because of this ambiguity, a particular image presented to the neural network can correspond to several
different surfaces (convex, concave, or saddle-shaped).

To resolve ambiguity in the signs of the two principal curvatures, two
assumptions were built into the network. The first assumption placed
restrictions on possible directions of illumination. It was assumed that
illumination always came from above (light tilt between 0° and 180°).
This was sufficient to fix the sign of one of the two principal curvatures. There is in fact evidence that biological systems do make this
assumption, coming from observations of the well-known "crater illu-
sion," in which craters come to be seen as mounds when the photograph
is turned upside down. The interpretation of the image, whether as a
crater or as a mound, is always consistent within the implicit assumption
that illumination is coming from above (Ramachandran 1988).

The sign of the second principal curvature in principle could have been
disambiguated by making further restrictions on illumination directions
(for example, not only does light always come from above, it always
comes from the left). However, there did not appear to be any plausible
justification for making this further restriction on illumination. Rather,
the assumption was built into the network that both principal curvatures
have the same sign. That is to say, the assumption was made that
the surfaces presented to the network were always convex or concave,
but never saddle-shaped. Possibly, this assumption may be relaxed in

more complex images where additional information is available from neighboring regions.

11.3.3   Constructing the Network Model

We used the "error back-propagation" learning algorithm as a design technique for constructing a network with the desired characteristics (Rumelhart, Hinton, and Williams 1986; Parker 1986; LeCun 1985; Werbos 1987). The details of the algorithm are given in Appendix 11.A. Essentially, the following was done. The network was presented with many sample images. For each presentation, responses were propagated up through several layers of neural-like units to a layer of output units. The actual responses of the output units were then compared with what the output for that image should have been. Based on this difference, synaptic weights throughout the network were slightly modified to reduce error, starting with synapses at the output layer themselves and then moving back down through the network (hence the name back-propagation). After thousands of image presentations, the initially random synaptic weights organized themselves into a set of receptive fields that provided the correct input/output transfer function. (In all cases, units could assume any level of activity over the range 0.0–1.0.)

It should be made clear at this point that the "back-propagation" algorithm was used purely as a formal technique for constructing a network with a particular set of properties. This is not a model of developmental neurobiology, and no claims are made about the biological significance of the process by which the network was created. The focus of interest here will be on the properties of the mature network.

As input for the network, we generated 2,000 images of elliptic paraboloid surfaces. Each paraboloid differed in the magnitudes of the principal curvatures, the orientation (principal direction) of the minimum curvature (the maximum curvature is always at right angles to this orientation), the slant and tilt of the illumination direction, and the location of the center of the surface within the overall image. Image parameters were all selected with a uniform random distribution. Principal curvatures were generated over the four-octave range $1/2°$ to $1/32°$. The direction of minimum curvature was between $0°$ and $180°$. Light tilt was also between $0°$ and $180°$, and light slant was between $0°$ and $60°$. The center of the paraboloid surface could lie anywhere within a circular disk comprising the central third of the image. These 2,000 images served as the training corpus for the neural network learning algorithm.

The particular network we used had three layers: an input unit layer, an output unit layer, and a hidden unit layer between them (fig. 11.3a).

There are no lateral interactions between units within a layer, nor any feedback connections. Each unit in a layer is connected to every unit in the subsequent layer. The overall organization of the network is seen in fig. 11.4c, which shows the response of the fully developed network to a typical input image. The two hexagonal regions at the bottom represent responses of the 122 input units. Responses of the 27 units in the hidden layer are represented in the 3 x 9 rectangular array above the hexagons. Finally, the responses of the 24 units in the output layer are represented in the 4 x 6 array at the top. In all cases, areas of the black squares are proportional to the activity of a particular unit. These three layers will be more fully described below.

The response properties of the input and output units were predefined for the network, based on what operations we wanted the network to perform, as well as being constrained by biological plausibility. Through the learning algorithm, the network proceeded to develop connections between the input units and the hidden units (the receptive fields of the hidden units), and connections between the hidden units and the output units (the projective fields of the hidden units). These hidden unit response properties essentially act as a mapping, or transform, that converts the inputs to the desired outputs. Before further considering the hidden units and their receptive fields, we describe the properties of the input and output units. The input layer consisted of two hexagonal spatial arrays of units, called the on-center units and off-center units (for an explanation of these cell types see chapter 10; only the spatial and not the temporal aspects of the receptive fields were incorporated into our model). A hexagonal array was chosen over a square array because we were interested in determining stimulus orientations, and a hexagonal array has a greater degree of rotational symmetry than a square one (biologically, there is too much scatter in the positions of retinal ganglion cells to readily classify them as falling into a simple geometrical lattice, whether square or hexagonal (Wässle, Boycott, and Illing 1981). The two input arrays (off-center units and on-center units) were superimposed on each other, so that each point of the image was sampled by both an on-center unit and an off-center unit. Each of these arrays consisted of 61 units, for a total of 122 units in the input layer (61 happens to come out to an even number on a hexagonal array). The receptive field of each input unit was the Laplacian of a two-dimensional Gaussian, or in other words the classic circularly symmetric center-surround receptive field found in the retina and lateral geniculate nucleus. This receptive field organization is illustrated in fig. 11.3b, which also shows that the receptive fields of the input units were extensively overlapped

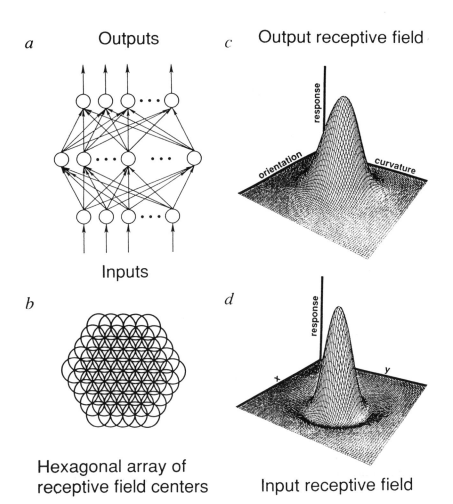

a — Outputs

Inputs

b

Hexagonal array of
receptive field centers

c — Output receptive field

d — Input receptive field

Figure 11.3
(a) Schematic diagram of network used here, having three layers: an input layer
(122 units), a middle "hidden" layer (27 units), and an output layer (27 units).
(b) Receptive field of an input unit, defined as the Laplacian of a Gaussian. This
figure shows an on-center unit. The network also included off-center units, in which
excitatory and inhibitory lobes were reversed. (c) Input units were organized into
hexagonal arrays. Circles represent receptive field centers. The input image was
sampled by two superimposed hexagonal arrays, representing on-center and off-center
cells. (d) Output units had two-dimensional tuning curves in a parameter space
defined by curvature orientation and curvature magnitude. Each of the 24 output
units had peak responses at a different combination of orientation and magnitude.

(fig. 11.3c). The receptive fields of on-center units had excitatory centers and inhibitory surrounds, while off-center units had opposite polarity. Responses of the input units to an image were determined simply by convolving the image with the units' receptive fields. Aside from being biologically motivated, choosing these center-surround input receptive fields (Laplacian of a Gaussian) is advantageous from a computational viewpoint. Specifically, these receptive fields, acting as second-derivative operators, have responses that tend to reduce changes in image appearance arising from changes in illumination direction (Marr and Hildreth 1980).

Moving to the output units, they have responses tuned to both curvature magnitude and curvature orientation, as illustrated in fig. 11.3d. In other words, they have receptive fields tuned to a local region in a two-dimensional magnitude-orientation parameter space (in contrast to the input units, which are tuned to a local region of geometrical space). The equation defining output responses is:

$$R = A(m) \ B(o) \tag{11.1}$$

where $A(m)$ is Gaussian as a function of the logarithm of curvature magnitude (lognormal function), and $B(o)$ is a Gaussian function of curvature orientation. This sort of multidimensional response is typical of those found in cells of the cortex, although cells responding specifically to curvature have not been demonstrated. The output units had curvature tuning curves $A(m)$ with peaks of either $1/8°$ or $-1/8°$, depending on whether the unit responded to a convex or a concave surface. Half-width bandwidth of curvature tuning was one octave at $1/e$ height. Orientation tuning curves $B(o)$ had peaks set to $0°$, $30°$, $60°$, $90°$, $120°$, and $150°$, with half-width bandwidth of $30°$ at $1/e$ height.

However, the problem with having a nonmonotonic, multidimensional response is that the signal from a single unit is degenerate. There are an infinite number of combinations of curvature and orientation that give an identical response. The way to solve this ambiguity is to have the desired value represented in a distributed fashion (distributed coding), by the joint activity of a population of broadly tuned units in which the units have overlapping receptive fields in the relevant parameter space (in this case curvature magnitude and orientation).

The most familiar example of this kind of distributed coding or representation is found in color vision. The responses of any one of the three broadly tuned color receptors is ambiguous, but the relative activities of all three allow one precisely to discriminate a very large number of colors. Note the economy of this form of encoding; it is possible to form fine discriminations with only a very small number of coarsely tuned units, as opposed to requiring a large number of narrowly tuned, nonoverlapping units (Hinton, McClelland, and Rumelhart 1986; Sejnowski 1988). The output representation of parameters in the model under consideration here will follow the coarse tuning approach. With this brief description of the concept of distributed representations, we can now examine the actual output representation used here, as illustrated in fig. 11.4. Again, the output units are represented by the 4 x 6 array at the top of the figure. The output units have tuning curves that are overlapping with peaks at different curvature orientations as one moves horizontally along a row. For the image used in this example, the curvature orientation was 10°. One can see from the size of the black squares for the output units along a row that the largest responses come from units that have peak responses close to 10°, and responses drop off as orientation tuning moves away from that value. The orientation value specified by any one unit is ambiguous, but the joint activities serve to precisely define orientation.

Moving vertically from top to bottom, the four rows represent different curvatures. The top two rows represent the value of the smaller of the two principal curvatures and the bottom two rows represent the larger principal curvature. Within each of those two pairs of rows, the top row responds if the curvature is positive (convex surface) and the bottom one responds if the curvature is negative (concave surface).

Unfortunately, this manner of representing curvature leaves the curvature magnitude ambiguous (unlike the situation in the orientation domain). For example, if a unit gives a small response, we don't know if it is because curvature is above or below the peak of the tuning curve. This is because there are no sets of output units tuned to different but overlapping ranges of curvatures, as there were units tuned to different but overlapping ranges of orientations (peak values of curvature are at either $1/8°$ or $-1/8°$, which are far enough apart so as not to overlap).

The way to remedy the situation would have been to introduce a greater number of output units, having overlapping tuning curves in the curvature domain. Having units sensitive to different ranges of curvatures is equivalent to making them sensitive to different spatial scales; surfaces with large curvatures have variations in reflected light intensities occurring at fine spatial scales, and small curvatures have variations occurring at broad spatial scales. Therefore, constructing a network whose outputs have overlapping curvature tuning curves would involve sampling the input image at different spatial scales (i.e., repeatedly convolving the input image with center-surround input receptive fields with

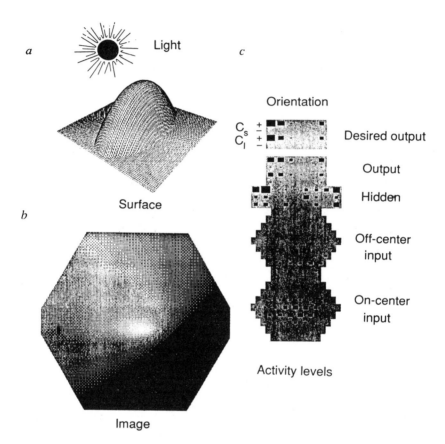

Figure 11.4
Typical input image and the resulting activity levels within a fully trained network.
(a) Example of elliptic paraboloid surface (flat base did not fall within input field
of the network). (b) Example of input image synthesized from light reflected off the
surface of an elliptic paraboloid surface. A set of 2000 such images were used to train
the network. (c) Responses of network to the image. Double hexagons show responses
of on-center and off-center input units. Area of a black square is proportional to a
unit's activity. Resulting activities in the 27 hidden units are shown in the 3x9 array
above the hexagons, and activities of the 24 output units are shown in a 4x6 array
at the top. This output should be compared with the 4x6 array at the very top
(separated from the rest), showing the correct response for the image. The 4x6 array
is arranged as follows. The six columns correspond to different peaks in orientation
tuning. Rows correspond to different curvature magnitudes.

different diameters, instead of a single diameter as has been done here). However, this has not been implemented here. The question of the integrating multiple spatial scales has been deferred until the neural network is presented with stimuli more complex than the smooth paraboloid surfaces used here.

11.3.4 Properties of the Fully Developed Network

A network containing 122 input units, 27 hidden units, and 24 output units was trained in the manner described earlier. The 2,000 input images were presented to the network one at a time, and after each presentation the connection strengths were changed slightly to make the values of the units on the output layer compare more closely with the desired output values. Around 40,000 trials were required before performance of the network reached a plateau at a median correlation of 0.88 between actual outputs and the correct outputs over the 2,000 input images used to train the network. The connection strengths developed by the network are presented in fig. 11.5, which will be fully described below. Learning curves (correlation as a function of number of trials) for different numbers of hidden units are shown in fig. 11.6, although only results for 27 hidden units will be discussed in detail below. The learning curves show that adding more hidden units improves performance up to a point, but beyond that, additional hidden units contribute nothing. This observation is corroborated by the finding that if there are too many hidden units, the superfluous ones fail to develop strong synaptic connections. Note also that a network with no hidden units (direct connections from the input to the output layers) performs better than a network with three hidden units. There is a bottleneck caused by the hidden layer, which reduces the total number of weights when there are only three hidden units. The network with no hidden units is essentially a perceptron and its performance is surprisingly good; this is probably a consequence of the on-center and off-center preprocessing stage, which is evidently a good input representation. However, the one-layer network fails badly at many images which would pose no difficult for humans. This indicates that some part of the problem is second-order or higher.

Ability of the network to generalize (produce the correct output when presented with patterns it had never seen before) was tested in the following manner. The set of 2,000 images was randomly divided in half. The network was trained on one set of 1,000 images, and then the mature network was tested (without learning) on the other half. The results are given in fig. 11.7, as histograms of all the correlation coefficients between actual and correct output for the 1,000 training images, and also

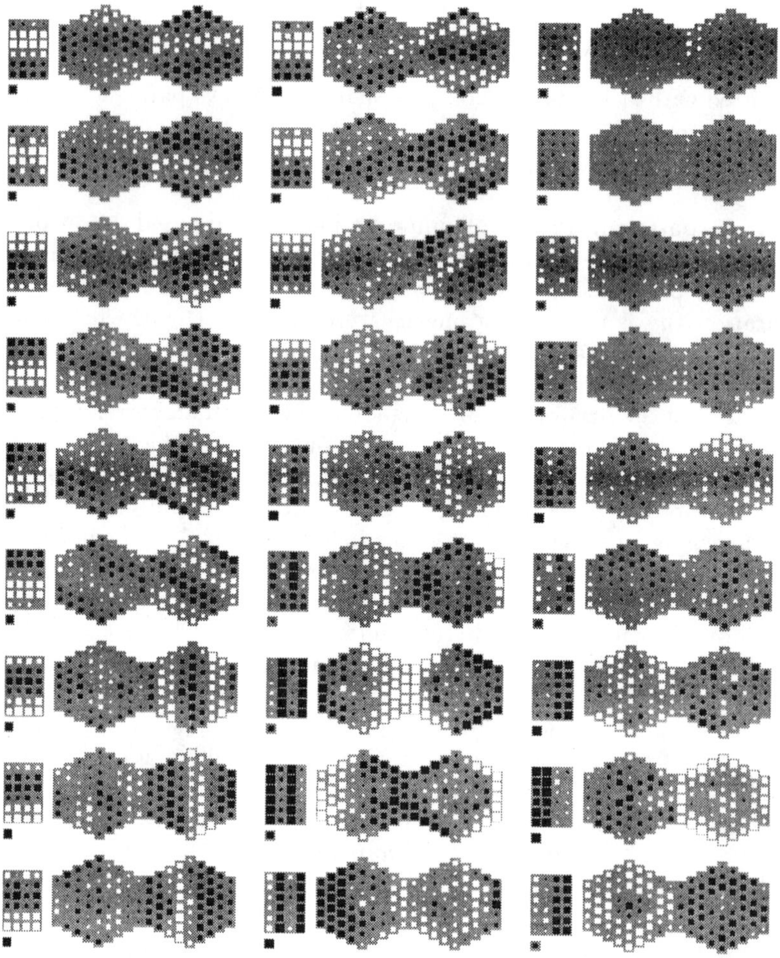

Figure 11.5
Hinton diagram showing connection strengths in the network. Each of the 27 hidden
units is represented by one hourglass-shaped icon, showing an input receptive field
from on- and off-center units (double hexagons), and an output projective field (4x6
array at the top). Organization of the 4x6 array is the same as described in fig. 11.3.
Excitatory weights are white, inhibitory ones are black, and the area of a square
is proportional to the connection strength it represented. Isolated square at the
upper left of each icon indicates the unit's bias (equivalent to a negative threshold).
Black horizontal lines group together units of the same type based on receptive field
organization.

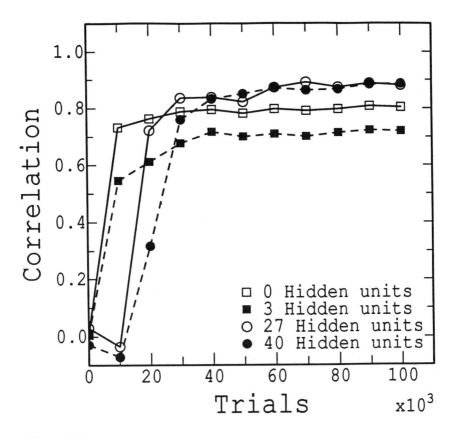

Figure 11.6
Learning curves for the network, showing correlation between actual and correct responses of the output units as a function of the number of learning trials. Learning curves for networks with different numbers of hidden units are shown here.

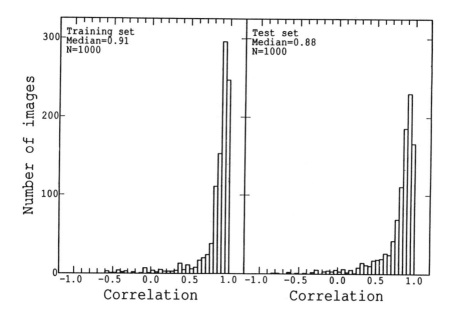

Figure 11.7
Demonstration of network's ability to generalize and give correct responses to images that were not part of its training set. The network was trained on a set of
1,000 images, and then tested on a different set of 1,000 images. (a) Distribution
of correlation coefficients between actual and correct outputs for the images of the
training set. (b) Distribution of correlation coefficients for images not part of the
training set.

the 1,000 test images. These histograms indicate that the network gen-
eralizes well to patterns that were not in the training set.

Figure 11.5 is of central importance in understanding the fully developed network. It is a Hinton diagram, showing all the connection
strengths between units in the fully developed network. Each of the
27 hidden units is represented by one of the grey hourglass-shaped figures. Connection strengths are represented as black and white squares
of varying size. The white squares are excitatory weights, the black
squares are inhibitory weights, and the area of the square is proportional to the magnitude of the weight. Within each hourglass figure two
sets of connections are shown. First, there are the connection strengths
from all input units to that particular hidden unit, and second, connection strengths from that hidden unit to all the output units. The two
hexagonal arrays on the bottom of each figure show the connections from

the on-center and off-center input arrays to the hidden unit (hidden unit receptive field), and the 4 x 6 rectangular array at the top are the connections from the hidden unit to units in the output layer (hidden unit projective field). Finally, the value of the bias, or negative threshold, is shown in the isolated square at the upper left corner of each hidden unit figure.

The pattern of excitatory and inhibitory connections in the two hexagonal input arrays can be interpreted as receptive fields of the hidden units. Most of the hidden units appear to be orientation-tuned to a variety of directions. These oriented fields have several excitatory and inhibitory lobes, which may occur in various phases. This is the pattern found in simple cells in cat and monkey visual cortex, which are often fit with Gabor functions (DeValois, DeValois, and Yund 1979; Kulikowski and Bishop 1981; Andrews and Pollen 1979; Wilson and Sherman 1976. See also fig. 10.5; the earlier studies of Hubel and Wiesel (1962, 1965) had focused on the central two or three lobes, which are the most prominent). In addition to units that were clearly orientation-selective, a few units had receptive fields that were more or less circularly symmetric.

Upon examining projective fields, three types become apparent. Type 1 has a vertical pattern of organization to the 4 x 6 array of weights, type 2 has a horizontal organization with alternate rows similar, and type 3 has a horizontal organization with adjacent rows similar. These classes of hidden units appear to provide information to output units about orientation of the principal curvatures (type 1), their signs (convexity/concavity) (type 2), and their relative magnitudes (type 3). A few hidden units were difficult to classify, and several failed to develop large weights.

Overall, then, we distinguish three types of hidden units: those providing orientation information, those providing information about the signs of principal curvatures, and those providing information about relative magnitudes of the two principal curvatures. It should be noted, however, that the receptive fields of some hidden units are somewhat irregular, and that combinations of units might be working together to provide information that is not apparent from examining single units. Incidentally, during construction of the network the three types of units always developed in a particular temporal sequence. Sign units came first, followed by orientation units, and finally magnitude units.

An interesting question is whether the hidden units in this network act as feature detectors or as parameter filters. By a feature detector we mean a unit that responds strongly when presented with an appropriate and specific stimulus and poorly to all other inputs, in essence

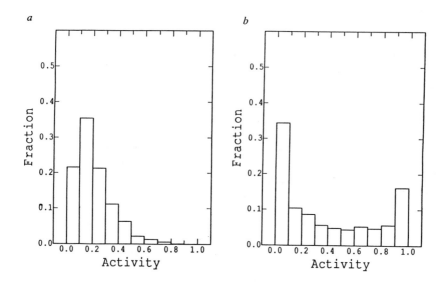

Figure 11.8
Distribution of responses of single units when the network was presented with a set of 2,000 images. (a) Unimodal distribution typical of a type 1 unit, selective for curvature orientation. Type 3 units, selective for the relative magnitudes of the two principal curvatures, also had unimodal distributions. We interpret units with this sort of response as filters indicating the values of particular parameters. (b) Bimodal distribution typical of a type 2 unit, selective for the signs of the principal curvatures (convexity/concavity). Units having this sort of response, which tended to be either fully on or off, are interpreted as feature detectors.

an all-or-nothing response. By a parameter filter we mean a unit that responds with a continuous range of activities when presented with various stimuli, a unit whose responses are defined by a rather broad tuning curve for a particular parameter. To investigate the matter, we looked at the responses of individual hidden units when presented with the corpus of 2,000 images. For each input image, the response of the unit fell between 0.0–1.0. By plotting a histogram of the unit's response levels when presented with many inputs we hoped to classify the unit, with the histogram of a parameter filter unit showing a unimodal distribution having a peak at some intermediate level of activity, and a feature detector unit having a bimodal response histogram with activities concentrated at either very high or very low levels.

We found examples of both kinds of behavior among the hidden units (fig. 11.8). Of the three hidden unit classes, the orientation units (type 1) and the magnitude units (type 3) had unimodal distributions, and we classified them as parameter filters. In contrast, the curvature sign units (type 2) invariably had bimodal distributions in which they tended to be fully on or fully off. We interpret type 2 as feature detectors that discriminate between surface convexity and concavity.

The results of the learning procedure shown in fig. 11.5 were representative of many training runs. Each started with a different set of random weights. Similar patterns of receptive fields were always found, and the same three types of units could be found by examining the connections to the output units. However, there was variation in the details of the receptive fields, and in the number of units that did not develop any pattern of connections. It appears that only a limited number of hidden units are needed to achieve the maximum performance, which always had an a correlation close to 0.88. The extra hidden units undergo "cell death" (occurring as a consequence of the weight decay term in the learning algorithm; see also Appendix 11.A), since they serve no useful role in the network and can be eliminated without changing the performance.

The term "receptive field" of a unit was used above to refer to the pattern of excitatory and inhibitory connections arriving from the preceding layer of units. However, the true receptive field is something different; it is not a pattern of synaptic connections, but the response of that unit to a stimulus, such as a spot or bar of light, as a function of spatial position. The stimulus response depends not only on the immediate synaptic inputs to a unit, but also on the filtering properties of units in the preceding layers.

To examine these true "receptive fields" we have explored the responses of units in the network to bars of light, in essence conducting "simulated neurophysiology." The bars were varied in position, orientation, width, and length. These bar stimuli were chosen because there is an extensive experimental literature using them, so that responses of real neurons are known.

The responses of hidden units to bars were easily predictable from the pattern of excitatory and inhibitory connections they received from the input units. Tuning curves were measured for all stimulus parameters (bar position, orientation, width, and length). Just by looking at the pattern of connection strengths in the weights diagram (fig. 11.5) it was possible to form a good estimate of what the optimal bar stimulus would be. The ease in understanding hidden unit responses is not surprising, since the only intermediary between the stimulus and the hidden units is the array of simple center-surround receptive fields of the input units.

The situation was quite different when measuring responses of output units to bar stimuli. Finding an optimal stimulus took extensive trial and error. Again, this is not surprising. The response of each output unit is determined by a weighted combination of the inputs from all 27 hidden units (although in practice a smaller number of hidden units tend to predominate). In other words, the response of each output unit is some combination of all the 27 patterns shown in fig. 11.5. It is therefore very difficult to grasp intuitively what the responses to a particular stimulus will be.

Despite the complex organization of receptive fields for output units, it was possible to obtain smooth tuning curves for the various bar parameters. Tunings were generally broader than in hidden units. One feature of some output unit responses was the presence of strong "end-stopped inhibition." Responses dropped off precipitously when bar length was extended beyond a certain point. Also, as the bar was swept across the network in a direction transverse to the optimal orientation, the output units responded over a broader region than the hidden units did (about 1.5–2.0 times as wide). This is as expected, since output units receive convergent input from a number of hidden units.

The responses of units in the hidden and output layers are reminiscent of the behavior of some units that have been found in primary visual cortex (Hubel and Wiesel 1962, 1965). It is possible to think of the hidden units as having simple cell-like properties, and output units as behaving like some types of complex cells. However, in drawing this analogy it should be kept in mind that the relationship between hidden units and output units is strictly hierarchical (in the sense that responses of output units are entirely synthesized from inputs from the preceding hidden units), while the extent to which such a hierarchical relationship holds for simple and complex cells has not yet been settled (Gilbert 1983; Bolz and Gilbert 1986).

A major point to make about the receptive field properties of units in this network, and perhaps the most important lesson to be drawn from this entire modeling study, is the following. Knowledge of the receptive field of a unit does not appear sufficient to deduce the function of that unit within a network. The receptive fields shown in fig. 11.5 can easily be interpreted as bar detectors, or edge detectors (or from another point of view, spatial frequency filters). What they are in fact doing is extracting principal curvatures from shaded surfaces. Yet it seems unlikely that this interpretation would have occurred to someone. The questions this network raises for standard interpretations of receptive fields of real neurons are obvious. While we can determine the receptive field of a neuron, there is at present no practical method of determining its projective field. Yet it would appear that the projective field is as important as the receptive field in determining the function of a neuron. The network model provides an alternative interpretation of the observed properties of cortical cells, namely that they can be used to compute shape from shading rather than, or in addition to, detecting edges. The information contained in the shaded portions of objects in images can partially activate the simple and complex cells in visual cortex, and these responses can be used to extract curvature parameters from the image. It might prove interesting to test the response properties of cortical cells with curved surfaces similar to those used here.

Although the response properties of the processing units in our model were similar in some respects to the properties of neurons in visual cortex, the way that these response properties arise could be quite different. For example, projections from the lateral geniculate are all excitatory, but we have allowed feedforward connections that are both excitatory and inhibitory. Also, the oriented responses of cells in visual cortex may arise in part from inhibitory interneurons, as discussed in detail in chapter 10 (see also Sillito 1985). However, our network is not meant to be a literal model of actual cortical circuitry, which is certainly much more complex, but rather a model of the representation in visual cortex of information about surfaces in the visual field. The same representations could be constructed differently in different systems, as indeed the orientation tuning of neurons in different species might also have different origins though they might serve the same function.

Nonetheless, we believe that our model can evolve toward a more detailed account of real cortical circuitry as more information is found about detailed patterns of connectivity between different cell types in cortex. As a first step towards creating a more realistic network, we constructed one that constrained all the connections from the on-center and off-center cells in the input layer to be excitatory, as found for principal cells in the lateral geniculate nucleus. The average performance of the network was nearly identical to the previous network, and same response properties were found for the hidden units as before. Evidently, the off-center cells were able to substitute for the on-center inhibition, and vice versa.

As was mentioned earlier, the network model handles shape from shading as a problem in pattern recognition, looking for particular configurations of light and dark over an extended region. In this respect the network resembles the model of Koenderink and Van Doorn (1980) (which they described but never implemented) and a more recent model by

Pentland (1988) that uses the sums of filters much like our hidden units. The information about the curvature parameters of a particular patch of image was contained in the distributed pattern of activity in hidden unit layer. Whatever precision the network loses by adopting such a delocalized analysis may be compensated by increased robustness.

Humans are only able to extract an approximate estimate of the curvature from local shading information, and it will be interesting to compare the accuracy of the network constructed here with that of humans under controlled psychophysical conditions (Mingolla and Todd 1986; Ramachandran 1988). It is also clear that humans use other cues to estimate curvatures, such as the outline of bounding contours. This suggests that the network presented here should be considered only a small part of a much more complex system that uses multiple cues.

11.4   Conclusions

It is clear that the present generation of neural models cannot begin to reflect the complexity of the real nervous system. From anatomy and physiology we know that the visual system is a tangled web of multiple inputs, feedback loops, and lateral interaction, and moreover that each unit within that web is a complex entity in itself, with the various nonlinear temporal and spatial integrative aspects of the dendritic tree being one part of that complexity. It is from a confrontation with this complexity, from a desire to see some pattern to it, that one is led to attempt the extraction of essential features and incorporate them into a simple model. This leads to the most difficult part in constructing a model, which is to decide what is an "essential feature" and what is "simple." These are ultimately matters of intuition and judgment, although of course the choices are related to the types of questions being asked (whether they concern psychological phenomena or biophysical problems).

The proposed network model of rivalry is intended as a functional description rather than a realistic model, and the "equivalent circuit" in the model may eventually translate into a much more complex network in the real nervous system. For example, the individual neurons in the model are likely to represent populations of real neurons that have some functional properties in common. Another limitation of the model is the difficulty in precisely specifying where in the system the neurons should be found. However, the model indicates places to look and predictions for what might be found there. The model suggests that it is worthwhile to investigate sites of reciprocal inhibition prior to the site of binocular convergence. This suggestion depends on both the psychophysical data and knowledge of mechanisms that are known to exist in the nervous system in the areas of interest. All of this provides experimentalists some justification to embark on a line of investigation that they might not otherwise have thought interesting.

An electrical circuit analog was used to study the nonlinear dynamics of the underlying neural model of binocular rivalry. It might be objected that the electrical circuit, which is made of transistors and resistors, is not relevant to the biological problem, because neurons have properties that are different at the biophysical level. Many of the qualitative features of the electrical analog circuit are insensitive to the detailed biophysical properties of the nonlinear summing elements; when such properties are important, then provision must be made for incorporating these properties into the electrical analog. In the case of the simple circuit for binocular rivalry, we can verify by simulation that a neural model with plausible biophysical properties displays the same qualitative properties as the electrical circuit. The value of the electrical circuit model is that it can be physically built and studied under real-time conditions, which is usually not possible with digital simulations. With analog VLSI technology (Mead 1989) it is possible to build many thousands of such circuits and to study their properties under conditions that would be difficult or impossible otherwise.

In the proposed network for extracting curvature parameters from shaded images, the receptive field properties needed at the intermediate level of hidden units were similar to the properties of simple cells in primary visual cortex. These properties were not determined by the intuition of the model builder, but by the learning algorithm. The modeler specified the function that the network was required to perform only by giving examples of inputs and the desired outputs. Once trained, the network model was able to compute curvature parameters for new images nearly as well as for the ones it was trained on. The learning algorithm that was used to construct the model need not have a counterpart in the nervous system for the resulting model to have validity; the process is not intended as a model of development but simply as a technique for generating hypotheses for what might be found in the nervous system.

It might be instructive to compare our approach with that taken in chapter 10, where a realistic model of the retina, LGN and layer IV of visual cortex were simulated. The questions that motivated that model were structural ones such as the projection patterns of LGN cells in cortex and the origin of orientation selectivity. The question of what

function the oriented simple cells had was not raised—it was enough
for the model to mimic the actual responses of simple cells under a
variety of conditions. In contrast, the questions that motivated our
model related to the properties of the images and the information that
could be extracted by the network. In our model of binocular rivalry, we
were led to the hypothesis that feedback connections to the LGN are able
to gate incoming sensory information. In our cortical model of shape-
from-shading, we found units in the hidden layer of our network that
were similar to simple cells; our primary concern was in interpreting
the function of these cells and not in their genesis. It was only after
examining the outputs of these cells—their projective fields—that we
were able to understand their function in the network. In the realistic
simulation of oriented cortical neurons presented in chapter 10, the cells
had no output projections, and hence could not have any function. It
is clear that these two models are complementary in their strengths and
weaknesses. Both types of models are needed if we are to understand
the visual cortex at all levels.

Neural network modeling is still at an early stage of development,
but it is already clear that new principles are emerging concerning the
representation of information in neural populations, and transformations
that are possible with these coding schemes. For example, Georgopoulos,
Schwartz, and Kettner (1986) have shown that in motor cortex, information about the intended direction of arm movement is distributed in
populations of neurons that are broadly tuned to the direction. Lee et
al. (1988) have presented evidence for the coarsely coded representation
of eye movements in the deeper layers of the superior colliculus. Zipser
and Andersen (1987) have applied the same approach used here to the
problem of transforming from retina-based coordinates to head-centered
coordinates. They report that the properties of the hidden units in their
model are similar in essential respects to those of some neurons in parietal cortex. The success of their model and ours depended to a large
extent on incorporating what was known about the single-unit properties and the style of representation found in cerebral cortex into the
models. Learning algorithms provide a new technique for drawing out
the implications of these assumptions and exploring some of the principles of distributed processing in sensory and motor systems. Ultimately,
evaluation of this claim rests upon the ability of the models to provide
results useful in organizing data and suggesting new experiments.

This work was supported by a Presidential Young Investigator Award to Terrence J. Sejnowski and grants from the National Science Foundation, Sloan Foundation, General Electric Corporation, Allied Corporation Foundation, Richard Lounsbery Foundation, Seaver Institute, Air Force Office of Scientific Research, and Office of Naval Research. The address of Sidney Lehky is Department of Biophysics, Johns Hopkins University, Baltimore, Maryland 21218. The address of Terrence Sejnowski is The Salk Institute, P. O. Box 85800, San Diego, California 92138. Electronic mail should be addressed to terry%sdbio2@ucsd.edu.

Appendix 11.A: Back-Propagation Learning Algorithm

Back-propagation is a learning procedure that modifies connection strengths throughout a neural network to reduce the error between the actual output of the network and the correct output. This adjustment occurs as the network is presented with many examples of the task at hand. It works on networks with multilayered feedforward architectures. Although the network described in this chapter only had three layers, the algorithm allows more. Also, in this network each layer only connected to the immediately subsequent layer, but in general there can be direct connections between the input layer and the output layer as well as through the hidden units. Finally, in this network connections between layers were global, which means that each unit in a layer connected to every unit in the subsequent layer. The algorithm does not require that connections be global.

We used the back-propagation algorithm in the form introduced by Rumelhart et al. (1986). (See also similar algorithms in Parker (1986), LeCun (1985) and Werbos (1987).) The properties of the nonlinear processing units in the model network include (1) the integration of diverse low-accuracy excitatory and inhibitory signals arriving from other units, (2) an output signal that is the nonlinear transform of the total integrated input, including a threshold, and (3) a complex pattern of interconnectivity. The output of a unit is formed by linearly summing all inputs from units of the previous layer, both excitatory and inhibitory, each weighted by a connection strength, and then passing this sum through a nonlinear function, as shown in fig 11.8. This function monotonically increases with input and has a sigmoid shape: it approaches 0.0 for large negative input, and it approaches 1.0 as the input becomes large. This roughly describes the firing rate of a neuron as a function of its integrated input: if the input is below threshold there is no output, the firing rate increases with the input, and it saturates at a maximum firing rate.

The sigmoid function that we used is given by

$$s_i = P(E_i) = \frac{1}{1 + e^{-E_i}} \tag{11.2}$$

where s_i is the output of the ith unit and the total input E_i is

$$E_i = \sum_j w_{ij} s_j \tag{11.3}$$

where w_{ij} is the weight from the jth unit in the preceding layer to the ith unit. These model units are identical to those used in chapter 7. The weights can have positive or negative real values, representing an excitatory or inhibitory influence (the behavior of the network does not depend critically on the exact mathematical form of the sigmoid function, and only needs to be a monotonically increasing function bounded from above and below). It is possible to place restrictions on the signs of the weights from a single neuron; for example, all of the weights from an inhibitory interneuron could be restricted to negative values.

In addition to inputs from other units, the activity of a unit depends on its threshold. In some learning algorithms, including this one, thresholds are variable and are continuously modified during training. To make the notation uniform in eq. 11.3, the threshold is treated as a bias arising from a special imaginary unit, called the true unit, which always had an activity level of 1.0 (in eq. 11.3 the true unit is the unit $j = 0$). The value of a unit's bias is determined by the weight of the connection from the true unit. This bias acts like a threshold whose value is the negative of the weight.

The goal of the learning procedure is to minimize the average squared error between the computed values of the output units and the correct pattern, s_i^*, provided by a teacher:

$$Error = \sum_{i=1}^{J}(s_i^* - s_i^{(N)})^2 \tag{11.4}$$

where J is the number of units in the output layer. The first step in the back-propagation procedure is to compute the output of the network for a given input using the procedure described above on successive layers. Once this is accomplished, the error gradient on the output layer is computed:

$$\delta_i^{(N)} = (s_i^* - s_i^{(N)})P'(E_i^{(N)}) \tag{11.5}$$

and then the error gradient is propagated backward through the network, layer by layer:

$$\delta_i^{(n)} = \sum_{j} \delta_j^{(n+1)} w_{ji}^{(n)} P'(E_i^{(n)}) \tag{11.6}$$

where $P'(E_i)$ is the first derivative of the function $P(E_i)$.

These gradients are the directions in which each weight should be altered to reduce the error for a particular item. To reduce the average

error for all the input patterns, these gradients must be averaged over
all the training patterns before updating the weights. In practice, it is
sufficient to average $\delta_i^{(N)}$ over several inputs before updating the weights.
Another method is to compute a running average of the gradient with
an exponentially decaying filter:

$$\Delta w_{ij}^{(n)}(new) = \alpha \Delta w_{ij}^{(n)}(old) + (1-\alpha)\,\delta_i^{(n+1)} s_j^{(n)} \qquad (11.7)$$

where $\alpha = 0.95$ is a smoothing parameter. In practice these weight
gradients were first averaged over 5 images before the smoothing was
performed, and the smoothed weight gradients $\Delta w_{ij}^{(n)}$ were then used to
update the weights:

$$w_{ij}^{(n)}(new) = (1-\beta)w_{ij}^{(n)}(old) + \epsilon \Delta w_{ij}^{(n)} \qquad (11.8)$$

where $\beta = 0.0001$ is a small number that produces decay of the weights
and $\epsilon = 10.0$ is the learning rate. The purpose of the weight decay is
to gradually reduce the size of any weight that is not serving a useful purpose. Supernumerary weights can make the patterns of weights
more difficult to interpret. When learning has reached an asymptote,
the "forces" of learning and decay are balanced. The values of these
parameters are chosen to optimize the final performance of the network
and minimize the learning time. They are problem-dependent and may
also be varied during the course of learning. The learning rate should
be large at the start of learning and can be reduced (along with the
weight decay) later when the learning curve is reaching an asymptote.
The error signal was back-propagated only when the difference between
the actual and desired values of the outputs was greater than a margin
$(= 0.03)$. This insures that the network does not overlearn on inputs
that it is already getting correct. This learning algorithm can be generalized to networks with feedback connections (Pineda 1987), but this
extension will not be discussed further.

The definitions of the learning parameters here are somewhat different
from those in Rumelhart et al. (1986). In the original algorithm ϵ is used
rather than $(1-\alpha)$ in eq. 11.7. Our parameter α is used to smooth the
gradient in a way that is independent of the learning rate, ϵ, which
only appears in the weight update, eq. 11.8. Our averaging procedure
also makes it unnecessary to scale the learning rate by the number of
presentations per weight update.

A simulator including source code for the back-propagation algorithm
written in the programming language C is included in McClelland and
Rumelhart (1988).

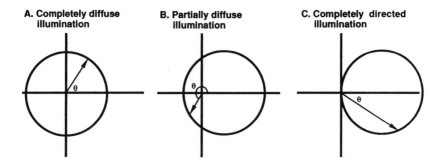

Figure 11.9
Geometrical illustration of illumination and reflectance model under three illumination conditions. Partially diffuse illumination was the condition actually used in
the shape-from-shading model. The angle between the surface normal and the predominant direction of illumination is indicated by θ, and the length of the vector
extending from the origin to the circle indicates the intensity of light reflected for a
surface oriented at that angle. The vectors shown in the figure are arbitrarily chosen
examples.

Appendix 11.B: Illumination and Reflectance Model

The surfaces used in the shape-from-shading model had matte, or diffuse reflectance properties, as opposed to being shiny or specular. The
illumination upon the surfaces was also diffuse, by which we mean that
although light came predominantly from a particular direction, there
were also components from all directions arising from scattering and reflections. This diffuse illumination was used in order to eliminate sharp
shadow edges upon the paraboloid surfaces (for a general discussion of
these issues within the context of computer vision, see Horn 1986). The
properties of illumination and reflectance used here are illustrated geometrically in fig. 11.9. The value of θ indicates the angle between the
surface normal vector and the predominant direction of illumination.
The intensity of light reflected from a surface is indicated by the length
of the vector with its tail at the origin and tip lying on the circle.

Three illumination conditions are shown in fig. 11.9: (A) completely
diffuse, (B) partially diffuse, and (C) completely directed, of which we
used the second. For the completely diffuse situation, the surface is
uniformly illuminated from all directions and there is no shading. This

is represented in fig. 11.9A by a circle centered on the origin, in which the
reflection vector has constant length independent of orientation. Going
to the other extreme, the situation for completely directed illumination
(fig. 11.9C) is represented by a circle tangent to the ordinate. Here
the length of the reflection vector is $\cos(\theta)$, as in normal Lambertian
reflection, provided $-90° < \theta < 90°$. Those limits correspond to the
occurrence of sharp shadow edges, since the reflectance vector is zero
beyond them. Because we wanted illumination properties between the
two extremes just described, we modeled it by simply shifting the circle
to an intermediate position, as shown in fig. 11.9B. The equation for this
is:

$$R = \cdot \cos(\theta) + \sqrt{(\cos^2(\theta) - 1) + b^2}, \tag{11.9}$$

with $a = (1-R_{min})/2$ and $b = (1+R_{min})/2$. This is the equation for a
circle in polar coordinates, where b is the radius of the circle whose center
has been shifted by a from the origin. R_{min} is the minimum intensity of
light reflected from the surface (the left edge of the circle), which occurs
when the surface is oriented at 180° from the predominant illumination
direction. The parameters a and b both depend on R_{min}. Intuitively,
a determines the relative contribution of scattered illumination, while
b is essentially a normalization factor that keeps maximum reflectance
equal to 1.0 (i.e., expands or contracts the circle so that its right edge
lies a unit distance from the origin). This normalization is not shown in
fig. 11.9, where all circles are of equal diameter.

If $R_{min} = 0$ then eq. 11.9 reduces to Lambertian reflectance $R = \cos(\theta)$, with light coming entirely from one direction. At the other extreme, if $R_{min} = 1.0$ then eq. 11.9 reduces to the constant $R = 1.0$
(which is a circle centered at the origin). In this case there is no predominant light direction. The illumination is entirely isotropic, and there is
no shading. By setting $0.0 < R_{min} < 1.0$, the degree of anisotropy in
the illumination (relative amounts of direct and scattered light) can be
continuously varied. For the work presented here $R_{min} = 0.05$.

This model of illumination and reflectance is a purely empirical approximation for handling diffuse illumination; it appears to be simple
and sensible but is not based on a quantitative consideration of the
physics of the situation. The specifications of both reflection and illumination properties are intertwined within a single equation (eq. 11.1).
Scattered light is handled through the mathematical fiction that there
is non-zero reflectance for the directly incident light when θ lies outside
the range $-90°$ to $90°$, conditions for which in reality the surface is not
at all exposed to the illumination.

CHAPTER 12

Simulating Neurons and Networks
on Parallel Computers

MARK E. NELSON, WOJTEK FURMANSKI, and JAMES M. BOWER

12.1   Introduction

Earlier chapters in this book have stressed the importance of constructing neural models which attempt to capture relevant aspects of the structure and function of biological neural networks. However, limitations in
computing power often restrict the size of a simulation and the amount
of physiological and biophysical detail that can be included. Particularly when a model is in its development phase, the execution time of
the simulation becomes a crucial factor, since the modeling process involves repeatedly running the simulation, evaluating the results, adjusting parameters, and rerunning the simulation. If faster, more powerful
computers were available, then researchers could model larger networks
of neurons or include more of the structural detail relevant to the system
being modeled.

Traditionally, the fastest and most powerful state-of-the-art supercomputers have been relatively inaccessible, and thus of little practical
use to most neural modelers. This situation is beginning to change as
a result of programs such as that sponsored by the National Science
Foundation (NSF) which established a nation wide network to give university researchers access to several NSF-sponsored supercomputing facilities (Jennings et al. 1986). Even so, these facilities are shared among
hundreds of users, so an individual user only gets a small fraction of
the total available computing power. Recently, however, the computer
science community has been exploring an alternative means of achieving
supercomputer-level performance by employing many relatively modest
processors simultaneously to solve a single problem (Dongarra 1987a;
Fox and Messina 1987; Messina 1987). Research has shown that this
"concurrent" or "parallel-processing" approach is a very cost-effective
way of obtaining high computing performance. This technology will
allow single users or small groups of users to purchase dedicated par-

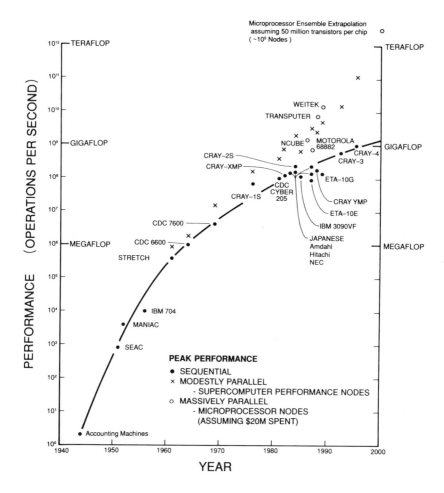

Figure 12.1
Projected peak performance values for sequential and parallel supercomputers. Actual achievable performance on specific problems may be significantly lower. This chapter will explore how to use parallel machines efficiently for modeling neurons and networks.

allel machines for their research, which will give them more integrated computing power than they could obtain through limited access to traditional supercomputers. Furthermore, because computing power can be extended in parallel computers by adding additional processors, these machines are projected to soon surpass traditional sequential supercomputers in terms of peak computing performance, as shown in fig. 12.1 (Fox and Walker 1988). In summary, the cost effectiveness of parallel machines and their considerable computing power makes this technology very attractive for modeling large complex systems.

The availability of affordable supercomputer-level performance via parallel processing is thus good news for neural network researchers, particularly given the ability to extend computing power by adding processors, as knowledge of neural systems and the resulting simulations become more complex. However, there is also a cost associated with using parallel machines, namely that of modifying traditional sequential modeling algorithms to run in parallel on many processors. For some classes of problems that are inherently sequential, this conversion is difficult or impossible. However, as we will show in this chapter, we have found it relatively straightforward to construct efficient concurrent implementations for many neuronal and neural network algorithms (Fox and Furmanski 1987).

In this chapter we will introduce the fundamental concepts of concurrent computing on parallel machines and consider some of the specific technical issues involved in efficiently simulating neurons and neuronal networks. We then outline a general framework for addressing such problems and illustrate our approach by presenting two specific examples that we have implemented on an NCUBE parallel computer: a multicompartment model of a single neuron and a large-scale network model of piriform cortex (described in detail in chapter 9). These two examples were chosen because they represent two extremes in neural modeling on parallel machines. In the first case, the computation for a relatively complicated single neuron is distributed over all the available processing nodes, while in the latter case, each node is responsible for many simpler neurons.

As stated above, our principal motivation for this work has been to increase the capabilities of neural network modeling by exploiting a new computer technology. We were gratified to find that neural models lend themselves to mathematical descriptions that are easy to embody in concurrent algorithms, but were not particularly surprised; after all the nervous system would seem to be "naturally parallel." In fact, this work has also provided an opportunity for considering the possible relationships between parallel processing on computers and parallel processing in the nervous system. We will take up this somewhat more speculative topic in the final section of this chapter.

12.2   Parallel Computers

Before we discuss the specifics of how to solve neural network-related problems on parallel machines, we will first characterize the potentialities as well as the limitations of the machines themselves. Thus we embark on a brief overview of the "comparative anatomy and physiology" of currently available parallel computers.

All computers, serial or parallel, consist of three basic components: processors, memory, and communication channels. Traditional sequential computers consist of a single central processing unit (CPU), some memory for program and data storage, and I/O channels for communicating between the CPU and memory, and with the outside world (terminals, mass storage devices, data buses, etc.). Parallel computers, on the other hand, consist of a number of distributed processing units (DPUs),[1] memory that can be either shared or distributed among the processors, and channels for communicating among processors and memory as well as with the outside world. A particular parallel machine is, therefore, characterized by its particular array of features, including those of the individual processors (instruction set, instructions per second, floating-point operations per second, etc.), those of its memory (number of bytes, access time, shared vs. distributed), and the nature of the communication channels between processors (communication speed, topology of connections, communication protocols). We will now explore each of these characteristics in more detail.

12.2.1   Processors

The computing power of individual processing units varies widely among existing parallel machines, from small units with single-bit arithmetic capabilities, as in the 65536-node Connection Machine, to large powerful units as in the 4-node Cray-XMP. As a general rule, the smaller and simpler the individual processors, the more that can be accommodated in a particular machine. This trend provides the basis for classifying parallel machines in two broad categories: fine-grained and coarse-grained, with

---

[1] This is not standard terminology. Most people still refer to individual processors in a parallel machine as CPUs, even though they are no longer "central" in the same sense.

fine-grained machines having a very large number of relatively simple processing nodes and coarse-grained machines having a smaller number of more powerful processors.

Probably the most familiar contemporary fine-grained machine is the Connection Machine from Thinking Machines Corporation (Hillis 1985, 1987), which in its first incarnation (CM-1) had up to 65536 single-bit processing nodes, with 4 Kbits of memory storage per node.[2] These fine-grained machines usually operate in the SIMD mode, which stands for Single-Instruction Multiple-Data. This mode of operation is synchronous in that each processor in the machine executes the same instruction simultaneously, but with the outcome dependent on data that is stored locally at each node. Although this programming approach is somewhat limited, it turns out to be quite efficient for certain classes of problems (Bowler et al. 1987; Hillis 1985; Wallace 1987). In addition to multipurpose SIMD machines like the Connection Machine, there are also classes of fine-grained machines that are dedicated to solving particular classes of problems like image processing or matrix calculations. These dedicated machines have custom tailored nodes and connections, making them very efficient at solving their particular problem, but of little use outside that domain.

Coarse-grained machines typically employ conventional sequential processors at each node, such as those commonly found in personal computers and workstations (e.g., Motorola 680xx, Intel 80x86, etc.). In some cases however, coarse-grained machines use custom processors that have been designed specifically for parallel processing, as in the case of the NCUBE hypercube (Palmer 1986) and the INMOS transputer (Barron et al. 1983). At the top end in terms of power and complexity of individual nodes are those found in machines like the four-node Cray-XMP and Cray-2 computers. Unlike the fine-grained machines discussed above, most coarse-grained machines are able to store individual programs at each node. Such machines usually operate in the MIMD mode, which stands for Multiple-Instruction Multiple-Data. This mode provides more flexibility than SIMD and allows individual processors to operate asynchronously. Of course, since processors working on the same problem must eventually interact, it is often desirable to establish certain temporal relationships between the processing on different nodes. The degree of temporal coordination can vary from loosely synchronous to essentially fully synchronous. The loosely synchronous mode, which turns

---

[2] A more recent version, CM-2, has up to 65,536 single-bit processors, 2048 Weitek floating-point units, and 64 Kbits of memory per processor.

out to be useful for many applications (Fox et al. 1988) including neural
network models, will be discussed in more detail in later sections.

12.2.2   Memory

Memory in a parallel machine can be classified as either shared (also
called global) or distributed (also called local). Shared memory is memory that can be directly accessed by any processor in the machine whereas
distributed memory can only be directly accessed by a single local processor. Almost all parallel machines have some amount of distributed
memory, ranging from small caches, providing fast access to frequently
used variables, up to large blocks at each node that store the complete
program and local data for the node. Shared memory, on the other hand,
is not found in all machines due to limitations that will be discussed below. Some parallel machine designs strike a compromise by including
both types of memory, or by implementing partially shared memory in
which blocks of memory are accessible by a subset of the processors and
these shared blocks are distributed throughout the machine.

Shared memory on a parallel machine provides two principal benefits.
First, it provides a convenient and efficient means for storing common
data that is needed by all of the processors to carry out a computation.
Second, it provides a means for communicating information between processors, without requiring additional dedicated communication channels.
This is accomplished by simply storing the result at an "agreed" location in shared memory where other processors can access it.[3] One of
the most popular architectures for sharing memory among several processors is the common bus design shown in fig. 12.2a. This architecture
works well for small numbers of processors and is well suited for both
multi-tasking (many jobs on one machine, with individual jobs assigned
to different nodes) and parallel processing (one job spread over many
processors). Machines of this type are manufactured by Alliant, Cray,
Elxsi, Encore, Eta, Flex, Sequent, and Warp among others.

The major disadvantage of shared memory is that contention results
if too many processors try to access memory simultaneously. This situation is analogous to the traffic slowdowns that occur at rush hour,
when the capacity of a limited-access freeway is exceeded. Although the
operating system can implement protocols for handling the pileup (i.e.,
deciding who has the right-of-way), machine performance can degrade
dramatically if processors must give up valuable calculation time waiting for memory access. The memory contention problem becomes worse

---

[3] Note that such communication still requires a protocol for handling the temporal
aspects of the communication.

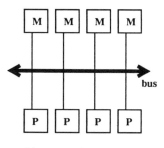

(a) common bus

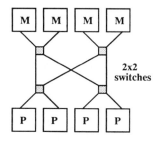

(b) omega (butterfly) switch

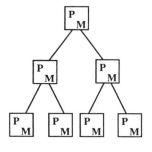

(c) tree

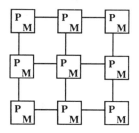

(d) grid

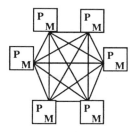

(e) fully-connected

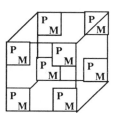

(f) hypercube

Figure 12.2
Memory architectures for parallel computers: (a) shared – common bus, (b) shared – omega (butterfly) switch, (c) distributed – tree, (d) distributed – grid, (e) distributed – fully-connected, (f) distributed – hypercube. (P = processor, M = memory)

as more processors are added. Thus, shared memory machines have
limited scalability, in that they cannot effectively accommodate a large
number of processors. One partial solution to the contention problems
of a shared memory design is shown schematically in fig. 12.2b. This
omega network switch connects several processors to a bank of shared
memories via a number of alternative routes. This design is used in the
BBN Butterfly machine (Schmidt 1987), and the switch is often referred
to as a butterfly switch. Existing designs allow up to 256 processors to
be switched in this way, and work is underway to extend this technique
to 512 processors.

A distributed memory architecture does not suffer from memory contention, because each processor only directly accesses its own local memory. Thus, in principle, these machines have an advantage over shared
memory machines, in that they can accommodate an arbitrarily large
number of processors. However, the tradeoffs are that data that are
common to all processors must be stored redundantly in each node of
the machine and that passing information between processors becomes
more complicated because shared memory is no longer available for interprocessor communication. In order to allow the exchange of information among processors, distributed memory machines must implement
direct connections between processors, called communication channels,
and data must be sent over these channels via message passing. Examples of distributed memory machines are the Connection Machine, the
Caltech/JPL hypercubes, and machines manufactured by Ametek, FPS,
Intel, and NCUBE, among others.

12.2.3   Connection Topology and Communication

As pointed out above, processors in a distributed memory machine must
communicate via physical communication links or wires. For these machines, physical limitations make it impractical to establish direct connections between all pairs of processors. Thus distributed memory machines are characterized, in general, by limited-connectivity architectures in which each processor communicates directly with only a subset
of the others. A particular pattern of connectivity is referred to as the
connection topology. Figure 12.2c–f shows some examples of common
connection topologies for distributed memory systems.

The best choice of connection topology is related to the nature of the
problem being solved. However, present-day parallel computers have
a limited ability to adapt their connection topologies to suit specific
problems. Reconfiguration of connection topologies in present-day machines is often limited to neglecting preestablished connections between

certain processors. For example, by "cutting" certain connections, a hypercube can be "unfolded" into a rectangular grid or a linear array. Some machines can be physically rewired by the user to achieve different topologies and a few machines are beginning to appear that allow connections to be dynamically established under software control. However, by far the most common situation is for parallel machines to have a preestablished connection topology that has been chosen to be a near-optimal configuration for the widest variety of problems. The most common general-purpose topology found in parallel machines today is the "hypercube" topology illustrated in fig. 12.2f and fig. 12.3. A hypercube, which is the generalization of an ordinary three-dimensional cube to an arbitrary number of dimensions, fulfills the principal design goals for a general-purpose parallel machine topology, namely that the total number of connections between processors grows relatively slowly with an increasing number of processors and that the average number of communication steps involved in passing a message between any pair of nodes is relatively small. Section 12.4.3 will analyze hypercube communication algorithms in more detail.

In addition to the connection topology, the other important characteristic of interprocessor communication is the communication speed. This is commonly specified in terms of the time required for the "typical" transfer of data between two processing nodes that are directly connected by a hardware link. This value turns out to be highly dependent on the operating system software, with the general trend being that the more flexible and functional the communications software, the longer the average communication time. In comparing parallel machines, one should be wary of quoted communication speeds, which often reflect the maximum speed supported by the hardware, as opposed to the actual speed measured under normal conditions within the context of a full operating system. Also there is often a sizable startup overhead, such that the time required to transmit a single data word is much longer than the average time per word for a large data packet.

12.2.4   Evaluating Overall Machine Performance

It is a troublesome task to summarize the performance of even a traditional serial computer in the form of one or two "performance values." This task becomes even more difficult for parallel processors where the added complexities of machine topology and interprocessor communication make the result even more dependent on the nature of the problem being solved. Nevertheless, two values for quantifying machine performance that are industry standards for sequential machines can also be

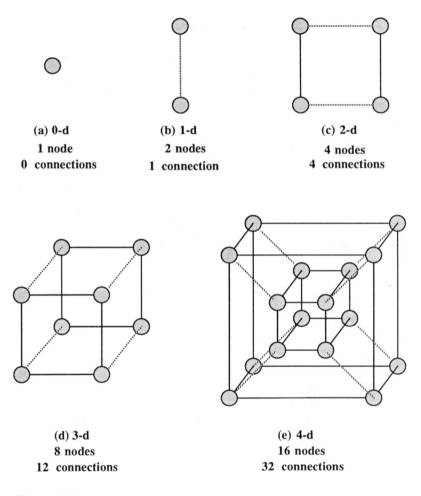

(a) 0-d

1 node

0 connections

(b) 1-d

2 nodes

1 connection

(c) 2-d

4 nodes

4 connections

(d) 3-d

8 nodes

12 connections

(e) 4-d

16 nodes

32 connections

Figure 12.3
Hypercubes are generalizations of ordinary cubes to higher (and lower) dimensions.
Hypercubes can be defined inductively, starting with a 0-dimensional hypercube,
which is just a single node. To form a cube of dimension d, start with 2 cubes of
dimension $d - 1$ and connect the "corresponding" nodes of each cube together.

applied to parallel machines. The first is the rate at which instructions are executed, usually quoted in MIPS (millions of instructions per second). The second, and generally more useful for scientific and engineering applications, is the rate at which floating-point operations such as addition or multiplication are executed, usually quoted in MFLOPS (millions of floating-point operations per second). Again, one must be wary of the many pitfalls in attempting to distill the complexities of machine performance down to one or two numbers. For example, the MIPS rating is difficult to interpret when comparing across machines that use different processors, due to potentially significant differences in instruction sets, especially with the current popularity of both RISC (reduced instruction set computer) and non-RISC processors. Likewise, the MFLOPS rating should not be relied upon blindly because the actual performance obtained on a particular machine is extremely problem-dependent. Vendors, quite understandably, like to quote the peak-performance values, but these values are usually based on purely theoretical estimates involving the cycle time of the machine and the minimum number of cycles required per floating-point operation. Actual measured performance values can be lower by an order of magnitude or more, depending on the problem (Dongarra 1987b). One should thus view theoretical MFLOPS ratings as the performance that the machine is guaranteed never to exceed. Some vendors should be commended for quoting the results of standardized tests such as the Linpack benchmark developed by Argonne National Laboratories (Dongarra 1987a). Still, such standardized benchmarks may not reflect the actual performance that will be achieved on a specific problem of interest.

As alluded to above, parallel machines are particularly bedeviled by differences between their peak and measured performance values. One of the reasons for these discrepancies is that real-world programs (as opposed to ones designed to achieve high performance ratings) often have to spend a good deal of time moving data around, and this overhead can significantly reduce the calculational throughput of a parallel machine. Often, for parallel machines, this can be attributed to the effects of interprocessor communication. However, another source of communication overhead that is often overlooked and sometimes of greater impact is the overhead in communicating with the "outside world," that is, in getting data in and out of the computer. For supercomputers in general and parallel computers in particular, the capability of generating massive amounts of data makes this a potentially very serious problem. In fact, if external communication is necessary frequently during the execution of a program (e.g., for saving or displaying the time course of a simulation), the external communication overhead can become a major bottleneck and the effective machine performance can degrade dramatically.

In summary, in evaluating the performance of different parallel machines, it is especially important to look beyond the basic performance figures and consider the details of the underlying architecture in relation to the nature of the problem that will be solved on the machine. Of course, the best measure of performance is the actual measured execution time for a problem of interest (and perhaps a measure of the development time, which can be significant if a machine is difficult to program), but in order to make this measurement one needs first to know how to go about solving problems on these machines.

12.3   Solving Problems on Parallel Machines

The fundamental idea of parallel processing is to distribute the workload for solving a problem onto many processors that carry out different parts of the task simultaneously. If the parallel implementation is perfectly efficient, then program execution is faster by a factor equal to the total number of parallel processors employed; in other words 1000 processors could complete a task in 1/1000 of the time required by a single processor. If the implementation is less efficient, due to overheads associated with the parallel implementation itself, then of course the speed-up will be less. Thus, given a particular parallel machine with a fixed number of processors and a particular architecture, the parallel programming task can be thought of as a process of finding an efficient implementation to result in as large a speed-up as possible. In practice, this speed-up has two beneficial effects. First, for a fixed problem size, it will significantly decrease the amount of time devoted to program development and evaluation, which involves repeatedly running, adjusting, and rerunning the program. Second, and of particular importance for neural network models, it will allow larger or more complex problems to be handled in the same amount of time as the original problem (e.g., larger numbers of simulated neurons).

Considerable effort has been expended over the last several years in understanding how to develop efficient implementations of many different kinds of algorithms on parallel machines (Fox et al. 1988). In the following discussion of the general concepts that have emerged from this effort, it is useful to keep in mind an analogy between the management of a large number of employees working on the same project and the management of a large number of computer processors working on a single problem. In both cases, one needs to consider how to divide up the task among the available workers (decomposition), how to keep everyone busy (load balancing), how to make sure everyone has the information they need to do their job (communication), and how to keep everyone in step if their work is interdependent (synchronization). These four basic concepts of decomposition, load-balancing, communication, and synchronization are fundamental to any concurrent process and will now be discussed briefly. Finally in this section we will outline how to quantify the effectiveness of a particular parallel implementation.

12.3.1   Decomposition

As we have stated before, the power of parallel processing arises from being able to distribute a single problem across a number of processors. In this context, the specific distribution of the problem is referred to as its decomposition. The first step in decomposing a problem is to choose a "problem domain" or "problem space" along which a problem can be broken up and distributed. This choice is, of course, problem-dependent and difficult to characterize in general, but it is often fairly obvious. For example, in the case of a large neural network, it would probably be the individual neurons, while for a multicompartment neuron model it would be the compartments, and for a matrix operation the matrix elements. In general it is some aspect of the problem that is repeated a number of times, possibly in different spatial locations.

For problems involving the modeling of physical systems, it is natural to think of the "domain" of the problem as the spatial area or volume that is being modeled. One natural way to consider distributing such a problem is by dividing it up into smaller contiguous subdomains (e.g., groups of neurons or compartments) and then assigning each subdomain to a different processor. This technique is called domain decomposition, and it is illustrated in fig. 12.4a–b. This type of decomposition can be generalized to a wide variety of problems, where the space being represented is not physical space, but some more abstract "problem space." In either case, this type of decomposition preserves local relationships in the space, except at subdomain boundaries where local relationships may be disrupted by processor boundaries.

Another frequently used method of decomposition, but one that does not explicitly preserve local relationships, is called scattered decomposition. In this technique, the problem domain is the same as before, but it is initially divided into much smaller pieces that are "scattered" over the available processors. Figure 12.4c–d shows examples of scattered decompositions. This "scattering" of the problem might seem counter-intuitive at first, but it is motivated by the fact that, for certain types of problems, it does a better job of keeping the processors uniformly busy. We will now discuss this issue, which is one of the central concerns in finding an optimal parallel decomposition.

Load Balancing Defining the problem domain is only the first step in developing an efficient decomposition. One then needs to consider how different decompositions within the chosen domain will affect performance. The most obvious impact of a particular decomposition is that it assigns responsibility for different parts of the problem space to different processors. Although the decomposition may have assigned roughly equal amounts of the problem space to each processor, it may not have assigned equal computational loads. Again this depends on the nature of the problem being solved. For problems that are regular and homogeneous, such as the modeling of molecular interactions in a crystal lattice or the modeling of certain early vision algorithms, for example, equal volumes in the problem space (e.g., "lattice space" or "retinal space") usually correspond to equal computational loads. However, for irregular or inhomogeneous problems this is not the case. A classic example of an inhomogeneous problem is that of modeling the stresses around a crack developing in a piece of material. In this case calculating the stresses in an area near the crack where the stress gradient is large represents a much heavier computational load than that for an equal area far from the crack, where the stress gradient is much smaller. In neural network modeling, nonuniformity of computational load can result from an inhomogeneous distribution of neurons or from shifting patterns of activity in the network. If the decomposition of such problems was carried out without the inhomogeneities in mind, some processors could end up with a significantly larger computational load than the rest.

The task of making sure that the processors each carry approximately equal shares of the computational load is referred to as load-balancing. There are two general categories of load-balancing: static and dynamic. In static load-balancing, a particular decomposition is selected once at the beginning of a program and does not change during its execution. In dynamic load-balancing, the decomposition actually changes with time in order to adjust for changing patterns of computational load. Of course, in the latter case, there is some overhead involved in monitoring these changes and redistributing the problem among the processors, but for certain classes of problems this is more than compensated for by the overall increase in performance. In the case of neural network modeling,

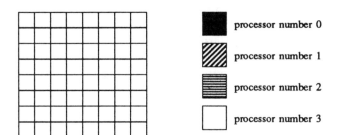

A 64-element problem domain

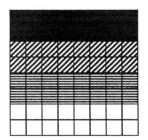

(a) domain decomp (strips)

(b) domain decomp (squares)

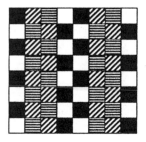

(c) scattered decomp (e=1)

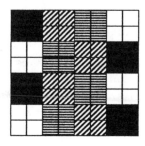

(d) scattered decomp (e=4)

Figure 12.4
Examples of the decomposition of a regular two-dimensional problem onto four processors: (a) domain decomposition into strips, (b) domain decomposition into squares, (c) scattered decomposition with 1 element per subdomain, and (d) scattered decomposition with 4 elements per subdomain.

one might expect to be able to accommodate inhomogeneities in neuron distribution with a static load-balancing technique, whereas inhomogeneities due to shifting patterns of activity might require a dynamic technique. However, as we will see for the piriform cortex model, shifting patterns of activity can often be handled with a static load-balancing technique such as the scattered decomposition.

The scattered decomposition technique, illustrated in fig. 12.4c,d, is "guaranteed" to result in a load-balanced decomposition if sufficiently small subdomains of the problem are scattered over the available processors. This is because computational "hot spots" get divided up and scattered uniformly over all the processors, resulting in balanced computational loads. Accordingly, the scattered decomposition, which always achieves a good load balance, would seem to be an ideal general-purpose solution to the decomposition problem. However, the cost associated with this decomposition technique is a potentially significant increase in interprocessor communication, since nearby elements in the problem space are now scattered among all the processors in the machine, rather than being on the same or nearby processing nodes, as they would be in a domain decomposition. As alluded to above, reducing interprocessor communication to a minimum is an important priority if one is to make efficient use of the computational powers of a parallel machine.

Communication   As mentioned previously, there are two distinct aspects of the computational load on a parallel machine. First, there is the irreducible amount of work or calculation that has to be done to "solve" the problem, whether it is solved on a sequential or a parallel machine. In addition there is a component of the workload that only applies to parallel machines arising from the overhead of communicating information between processors.

Interprocessor communication is necessary whenever a processor, in order to perform its calculation, requires information from another processor. Since this communication is usually costly in terms of time and resources, it is best avoided. However, for most "interesting" problems, including the simulation of neural networks, it is impossible to find a decomposition that completely eliminates this communication. In neural networks, and most other simulations of physical systems, the "coupling" between processors can be directly traced to the intrinsic couplings between elements in the problem space. It is the nature of these intrinsic couplings that affects the amount of interprocessor communication that will accompany a particular decomposition. Thus, in addition to achieving load balance, a good decomposition must also strive to minimize the interprocessor communication overhead, within the constraints imposed by the problem itself.

Any problem that involves interactions among elements in the problem space will pay a price in communication overhead for a decomposition in which these elements end up on different processing nodes. For example, as mentioned above, the scattered decomposition of a problem that is characterized by local interactions results in a large communication overhead, because information relevant to these interactions will have to be communicated to every node in the machine. In such cases the alternative of a domain decomposition often provides better performance because the locality of interactions in the problem is translated into a locality of interactions on the parallel machine, which minimizes interprocessor communication.

It should be pointed out here that the ideals of perfect load balance and minimal communication overhead cannot be achieved simultaneously. A good way to see the "push-pull" nature of these two factors is to consider that the communication overhead is minimized (zero) when all of the processing is assigned to a single node, a situation that represents the maximum load imbalance. Because of the problem-dependence, it is impossible to give a general prescription for how to find the decomposition that strikes the optimal balance between communication overhead and load imbalance. However, a good decomposition can often be found by inspection, or sometimes a simple analytic approach can be devised, or more generally it can be couched as an optimization problem, amenable to solution by a number of numerical techniques. We will explore some of these possibilities in more detail in section 12.5.

12.3.2   Synchronization

After decomposing a problem in such a way that it is reasonably well load-balanced and such that the communication overhead is reasonably small, we still have one more "managerial" task to attend to, namely that of keeping the computation synchronized across the multiple processors. Since processors need to communicate in order to reach a solution, one needs to make sure that they don't waste valuable time waiting for one another's results. There are several ways in which this can be accomplished. The simplest technique, and one that is especially well suited for fine-grained SIMD machines, is to run the processors in a completely synchronous mode in which all the processors execute the same instructions simultaneously. In this case, one always knows where every other processor is in its computation, and it is easy to arrange for the exchange of information on appropriate instruction cycles. The disadvantage of this mode is that it is not easy to accommodate irregular or inhomogeneous problems that would require that different processors perform different operations at different times. Such problems are better handled by coarse-grained machines operating in MIMD mode, in which the individual processors can run asynchronously. Asynchronous operation is very flexible, and can easily accommodate problems in which the temporal aspects of interprocessor communication are very irregular. However, for a large class of problems that includes discrete-time solutions of dynamical systems, the processors need to communicate with each other on a fairly regular basis. In such cases, a loosely synchronous mode of operation is preferred. This mode of operation is used for implementing the types of neuronal and neural network models, which we will discuss in section 12.4.

12.3.3   Quantifying Performance

We have described the parallel programming task as one of achieving the maximal speed-up by finding an efficient decomposition that is load-balanced and minimizes the communication overhead. We will now briefly quantify each of these aspects, so that meaningful comparisons can be made among different decompositions and among different machines. We consider specifically the loosely synchronous mode of operation, which is the one that we will use to implement our neural models. In this mode of operation, we can think of the program execution as consisting of "iterations." Each iteration is composed of two phases, first a calculation phase in which each processor runs asynchronously, performing the calculations necessary for its assigned problem domain, followed by a communication phase in which information is exchanged between processors. We define the following times associated with the execution of a single iteration of the algorithm: (1) the sequential computation time T_{seq}, which would be the time required by a single processor working alone, (2) the concurrent time T_{cc}, which is the time required by the full array of processors working together, (3) the calculation time for processor i, $T_{calc}(i)$, which is the amount of time that is spent in the first phase of the iteration, and (4) the communication time for processor i, $T_{comm}(i)$, which is the amount of time spent in the second phase.

We can now determine the average and maximum calculation and communication times for a single iteration:

$$T_{calc}^{max} = \max_i(T_{calc}(i)) \qquad\qquad (12.1)$$

$$T_{calc}^{avg} = \frac{1}{N} \sum_{i=1,N} T_{calc}(i) \qquad (12.2)$$

$$T_{comm}^{max} = \max_i(T_{comm}(i)) \qquad (12.3)$$

$$T_{comm}^{avg} = \frac{1}{N} \sum_{i=1,N} T_{comm}(i) \qquad (12.4)$$

We will now obtain approximate expressions for T_{seq} and T_{cc} in terms of these quantities. An approximation for T_{cc} is derived by using the fact that the time required for each of the two phases of an iteration is limited by the slowest processor.[4]

$$T_{cc} \approx T_{calc}^{max} + T_{comm}^{max} \qquad (12.5)$$

An approximation for T_{seq} is based on the fact that the sequential version involves only calculation time, since there is no interprocessor communication with a single processor. This sequential calculation time will be equal to the sum of the calculation times for all the concurrent processors, assuming that there was no additional calculation overhead in the concurrent version of the algorithm (there will be additional communication overhead).

$$T_{seq} \approx \sum_{i=1,N} T_{calc}(i) = N \cdot T_{calc}^{avg} \qquad (12.6)$$

We now define the following performance parameters:

$$\sigma = \frac{T_{seq}}{T_{cc}} \qquad (\text{speed} - \text{up}) \qquad (12.7)$$

$$\epsilon = \frac{\sigma}{N} \qquad (\text{efficiency}) \qquad (12.8)$$

$$\lambda = \frac{(T_{calc}^{max} - T_{calc}^{avg})}{T_{calc}^{avg}} \qquad (\text{load imbalance}) \qquad (12.9)$$

$$\eta = \frac{T_{comm}^{max}}{T_{cc}} \qquad (\text{communication overhead}) \qquad (12.10)$$

---

[4] This derivation of T_{cc} assumes that calculation and communication cannot be overlapped. Some overlap can be obtained on machines that use separate processors for calculation and communication at each node.

Using the relationships in eqs. 12.5-12.10, we obtain:

$$\epsilon \approx \frac{(1 - \eta)}{(1 + \lambda)} \tag{12.11}$$

When the overheads from load imbalance and communication are small,
they approximately sum up to the total inefficiency:

$$1 - \epsilon \approx \lambda + \eta \quad \text{(small } \lambda, \eta) \tag{12.12}$$

We will refer to these relationships frequently in the next two sections,
which will discuss specific issues pertaining to the modeling of neuronal
and neural networks on parallel machines.

12.4   Simulating Neurons and Networks

We begin our discussion of how to simulate neurons and networks on parallel machines by recapitulating our discussion up to this point. In order
to achieve an efficient parallel implementation of a particular model, one
must find a decomposition that minimizes the overheads from load imbalance and interprocessor communication. These two aspects of the
problem are coupled in such a way that both factors cannot be minimized simultaneously. Thus one needs to find a decomposition that
strikes a compromise between these two factors. In doing so, the structure of the underlying problem as well as the structure of the parallel
machine on which it will be implemented must be examined. Load imbalance is found to be related to the spatial and temporal patterns of
calculational load in the problem space and how it is distributed among
the processors. Communication overhead can be related to the underlying problem topology, the machine topology, and the communication
software. We will now describe how to go about analyzing the computational structure of single neurons and neural network models, and how
to use the resulting information to find a good decomposition.

12.4.1   A Generic Neural Model Description

In order to unify our discussion of these issues for a variety of neuronal
and neural network models, we will use the following generic description
of a neural model. The problem domain is assumed to consist of a large
number of elements, which represent the components of the problem that
will be distributed among the processors.[5] For example, these elements

---

[5] The elements are not required to be identical. In the derivations that follow, one
could easily include a subscript to distinguish among element types, but for the sake
of simplicity we will not do so.

might represent individual neurons in a large network model (e.g., piriform cortex, chapter 9), or compartments in a multicompartment neuron
model (e.g., α motoneuron, chapter 3). Figure 12.5b,c illustrates how
particular neural element types might map onto the generalized abstract
model element shown in fig. 12.5a. Of course, much more detailed neural
elements could easily be constructed within this general framework.

Model elements can communicate with each other via connections. In
a simple neural network model, the connections might represent axons,
while in a multicompartment neuron model they would represent the
axial couplings between compartments. The pattern of connections between elements defines the problem topology. The information that is
communicated between elements is assumed to take the form of messages, which can represent such things as action potentials, membrane
voltages, or ion concentrations.

The computational task in this general framework involves finding the
discrete-time approximation to the solution of a set of ordinary differential equations or update rules that describe how the elements evolve in
time. The simulation consists of a number of "time steps" or iterations
that conceptually can be divided into two phases, an update phase and
a communication phase. During the update phase, each element examines its input messages, updates its internal state variables, and decides
whether or not to generate output messages. During the communication
phase, the outputs are communicated to other elements, perhaps with
explicitly simulated delays between the generation of a message at one
element and its arrival at another.

12.4.2   Estimating Load Imbalance

As described in eq. 12.9, the load imbalance is related to differences in
the calculation time per iteration among the processors. Thus in order
to evaluate the load imbalance for a particular decomposition, we need
to be able to estimate the calculation load associated with each processor. The total calculation load includes everything that would need to
be computed to solve the problem on a traditional sequential computer.
Thus the calculation load includes the calculations involved in both the
element update and the inter element communication phases of an iteration. The fact that the simulation of communication between elements
is included in the calculation load is often a point of confusion. At first,
one might think that it should contribute to the communication load.
This confusion arises when one fails to make a clear distinction between
the simulation of interelement communication in the neural model and
the actual interprocessor communication that takes place when running

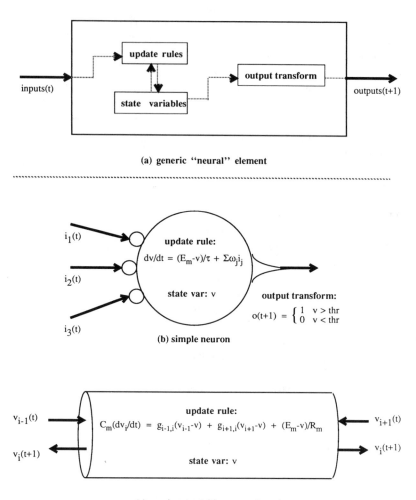

(a) generic "neural" element

(b) simple neuron

(c) passive dendritic compartment

Figure 12.5
Model computing elements for simulating neurons and networks: (a) a generic model
element, (b) an element for simulating simple neurons, and (c) an element for simulating simple dendritic compartments.

the simulation. Interelement communication is an intrinsic part of the modeling problem and is always present, even in a sequential implementation on a single processor. Interprocessor communication, however, is an overhead that arises only when the model is implemented on a parallel machine.

We can analyze the calculation load in terms of the contributions from the two phases of an iteration:

$$T_{calc} = T_{calc}^{update} + T_{calc}^{comm} \tag{12.13}$$

where T_{calc} is the total calculation time per iteration, T_{calc}^{update} is the calculation time devoted to updating the elements, and T_{calc}^{comm} is the calculation time devoted to interelement communication. The update phase of an iteration contributes to the calculation load in proportion to the number of elements that need to be updated, whereas the communication phase contributes in proportion to the number of messages that need to be processed. These scaling relations are expressed in the following equation:

$$T_{calc} = \alpha E + \beta M \tag{12.14}$$

where E is the number of elements, M is the number of messages, and α and β are proportionality constants that express the calculation time per element for the update and the calculation time per message for interelement communication.

For a particular decomposition, the number of elements and number of messages may vary from processor to processor. In this case, eq. 12.14 applies to each processor individually.

$$T_{calc}(i) = \alpha E(i) + \beta M(i) \tag{12.15}$$

where i is the processor number. Variations in $T_{calc}(i)$ contribute to the load imbalance as expressed in eqs. 12.1, 12.2, and 12.9, which we duplicate here for convenience:

$$T_{calc}^{max} = \max_{i}(T_{calc}(i))$$

$$T_{calc}^{avg} = \frac{1}{N} \sum_{i=1,N} T_{calc}(i)$$

$$\lambda = \frac{(T_{calc}^{max} - T_{calc}^{avg})}{T_{calc}^{avg}}$$

Given α, β, $E(i)$, and $M(i)$ it is easy to calculate the load imbalance λ from the above equations. A good way to estimate α and β is to actually time the update and communication phases of the simulation on a sequential machine. It does not matter if the sequential machine has a different kind of processor than the parallel machine, since the load imbalance is insensitive to the overall normalization of the calculation times. Thus performance differences between processors don't matter (to first order) when estimating load imbalance, although they do affect the overall calculation time. If one cannot actually time the two phases of an iteration (because the model has not been coded yet, for example), one can also estimate α and β by writing down the update and communication algorithms in detail and then counting the number of operations or floating-point calculations per element and per message. The determination of $E(i)$ is straightforward, since it simply involves counting the number of elements that end up on each node in a particular decomposition. The determination of $M(i)$ is equally straightforward if the elements send and receive messages on every iteration, as would be the case for communication between compartments in a multicompartment model. In this case, the number of messages per iteration is simply equal to the number of elements times the number of connections per element. This specific case is treated in section 12.5.1, where we discuss the implementation of a multicompartment neuron model.

It is more difficult to estimate $M(i)$ when communication does not take place on every iteration, as would be the case for communication between neurons via action potentials. In this case, one actually needs to take into account the spatial and temporal patterns of activity, which may change during the course of a simulation. If the neurons are uncorrelated in their activity, then one can simply modify the estimate of $M(i)$ to include the probability per iteration that an element will send a message.[6] If the neural activity is correlated (which is the case for many network models), then one also needs to factor in the correlations among the elements on each node. For example, if the activity in a network model is local and synchronous, then in a domain decomposition it would often occur that most of the elements on one or a few nodes would be active, while elements on other nodes would be relatively inactive. For a problem in which the calculation load was dominated by the simulation of communication, this would result in a large load im-

---

[6] There are usually different calculation loads associated with sending a message and with receiving one. A rigorous treatment would distinguish between these two cases. However, we will assume that on average an element sends and receives the same number of messages per iteration.

balance. In our discussion of the implementation of the piriform cortex model (section 12.5.2) we will see how this situation can be handled.

12.4.3   Estimating Communication Overhead

Estimating the load imbalance for a particular decomposition is only half the job. Now we come to the somewhat more involved task of estimating the interprocessor communication overhead. The reason that this is more involved is that it is dependent on the connection topology and communication software of the parallel machine that is being used. In this section we will confine our discussion to machines that use a hypercube topology, although our discussion could fairly easily be modified for other machine topologies. The hypercube topology is a particularly good example to use because it is relatively efficient for a wide variety of problem topologies, and it is easy to analyze due to the regularity of its structure. For these same reasons, it is also one of the most common topologies found in today's parallel machines.

We are interested in evaluating the communication overhead η, which can be expressed as (cf. eqs. 12.5, 12.10):

$$\eta = \frac{T_{comm}^{max}}{T_{cc}} = \frac{T_{comm}^{max}}{T_{calc}^{max} + T_{comm}^{max}} \tag{12.16}$$

We discussed how to estimate T_{calc}^{max} in section 12.4.2, so in order to evaluate η we only need to discuss how to estimate T_{comm}^{max}, which is the maximum time per iteration devoted to interprocessor communication. At first one might think that this would simply be a matter of finding the node with the maximum number of messages $M(i)$, and multiplying the number of messages by some "typical" time required to communicate a message. However, things are not so simple, because the communication time associated with each message depends on its source and destination node, which in turn depends on the nature and decomposition of the problem. For example, in the case of a problem with predominantly local connectivity, and a domain decomposition with many elements per node, numerous messages would be destined for elements that reside on the same processing node. Since these messages do not need to pass between processors, they would not contribute to the interprocessor communication overhead at all. An additional complication in analyzing the communication load arises from the fact that in a limited-connectivity machine like the hypercube, a message must often pass through intermediate nodes to get to its destination. This means that a processing node may incur a communication load even though no message originates or terminates there. Thus the task of evaluating the communication load on the hypercube cannot be carried out on a node-by-node basis but requires a global analysis of parallel communication algorithms.

We will now discuss some of these communication algorithms for the hypercube topology. In order to make our discussion more intuitive, we will use the following "post card" analogy. Imagine that each message travels through the hypercube on a post card that contains the "address" of the recipient and a "zip code" that is the binary representation of the hypercube node number of the recipient. In the case of neural models, the actual message being sent might be an action potential indicating that the originating neuron had fired, or it might be the membrane potential of the originating dendritic compartment. The interprocessor communication load involves getting all of these post cards delivered to the proper zip codes. In addition, of course, there is the task of getting the messages to the proper address once they arrive at the proper zip code, but, as discussed above, this task is local to each processor and therefore falls under the category of calculation load (see section 12.4.2).

When a message is mailed, it is repeatedly "forwarded" from node to node until it reaches its destination node. The maximum number of times that a message might need to be forwarded is equal to the maximum "distance" between two nodes, which is equal to the dimension of the hypercube, $d = \log_2 N$, where N is the total number of nodes. In the general case, we must assume that it will take a total of d forwarding cycles to insure that every message has had enough time to reach its destination. On each cycle, a "postmaster" at each node decides whether or not to forward messages to other nodes. There is a well-defined algorithm for each postmaster to follow that guarantees that all messages will be forwarded a minimal number of times and arrive at their destination nodes within d cycles. On the ith forwarding cycle each postmaster examines the ith bit of the zip code for each message and compares it with the ith bit of the local zip code. If they are the same, then the message is retained; if they are different, the message is forwarded to the neighboring node whose zip code differs from the local one in the ith bit. This same algorithm can also be applied to cases in which it is known that the communication distance is limited, such that the full d forwarding cycles are not required. The most common example is when messages only need to be sent between neighboring processors. In this case the communication can be accomplished in a single forwarding cycle instead of d cycles.

Due to the tremendous variety of possible problem topologies and possible decompositions, it is difficult to give a general expression for T_{comm}^{max}. It is more useful at this point to illustrate how to estimate T_{comm}^{max} for a couple of simple cases. First, consider the case of a nonbranching dendrite, modeled as a multicompartment cable that is divided into E_{tot} elements and is implemented on a d–dimensional hypercube that has $N = 2^d$ nodes. The update rules for this problem are such that each element of the cable only needs to communicate with its nearest neighbors. In a domain decomposition, the cable would be divided up into contiguous segments and each segment would be assigned to a different processor. The number of elements assigned to processor i would be $E(i) = E_{tot}/N$, and the number of messages per iteration on that processor would be $2E(i)$. However, of these $2E(i)$ messages, only the ones from the end of each segment would need to be sent to other processors. Thus the interprocessor communication load would consist of just two messages per node per iteration. This linear problem can be decomposed onto the hypercube in such a way that these messages only need to pass between neighboring nodes and thus require only one communication cycle per iteration.[7] The maximum communication time per iteration is thus

$$T^{max}_{comm} = 2t_{comm} \qquad \text{(linear array, domain decomp.)} \qquad (12.17)$$

where t_{comm} is the time required to pass a single message between two neighboring nodes.

In a scattered decomposition, processor i will still handle $E(i) = E_{tot}/N$ elements and $2E(i)$ messages. However, since the elements have now been scattered over the hypercube, the destination nodes for these messages have effectively been randomized. The maximum distance a message would have to travel is d nodes, and the minimum is 0. On average, the distance will be $d/2$. Thus the interprocessor communication time per iteration will be

$$T^{max}_{comm} = 2E(i)\left(\frac{d}{2}\right)t_{comm} \qquad \text{(linear array, scattered decomp.)} \qquad (12.18)$$

which is significantly longer than that for the domain decomposition.

The nonbranching cable problem represents a sparsely connected topology, since each element is connected to at most only two of the $E_{tot} - 1$ possible destination elements. For comparison, we now consider the class of fully connected problems that fall at the other end of the connectivity spectrum. In these problems each element connects to all of the $E_{tot} - 1$ other elements. Again we assume E_{tot} elements distributed over the

---

[7] A hypercube can be "unfolded" to form a variety of other topologies, including a linear array.

N nodes of a d-dimensional hypercube. Since the average distance a message needs to travel is $d/2$, the communication time works out to be

$$T^{max}_{comm} = E(i)E_{tot}\left(\frac{d}{2}\right) \qquad \text{(full connectivity, any decomp.)} \qquad (12.19)$$

Because of the symmetry of the fully connected topology, the communication time turns out to be independent of whether one chooses a domain or scattered decomposition.

We will refer to the above communication algorithm, which individually routes each post card to its proper destination, as the "router" algorithm. For decompositions that result in a fairly uniform message load across the processors, we can generalize the form of the communication time:

$$T_{router} = E(i)\langle m\rangle\left(\frac{d}{2}\right)t_{comm} \qquad (12.20)$$

where $\langle m\rangle$ is the average number of messages per element. (For a fully connected network, $\langle m\rangle$ is equal to E_{tot}, the total number of elements, and eq. 12.20 reverts to eq. 12.18.) Although the router algorithm is very simple, it is not very efficient for highly or fully connected problem topologies. We can see this by analyzing the interprocessor message traffic for the router algorithm in the fully connected case. Returning to our post card analogy, we observe that each element is sending out E_{tot} post cards, all with different addresses, but with the same message (e.g., the membrane voltage of the element, or the fact that the element just fired an action potential). A more efficient approach would be for each element to send a single post card with its message to the postmaster at each node with instructions to distribute that message to all of the addresses on that node. That would cut down tremendously on the interprocessor communication load, and the distribution by the postmaster would take no more time than it did to deliver all the messages in the original algorithm. In this new algorithm, which is called "index" for reasons that will be explained shortly, each element only sends N messages per iteration and the communication time is

$$T_{index} = E(i)N\left(\frac{d}{2}\right)t_{comm} \qquad (12.21)$$

The reason this algorithm is called "index" is because there is a trick that allows the zip code information to be carried as an array index in the message "vector." This allows the communication algorithm to be implemented without "post cards" in a very compact and efficient form (Fox and Furmanski 1988b). Based on eqs. 12.18 and 12.19, one would predict that the index algorithm would be more efficient that the router algorithm whenever the average number of messages per element was larger than the number of processing nodes (i.e., $\langle m \rangle \geq N$). In fact, because of the additional gain from using the "index trick," the crossover point is at an even lower value of $\langle m \rangle$.

There is one more improvement that can be made to our communication scheme in many cases. If the operations that are being carried out at the destination element on each iteration are stereotyped and if they are commutative and associative, that is, if it doesn't matter what order the messages arrive in on a particular time step or how they are grouped on that time step, then the interprocessor communication load can be reduced by having the postmasters perform this operation on any pair of messages heading for the same destination. The most common example of such a commutative and associative operation in neural models is simply the process of addition. If all of the messages arriving at an element are going to be summed together before further processing, then intervening postmasters can extract post cards that are headed for the same address and replace them with a single post card carrying a new message that is the sum of the original messages. The result of such a procedure is that the total number of messages traveling between processors decreases on each message-forwarding cycle of the communication phase of an iteration. In the fully connected case, it turns out that the number of messages is exactly halved on successive cycles. By carrying out this additional step during the communication cycle, the index algorithm is transformed into an even more efficient version, called the "fold" algorithm, which has a communication time of

$$T_{fold} = E(i)N \sum_{t=1}^{d} \frac{1}{2^t} t_{comm} \approx E(i)N t_{comm} \tag{12.22}$$

By comparing eqs. 12.21 and 12.22 we see that the fold algorithm is faster by a factor of about $d/2$ than the index algorithm. This modification can also be made to the router algorithm to turn it into the accumulator algorithm. The expression for the communication time in this case is not simple,

$$T_{accumulator} = E(i)N \sum_{t=1}^{d} \frac{1}{2^t} [1 - [1 - \frac{\langle m \rangle}{E_{tot}}]^{2^{(t-1)}}] t_{comm} \tag{12.23}$$

but it turns out to interpolate smoothly between the router formula in eq. 12.20 for small $\langle m \rangle$ and the fold formula (eq. 12.22) for large $\langle m \rangle$.

12.5   Examples

We will now discuss the implementation details of two specific examples
of neural models on the NCUBE hypercube: a multicompartment model
of a single neuron, and a large network model of piriform cortex.

12.5.1   Multicompartment Neuron Model

In section 12.4.3 we briefly discussed the decomposition of a simple nonbranching cable model on a hypercube machine. In this section we
extend this analysis to include the more interesting case of a generic
multicompartment model with an arbitrary number of branches (see
chapter 3 for a detailed discussion of such models). Instead of selecting
a particular dendritic morphology to analyze, we will consider the decomposition of a class of generic dendritic trees, whose morphology is
characterized by two parameters: the maximum branching depth and
the branching probability per node.

Our task here, of course, is to find a decomposition of the tree on
the hypercube that minimizes the sum of the load imbalance and the
communication overhead. It will facilitate our discussion of the general
case if we first discuss the results for the simple nonbranching cable.
Load balance is easy to achieve for the simple cable, where we assume
all elements represent equal computational loads. In this case, we only
have to assure that each node is responsible for the same number of
elements. Still, there will be a small residual imbalance due to the fact
that the total number of elements E_{tot} will not be an exact multiple of N,
so some nodes will have an extra cable element assigned to them. From
eq. 12.7, we see that the load imbalance due to this slight imbalance is
approximately $1/e$, where e is the number of elements per node.

$$\lambda = \frac{(T_{cc}^{max} - T_{calc}^{avg})}{T_{calc}^{avg}} \approx \frac{(1+e)t_{update} - et_{update}}{et_{update}} = \frac{1}{e} \qquad (12.24)$$

where t_{update} is the calculation time associated with updating each element. Thus the load imbalance gets smaller as the number of elements
per node increases.

Now we have to estimate the communication overhead for the simple cable problem. In section 12.4.3, we saw that a domain decomposition provides the least communication time per iteration, since only
two of the e cable elements assigned to each node need to communicate with other processors. The communication time for this cases is
$T_{comm} = 2t_{comm}$, where t_{comm} is the time required to pass a single mes-

sage between two neighboring nodes. The communication overhead is thus

$$\eta = \frac{T_{comm}}{T_{calc} + T_{comm}} = \frac{2t_{comm}}{et_{update} + 2t_{comm}} \tag{12.25}$$

In general, the update time involves a number of floating-point operations δ, where δ is typically on the order of 10–100 (depending on whether the element is active or passive, how many channel types it has, etc.). Thus $t_{update} = \delta t_{calc}$, where t_{calc} is the calculation time for a single floating-point operation. As mentioned earlier, for most present-day parallel machines the calculation time t_{calc} and communication time t_{comm} are usually similar in magnitude. Thus we see that, for the cable problem, the calculation time per iteration dominates the communication time, since $e\delta$ is always much larger than 2. We can now approximate the communication overhead as

$$\eta \approx \frac{2}{e\delta} \frac{t_{comm}}{t_{calc}} \tag{12.26}$$

Assuming $t_{calc} \approx t_{comm}$, and that the number of elements per node is large, then we can estimate the inefficiency of the decomposition:

$$1 - \epsilon \approx \lambda + \eta \approx \frac{1}{e} + \frac{2}{e\delta} \tag{12.27}$$

As we mentioned above, δ is usually relatively large so the communication overhead makes a negligible contribution to the inefficiency relative to the load imbalance.

This situation continues to hold when we generalize the problem to the arbitrary branching topology, since the problem is still sparsely connected and the number of messages that need to be communicated between nodes on each iteration is still very small. Thus the decomposition task should be weighted more toward finding a good load-balanced solution than to trying to minimize the communication overhead. We have used two different techniques to decompose the randomly generated dendritic trees. The first technique is referred to as recursive bisection (Fox 1987). As the name implies, the dendritic tree is repeatedly cut into two nearly equal subdomains until there are as many subdomains as processors. Each bisection splits the tree at the single point that results in the best balance between the two remaining halves. Figure 12.6a illustrates this procedure. Note that it is not alway possible to find a single cut that results in two pieces of exactly the same size, thus the load balance achieved using this approach is not perfect. Nevertheless, as shown in

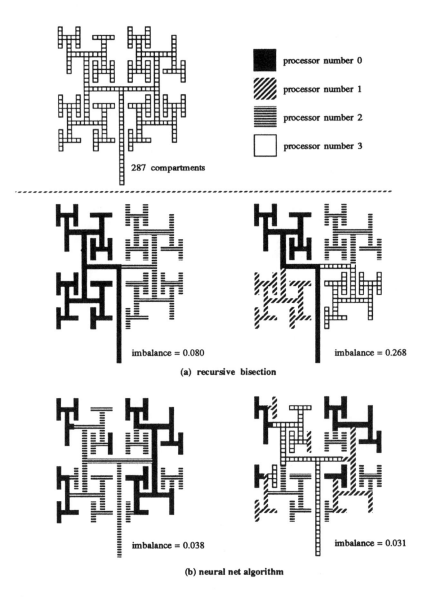

Figure 12.6
Load-balancing decomposition of a multicompartment neuron model onto 4 processors using (a) a recursive bisection technique, and (b) a neural net algorithm. The processor assignments of each compartment and the resulting load imbalance are shown.

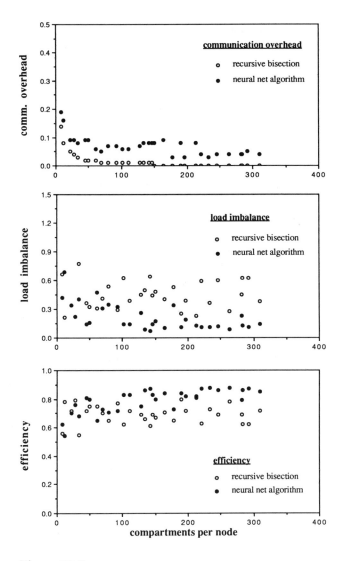

Figure 12.7
Communication overhead, load imbalance, and efficiency for the decomposition of many randomly generated multicompartment neurons vs. the average number of compartments per processor. The open points are for the recursive bisection technique and the solid points are for the neural net algorithm. Results are shown for a 16-node hypercube.

fig. 12.7, it does a reasonably good job, but it results in a solution that is too heavily weighted to reducing the communication overhead.

A better solution to the decomposition problem can be obtained by using an optimization technique to find a global efficiency maximum. Such an approach allows one to explicitly trade off load imbalance for communication overhead, whereas the recursive bisection technique, by its nature, always achieved a minimum communication overhead, at the cost of load imbalance. The optimization technique that we have used for this problem (Fox and Furmanski 1988a) involves expressing the inefficiency as an energy function of the processor assignments of each compartment and then simulating a Hopfield-type network to converge to a solution that is an energy minimum (Hopfield and Tank 1986). Figure 12.6b shows a typical example of the node assignments generated by this technique. Note that each processor tends to be assigned a number of contiguous regions of the dedritic tree, instead of just one contiguous region as in the recursive bisection technique. As a result, the communication overhead is larger, but the load imbalance is smaller. Thus, as shown in fig. 12.7, the overall efficiency of this neural-net technique is somewhat better than the bisection technique.

In summary, we see that one can usually obtain an efficiency of 80–90% for such problems. On a 64-node hypercube this translates into a speed-up of a factor of 50–60 over a sequential version. Of course, the actual execution time for any particular model will depend on the computational complexity of the individual compartments.

12.5.2 Piriform Cortex Model

The general structure of piriform cortex and of the model that we implemented are described in chapter 9. There are slight differences between the model that was implemented on the hypercube and the somewhat more detailed one that is described in chapter 9. This does not reflect limitations of the hypercube itself, but rather an effort to keep the hypercube implementation of the piriform cortex model as simple as possible in order to facilitate our analysis. In the following discussion we will point out these differences where relevant and will otherwise simply refer to the earlier chapter for additional background.

We start our analysis of the parallel implementation of the model by describing it in terms of the generic neural model formalism presented in section 12.4.1. The elements of the model are taken to be the individual pyramidal cells. In the hypercube implementation, the feedback interneurons are not modeled as separate elements but are "lumped" into the properties of the pyramidal cells. The elements of the model

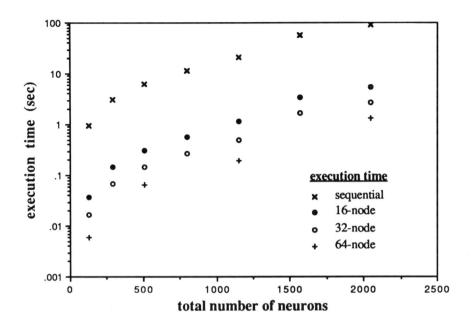

Figure 12.8
Execution time per iteration vs. total number of neurons, N, for the piriform cortex model (chapter 9). Results are shown for the sequential version, and for 16-, 32- and 64-node hypercubes. The sequential execution time is approximately proportional to N^2.

are fully connected, that is, every pyramidal element has connections to every other one.[8] The interelement messages in the model are single spikes, and there is an explicit propagation delay between elements (see section 9.4.1). The update rules that specify how the model evolves in time are outlined in sections 9.4.2–9.4.3. In the hypercube version, the synaptic connection weights were static.

As we discussed in section 12.4.2, the calculation load for any neural model simulation includes the calculations involved in both the update and communication phases of an iteration. In this particular model, the simulation of communication dominates the calculation load for large networks. This is due to the fact that in this implementation of the model, the network elements are effectively fully interconnected. Even

---

[8]Note that the piriform cortex itself is not fully connected. The full connectivity of the model elements results from the choice of representation. See section 9.2 and Appendix 9.D of chapter 9 for details.

though the spike events are discrete in time, the result of the combined effects of propagation delay and synaptic duration is that a single spike affects a progressively enlarging region around its point of origin at later times. Thus each discrete event affects a finite fraction of the whole cortex on each iteration of the simulation. Figure 12.8 shows the measured execution times per iteration as a function of the total number of neurons. The sequential time scales with the square of the number of elements, which is the expected result for an essentially fully-connected network. We will express this scaling relationship as

$$T_{seq} \approx \delta E_{tot}^2 t_{calc} \tag{12.28}$$

As reported in section 9.7.4, over 90% of the sequential computation time involves the distribution of information between elements, with the remaining time spent updating the states of individual elements.

Now we come to the task of choosing an efficient parallel decomposition for this problem so that the communication overhead is minimized and the processor workload is balanced. Because of the essentially full connectivity of the model, it turns out that the communication overhead is relatively insensitive to the choice of decomposition. This is because each event must eventually be communicated to every other element in the model, so, averaged over the number of iterations required for a simulated spike to propagate across the model cortex, the communication load is independent of where each element is located in the decomposition.[9] This leaves us with the problem of finding a decomposition that minimizes only the load imbalance. As we pointed out in section 12.3.1, the scattered decomposition handles this class of problem quite naturally, and it is the one we choose. If we had chosen a domain decomposition instead, we would find that there would be a substantial load imbalance due to the communication load associated with the characteristic "waves" of activity in the cortex (see chapter 9), which introduce spatial and temporal correlations in the communication load.

Having found a suitable decomposition, we have only to decide on a suitable communication algorithm. As discussed in chapter 9, the effect of a spike event on a destination element is a prolonged conductance change (eq. 9.5). The combined effect of several spikes, however, is just the summed conductance change of each individual spike; thus this process satisfies the requirements of commutativity and associativity

---

[9] Note that if the local interneurons were treated as individual elements, instead of being lumped into the pyramidal elements, the communication overhead would increase for decompositions that did not preserve the local structure.

that allow us to use the extremely efficient fold communication algorithm described in section 12.4.3.

Now that we have chosen both a decomposition and a communication algorithm, we can estimate the load imbalance, communication overhead, efficiency, and speed-up for this problem. First, we consider the communication overhead. Combining eqs. 12.16, 12.22, and 12.28, we find

$$\eta \approx \frac{1}{\delta} \frac{1}{(E_{tot}/N)} \frac{t_{comm}}{t_{calc}} \tag{12.29}$$

Thus we see that the communication overhead depends only on the number of elements per node, $e = E_{tot}/N$, and not individually on the total number of elements or the total number of nodes. As expected, it also scales with t_{comm}/t_{calc}, the ratio of the communication time to the calculation time for the particular machine. We can check the scaling with $1/e$ by running the simulation under a variety of conditions and then plotting the results as a function of e, as shown in fig. 12.9. The scaling curve in this figure can be parameterized as $3/e$, which means that the communication overhead is about 30% with 10 elements per node and about 3% with 100 elements per node. The load imbalance, which arises from fluctuations in the number of messages sent per node per iteration, also scales with $1/e$, as shown in fig. 12.9. From these two figures we see that the communication overhead and load imbalance are of similar sizes:

$$\eta(e) \approx \lambda(e) \approx \frac{3}{e} \tag{12.30}$$

When the number of neurons per node e is large, then these two contributions are small and the total inefficiency is just the sum of the two contributions (cf. eq. 12.10):

$$\epsilon \approx 1 - \eta - \lambda \approx 1 - \frac{6}{e} \tag{12.31}$$

Since each contribution scaled with e, so does the overall efficiency, as shown in fig. 12.9. As reported in section 9.7.4, a simulation of 1,500 pyramidal cells on a sequential computer (Sun 3/260 with floating-point accelerator) took about 10 $cpu\ sec$ per step. With a step size of 0.1 $msec$, the execution time for a 200 $msec$ simulation was about 5 hr. For a similar size model on the 64-node NCUBE, the execution time per iteration would be about one second, and the total time for a 200 $msec$ simulation would be about half an hour.[10]

---

[10]Note that the floating-point performance of a single NCUBE node is about a factor of five slower than a Sun 3/260 with FPA.

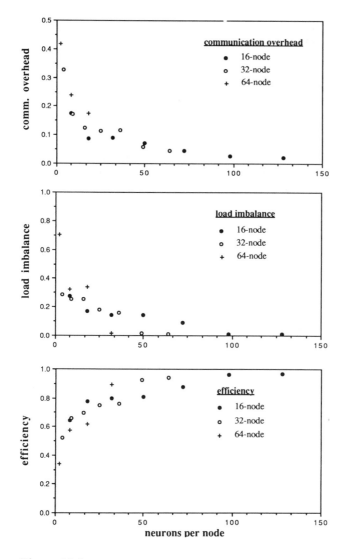

Figure 12.9
Communication overhead, load imbalance, and efficiency for the piriform cortex
model vs. the average number of neurons per processor. Results are shown for 16-,
32-, and 64-node hypercubes.

12.6 The Brain as a Parallel Computer

The main body of this chapter has focused on the technical issues involved in efficiently using the computing power of parallel machines to simulate realistic models of biological neural networks. However, as mentioned in the introduction, a second objective of this effort, and the subject of this brief section, is to consider whether or not any of the insights gained into the structural and functional relationships of parallel computers might be applicable to our attempts to understand the organizational principles of biological nervous systems. Bearing in mind that scientists have always used the most sophisticated machine of the day as a metaphor for the brain (C. Koch, personal communication), it seems natural to describe both nervous systems and parallel computers as collections of distributed processing elements that interact with each other over limited-bandwidth communication channels. Given this fundamental similarity, it is interesting to view the brain as a sophisticated parallel processor and to look for biological analogies to the principles of parallel processing outlined above.

Grain Size in the Nervous System   One of the first distinctions we made, when describing parallel computer architectures, was between coarse-grained and fine-grained machines. Thus it is natural to ask "what is the grain size of the brain?" Unfortunately grain size, at least as we have used it, is not well defined; it is just a relative measure within the range exhibited by present-day parallel computers, making it impossible to rank the brain on the same scale. One could try to argue that the nervous system is fine-grained because there are so many processors (neurons), which is, in general, a property of fine-grained computers. One could also argue that it is coarse-grained because individual neurons are often at least as complex and sophisticated as the microprocessors that characterize coarse-grained computers.

While it may not make much sense to try to compare grain size between computers and brains, it may make more sense to look at grain size within different parts of the brain, where we might expect tradeoffs between the number and complexity of neurons. For example, the most numerous cell type in the brain, the granule cells of the cerebellum, are structurally, and therefore presumably functionally, relatively simple, while the Purkinje cells they project to are far fewer but are structurally and functionally very complex. Thus it seems that both parallel computers and the nervous system may be subject to constraints that dictate tradeoffs within each system, and the nervous system may well optimize the grain size of different subsystems based on the nature of the computations that must be carried out.

Connection Topology   Almost all contemporary computers are characterized by a specific and uniform pattern of connections between their processors, such as the hypercube topology. In the nervous system, there is no such standardized connectivity pattern that spans all neurons in all structures. Instead, different brain regions have different characteristic patterns of cell-to-cell connectivity. Within regions, the uniformity of connections ranges from highly irregular (as in the reticular nuclei) to highly regular (as in the cerebellum).

The question of overall network topology, and why the nervous system does not adopt a uniform strategy, almost certainly reflects the fact that specific neural networks evolved within the context of particular sets of information-processing problems. Parallel computers, on the other hand, are usually designed to be general-purpose machines and to be able to handle a wide variety of problems. As described in the main body of this chapter, a parallel programmer tries to find the optimal decomposition of a particular problem for a fixed machine architecture. In the case of the nervous system, evolution has had the opportunity to optimize the machine architecture itself to fit the problem.

Communication Overhead   In earlier sections we described the task of parallel programming as an optimization problem in which both communication overhead and load imbalance must be minimized. It is likely that both of these selective pressures also operate in the nervous system. For example, consider the issue of communication overhead, which has two distinct aspects. First there is the "hardware" overhead associated with actually making the physical connections between processors. As we pointed out earlier, this constraint is significant for parallel computers; it is the principal reason for implementing limited-connectivity architectures. This communication-related overhead is almost certain to severely constrain nervous system design as well. The optimized-connection topology in the brain would probably be characterized by relatively large numbers of local connections and much sparser longer-range connections, which, judging from neuroanatomy, is characteristic of many parts of the nervous system, including neocortex.

There is also a software-related aspect of communication overhead, which we discussed in detail in the main body of this chapter. In parallel computers, this overhead results from the fact that processors must actually "wait" for information to arrive from other processors before they can proceed with their calculations. This decreases their efficiency in proportion to the fraction of time that they spend sending and receiving information. It seems that the nervous system has evolved a computational strategy that largely avoids this type of overhead, since neurons can simultaneously "calculate" (e.g., integrate synaptic inputs in the dendrites) and "communicate" (e.g., generate action potentials at the soma), without any loss of efficiency.

Load Imbalance When finding an optimal decomposition on a parallel computer, one strives to maintain a relatively uniform workload on all of the processors; otherwise valuable computational resources are wasted. The desire to have balanced effort across a network of neurons may also be a serious design objective for the evolution of the nervous system as well. The high metabolic rates of neural tissue and the resulting need to provide a steady flow of glucose and oxygen results in considerable evolutionary pressure to assure that, over the medium term, neural activity is relatively well balanced. This selective pressure may, in fact, result in individual neruons becoming incorporated into several different networks subserving a variety of processing tasks, as seen in visual cortex.

12.6.1 Conclusions

By considering structural and functional relationships in parallel computers, one is confronted with new and interesting ways of thinking about the nervous system, and vice versa. Thus, in addition to providing a powerful new computational tool for neural modelers, we suspect that a significant value of modeling neurons and networks on parallel computers lies in the interplay of ideas that it engenders between neurobiology, applied neural network research, and computer science.

The address of Mark Nelson and Jim Bower is Division of Biology 216-76, and of Wojtek Furmanski is Division of Physics 356-48, California Institute of Technology, Pasadena, California 91125. Electronic mail should be addressed to nelson@caltech.edu or nelson@caltech.bitnet.

CHAPTER 13

Numerical Methods for Neuronal Modeling

MICHAEL V. MASCAGNI

13.1 Introduction

In this chapter we will discuss some practical and technical aspects of numerical methods that can be used to solve the equations that neuronal modelers frequently encounter. We will consider numerical methods for ordinary differential equations (ODEs) and for partial differential equations (PDEs) through examples. A typical case where ODEs arise in neuronal modeling is when one uses a single lumped-soma compartmental model to describe a neuron. Arguably the most famous PDE system in neuronal modeling is the phenomenological model of the squid giant axon due to Hodgkin and Huxley. Finally, we will consider the problems associated with evolving in time a Hopfield-type neural network consisting of multilayered perceptronlike neural units that has explicit delays and/or temporal properties incorporated into the firing rules (Hopfield and Tank 1986).

The difference between ODEs and PDEs is that ODEs are simply equations in which the rate of change of an unknown function of a single variable is prescribed, usually the derivative with respect to time. In contrast, PDEs involve the rates of change of the solution with respect to many independent variables. For the PDE models we will discuss the independent variables of time and space. The numerical methods we will discuss for both ODEs and PDEs involve replacing the derivatives in the differential equations with finite difference approximations to the derivatives. This reduces the differential equations to algebraic equations. The two major classes of finite difference methods we will discuss are characterized by whether the resulting algebraic equations explicitly or implicitly define the solution at the new time value. We will see that the method of solution for explicit and implicit methods will vary considerably, as will the properties of the solutions to the resulting finite difference equations.

To simplify our exposition, we will use the Hodgkin-Huxley equations as illustrative examples for the numerical methods we will consider for differential equations. Recall that if one space-clamps a section of a squid giant axon by longitudinally inserting a silver electrode, the membrane potential will no longer depend on the spatial location within the clamped region. This reduces the original PDE to a system of ODEs and leads us to model the membrane potential with the following system of ODEs that describe the balance between the ionic and capacitive currents in the clamped region of the squid axon:

$$C\frac{dV}{dt} = -\overline{g}_{Na}m^3h(V - E_{Na}) - \overline{g}_K n^4(V - E_K) - \overline{g}_{leak}(V - E_{leak}) \quad (13.1)$$

where

$$
\begin{aligned}
\frac{dm}{dt} &= (1 - m)\alpha_m(V) - m\beta_m(V) \\
\frac{dh}{dt} &= (1 - h)\alpha_h(V) - h\beta_h(V) \\
\frac{dn}{dt} &= (1 - n)\alpha_n(V) - n\beta_n(V)
\end{aligned}
\qquad (13.2)
$$

In addition to this relation for current balance, Hodgkin and Huxley provided expressions for the functions $\alpha_m(V)$, $\alpha_h(V)$, $\alpha_n(V)$, $\beta_m(V)$, $\beta_h(V)$, and $\beta_n(V)$ based on empirical observation as well as an empirical method for incorporating differences in the ambient temperature into their model (Hodgkin and Huxley 1952).

If instead of space-clamping the *Loligo* giant axon one allows the voltage across the membrane of the axon to vary with longitudinal distance along the axon, x, as well as time, then the membrane potential satisfies a PDE similar to the space-clamped case, except that eq. 13.1 is replaced with

$$
\begin{aligned}
C\frac{\partial V}{\partial t} = & \frac{a}{2R}\frac{\partial^2 V}{\partial x^2} - \overline{g}_{Na}m^3h(V - E_{Na}) - \\
& \overline{g}_K n^4(V - E_K) - \overline{g}_{leak}(V - E_{leak})
\end{aligned}
\qquad (13.3)
$$

Below we will consider the complete mathematical description of these two problems related to the squid giant axon and their numerical solution beginning with the space-clamped ODE model. It is important to note that the Hodgkin-Huxley systems are useful examples for numerical computation in two complementary ways. First, the Hodgkin-Huxley models are very complex and so provide a realistic and challenging system to test our proposed numerical methods. Numerical methods that work on the Hodgkin-Huxley systems should work equally well on other equations the neuronal modeler may wish to explore. Second, the Hodgkin-Huxley equations are basic expressions of current conservation, so the modification of our formulas for the numerical solution of the Hodgkin-Huxley system to accommodate other neuronal models is straightforward, provided the models are also explicitly based on the electrical properties of nerves, and the kinetics associated with the individual ionic currents can be described with first-order kinetic equations as in eqs. 13.2.

13.1.1   Numerical Preliminaries

Before we discuss specific methods for ODEs and PDEs, there are three general concepts associated with these differential-equation numerical methods that should be introduced. These are the concepts of stability, consistency, and convergence for a numerical method. The most fundamental of these concepts is convergence. We say a numerical method is convergent if the error between the solution via the numerical method and the exact solution can be made as small as we please. Because we will be discussing finite-difference methods where space and time will be discretized with numerical time step Δt and a spatial mesh size Δx, convergence for a finite-difference method amounts to showing that the numerical solution differs from the exact solution by a term that goes to zero as Δt and Δx go to zero in some way. In essence, the mathematical analysis of numerical methods amounts to the rigorous establishment of convergence for proposed numerical methods for the solution of particular problems.

In the establishment of general convergence theory, the concepts of stability and consistency of a numerical method have emerged as fundamental. As the name implies, consistency of a numerical method ensures that the numerical solution solves a discrete problem that is consistent with the desired continuous problem. For finite-difference methods for differential equations, this amounts to determining if the difference equations, when applied to the exact solution of the continuous problem, result in only a small approximation (truncation) error. If this truncation error goes to zero as Δt and Δx go to zero in some way, then the numerical method is consistent because the exact solution approximately satisfies the equations for the numerical solution. This definition for consistency sounds suspiciously like the above definition for convergence; however, a method can be consistent and yet not convergent. This is because consistency demands only that the exact solution satisfy the finite difference equations with a truncation error that formally goes to zero with the grid parameters. Convergence demands that

the numerical and exact solutions can be made to differ by an arbitrarily
small amount at every point in time and space. Convergence is a more
restrictive definition.

Stability is the concept that fills the definitional gap between consistency and convergence for a wide class of problems. We call a finite-
difference method stable if the solution to the finite difference equations
remains bounded as the grid parameters go to zero. It is a notable fact
that some consistent finite-difference methods are not stable. In these
cases the numerical solution may grow without bound even when the
analytical solution to the same problem might actually be quite small.
A method with this type of behavior is obviously not convergent. We
should note that some stable finite-difference solutions can exhibit small
oscillations about the exact solution and still be of great utility. Therefore we can appreciate the importance of using finite-difference methods
that give solutions that do not grow without bound. A more precise
definition of stability is beyond the scope of this chapter; however, an
accurate analogy of stability for finite-difference methods can be made
with the Hadamard's concept of a well-posed problem for differential
equations (Courant and Hilbert 1962). It is important to add that certain finite-difference methods are stable with certain combinations of the
grid parameters, or for differential equations with particular properties,
but not for some others. For these reasons, the concept of stability is often weakened to permit discussion of particular methods and equations.
Thus there may be several progressively less restrictive definitions of
stability presented in a discussion of a class of numerical methods. This
is especially so for finite-difference methods for ODEs.

One of the most remarkable results in the analysis of finite-difference
methods for differential equations is the relationship between consistency, stability, and convergence for linear differential equations. This
result is known as the Lax equivalence theorem (Lax and Richtmeyer
1956) and states that a finite-difference method for linear ODEs or PDEs
is convergent if and only if it is both consistent and stable. Thus for
these linear problems, the two concepts of consistency and stability are
exactly complementary. Because of this elegant relationship between
these three concepts for linear problems, numerical methods for nonlinear problems also discuss consistency and stability in the context of
establishing numerical convergence; however, in these nonlinear cases
it is important to remember that there is no general Lax equivalence
theorem. Thus one must use mathematical tools of one's own design to
prove convergence in these nonlinear situations.

For those interested in a more detailed discussion of the Lax theory and the concepts of consistency, stability, and convergence, the introduction to the chapter on methods for PDEs in the classic text by Isaacson and Keller (1966) gives a very lucid and elegant presentation of this material with a minimum of mathematical machinery. The same material can also be found as introductory material in the standard reference of Richtmeyer and Morton (1967) for the reader familiar with the elements of functional analysis. A modern summary can be found in the introductory chapter in Sod's monograph on finite-difference methods (Sod 1985). Here terminology and notation consistent with the modern numerical analysis literature is used.

13.2   Methods for ODEs

The theory for the numerical solution of ODEs is very well established, and the rigorous analysis of many classes of numerical methods has an extensive literature (see, for example, Collatz 1960; Gear 1971a; Henrici 1962; Lambert 1973). For practical purposes it is convenient to distinguish numerical methods for ODEs based on a property of the ODEs known as stiffness. Stiffness is a measure of the difficulty in solving an ODE numerically, much in the same way as the condition number of a matrix measures the difficulty of numerically solving the associated system of linear equations (see Appendix 13.A).

Before we begin our discussion on numerical methods for ODEs, let us lay out the usual mathematical setting for discussing the numerical solution of ODEs. The Hodgkin-Huxley ODE model, eqs. 13.1 and 13.2, is a system of four first-order ODEs. We can define the four-dimensional vector of functions, $\vec{U} = (V, m, h, n)$, and rewrite eqs. 13.1 and 13.2 to obtain the single vector-differential equation

$$\frac{d\vec{U}}{dt} = \vec{F}(\vec{U}, t) \tag{13.4}$$

Here $\vec{F}(\vec{U})$ is a vector-valued right-hand side corresponding to the right-hand sides in eqs. 13.1 and 13.2 with eq. 13.1 rewritten by dividing through by C. In general, it is always possible to rewrite any system of ODEs as a single system of first-order ODEs, even when we begin with ODEs that have second- or higher-order derivatives (John 1965). It is important to recognize this fact because as this unity of form for all ODEs is often exploited in the numerical analysis literature by only presenting numerical methods for first-order systems of ODEs.

Having rewritten our equations in the form of eq. 13.4, one more piece of mathematical information is needed before we can begin solving the ODEs. Equation 13.4 tells us only how the unknown functions change with time; we must know at which values these functions start to compute a particular solution. This first-order system of ODEs is commonly thought of as part of an initial value problem (IVP), where given some initial values, the solution is thereafter uniquely determined. Thus, for the numerical solution of the IVP of eq. 13.4, we must likewise specify initial conditions to begin our computation. Thus when modeling neuronal elements with ODEs, remember that not only is a tractable functional description of the ODEs required, but reasonable initial conditions are also necessary to obtain meaningful solutions.

13.2.1   Qualitative Definition of Stiffness

Given that we have completely defined the IVP for our ODE model, the choice of a numerical method and the time-step size Δt depends on whether this IVP is stiff or not. There are, in fact, many ways of quantitatively expressing the concept of stiffness for ODEs. A useful qualitative definition is that a system of ODEs, or a single ODE for that matter, is said to be stiff if the solution contains a wide range of characteristic time scales. The problem with a wide range of time scales can be appreciated through a simple illustration. Suppose the fastest time scale in an ODE has duration λ, whereas the slowest has γ. If γ/λ is large, then a numerical time step, Δt, small enough to resolve phenomena on the λ time scale, requires γ/λ steps to resolve phenomena on the γ time scale. This is not a problem if the phenomena on the λ time scale are of interest; however, if the λ time scale is of little interest it would seem an obvious strategy to choose $\Delta t \approx \gamma$. For certain numerical methods, generally explicit methods, this turns out to be a numerical disaster, because the inaccuracy in resolving the λ time scale leads to catastrophic numerical instabilities often resulting in wild oscillations in the computed solution. This is the primary manifestation of stiffness.

Basically, then, we should distinguish between methods that are acceptable when the ODEs are stiff and methods that can be used when the ODEs are not stiff. Fortunately, this is well understood; moreover, the ODEs that arise in most neuronal modeling contexts are readily identified as being stiff or not. The other important discriminant for choosing a particular numerical method is the quality of the numerical solution produced. For ODEs, the accuracy of a numerical method depends on the particular ODE to be solved and on the step size Δt. This quality is usually expressed in "big Oh" notation. Thus if we say that method A is $O((\Delta t)^2)$ accurate, we mean that the numerical solution to an ODE obtained with method A differs from the exact solution to the ODE by an amount that goes to zero like $(\Delta t)^2$ as Δt goes to zero. Thus if we halve Δt from one computation to another still using method A, the error decreases by a factor of $(\frac{1}{2})^2$. Higher-order methods are much more accurate, but in general they are much more complicated to implement than lower-order accurate methods, so there is a practical decision to be made concerning the numerical accuracy requirement versus the overall cost in implementing and using a particular method when choosing an ODE method for a given computation.

Two important concepts that relate to the numerical errors involved in solving an ODE numerically are called local and global truncation (or discretization) errors. The local truncation error is the error between the numerical solution and the exact solution after a single time step. If we recall the definition of consistency from before, it is the local truncation error that must go to zero as Δt goes to zero for the consistency of an ODE method. For most finite-difference methods, it is elementary to compute this local truncation error with the help of the Taylor series expansion of the solution. The global truncation error is the difference between the computed solution and the exact solution at a given time $t = T = n\Delta t$. This is the error that must go to zero as Δt goes to zero to give us convergence. In general, one cannot merely use the Taylor series to calculate the global truncation error explicitly, but it can be shown that if the local truncation error is $O((\Delta t)^p)$, then the global truncation error will also be $O((\Delta t)^p)$ (Stoer and Bulirsch 1980). In the literature one speaks of a p-ordered method to mean that the local truncation error is $O((\Delta t)^p)$.

13.2.2 Methods When Stiffness Is Unimportant

A large class of well-studied numerical methods that yield high-accuracy solutions are called the linear-multistep methods (Miranker 1975). These methods include, among others, the methods of Adams, Newton-Cotes, Nystrom, and backward differentiation. The linear-multistep methods include both explicit and implicit variations, as well as variations of differing numerical accuracy. Another popular family of finite-difference methods are the Runge-Kutta methods. These methods also come in explicit and implicit varieties and versions with different accuracy. Yet another class of numerical methods for ODEs is called predictor-corrector methods, because they consist of two steps: an initial prediction of the solution at the new time value, usually with a simple low-order method, followed by iterative correction of this prediction with another, usually high-order, method.

To clarify the difference between explicit and implicit methods, let us consider the simplest methods for the numerical solution of eq. 13.4. These methods are the forward- and backward-Euler methods and are the most basic explicit and implicit linear-multistep methods. Let us denote $t^n = n\Delta t$ and $\vec{U}^n = \vec{U}(n\Delta t)$; then the forward-Euler method is simply

$$\frac{\vec{U}^{n+1} - \vec{U}^n}{\Delta t} = \vec{F}(\vec{U}^n, \; t^n) \tag{13.5}$$

and the backward-Euler method is

$$\frac{\vec{U}^{n+1} - \vec{U}^n}{\Delta t} = \vec{F}(\vec{U}^{n+1}, \; t^{n+1}) \tag{13.6}$$

If we rewrite eq. 13.5 as $\vec{U}^{n+1} = \vec{U}^n + \Delta t \vec{F}(\vec{U}^n, \; t^n)$, we see that the forward-Euler method gives us an explicit formula to evaluate for $\vec{U}^{n+1}$ in terms of the known $\vec{U}^n$. If we rewrite eq. 13.6 with the known quantities on the right and the unknowns on the left, we get $\vec{U}^{n+1} - \Delta t \vec{F}(\vec{U}^{n+1}, \; t^{n+1}) = \vec{U}^n$. This is not an expression that can be simply evaluated to obtain $\vec{U}^{n+1}$; instead, this is an equation whose solution implicitly defines $\vec{U}^{n+1}$. This illustrates the difference between explicit and implicit methods. In addition, this shows us that with an implicit method we must know not only the method's difference formula but also a numerical method to solve the equations that arise at each time step.

All these methods work well when stiffness is not an issue, and the primary criterion one should use to choose between them is that the chosen method should require as little computational work as possible while still providing the required solution accuracy. There are no hard and fast rules for making this comparison, but a few rules of thumb can be used to guide us. A convenient measure of the computational work required in an ODE calculation is the total number of evaluations of the right-hand-side functions, as in the space-clamped Hodgkin-Huxley model, eqs. 13.1 and 13.2. Suppose we wish to solve the IVP for this Hodgkin-Huxley system, with initial conditions given at $t = 0$ up to a time $t = T$. If we call $M = T/\Delta t$, which is the number of time steps, and define K to be the number of function evaluations per time step for a given numerical method, then the most efficient choice of numerical method minimizes the product MK. In general, the number of function evaluations per time step for a finite-difference calculation is roughly

proportional to the order of accuracy one obtains in the numerical solution. Thus, minimizing MK involves the trade-off between using as
large a step size as possible to minimize M and as low an accuracy
method as is acceptable to minimize K. Practically, software for the
numerical solution of ODEs is readily available or fairly easy to write,
as long as the method is not of very high accuracy order. An accuracy
of $O((\Delta t)^2)$ or $O((\Delta t)^4)$ is sufficient for most purposes, so one may first
choose a particular method that is practically convenient with sufficient
accuracy and then decide on the step size Δt based on M.

The Runge-Kutta methods have popular variants that are second- and
fourth-order. If we consider the solution to eq. 13.4, the second-order
method is summarized by

$$
\begin{aligned}
\vec{U}^{n+1} &= \vec{U}^n + \frac{\Delta t}{2}[\vec{k}_1 + \vec{k}_2], \text{ where} \\
\vec{k}_1 &= \vec{F}(\vec{U}^n, \, t^n) \\
\vec{k}_2 &= \vec{F}(\vec{U}^n + \Delta t\vec{k}_1, \, t^{n+1})
\end{aligned}
\tag{13.7}
$$

The fourth-order method is

$$
\begin{aligned}
\vec{U}^{n+1} &= \vec{U}^n + \frac{\Delta t}{6}[\vec{k}_1 + 2\vec{k}_2 + 2\vec{k}_3 + \vec{k}_4], \text{ where} \\
\vec{k}_1 &= \vec{F}(\vec{U}^n, \, t^n) \\
\vec{k}_2 &= \vec{F}(\vec{U}^n + \tfrac{1}{2}\Delta t\vec{k}_1, \, t^{n+1/2}) \\
\vec{k}_3 &= \vec{F}(\vec{U}^n + \tfrac{1}{2}\Delta t\vec{k}_2, \, t^{n+1/2}) \\
\vec{k}_4 &= \vec{F}(\vec{U}^n + \Delta t\vec{k}_3, \, t^{n+1})
\end{aligned}
\tag{13.8}
$$

In eq. 13.8, $t^{n+1/2} = (n + 1/2)\Delta t$. We notice that eq. 13.7 requires two
evaluations of $\vec{F}$ and is a second-order method, and eq. 13.8 requires
four function evaluations for this fourth-order method.

13.2.3   Methods with Adaptive Step Size

Suppose that one is interested in understanding the repetitive firing
behavior of the Hodgkin-Huxley system in response to a steady input
current. Then the calculation must be carried out until either periodic
repetitive firing is observed or the system reaches some other stable
steady-state solution. The phenomenon of interest is some function of
the long-time behavior of the system, which is only obtained after an
initial system transient has subsided. Therefore, the length of time to

be calculated is not known beforehand. This lack of knowledge of T prevents us from using the heuristics of the previous section to guide us in a choice of Δt for this particular computation.

A clever variation on the above methods that removes the necessity for *a priori* knowledge of T is the above methods augmented with an algorithm that adaptively varies the numerical step size Δt. All the ODE methods mentioned thus far are well understood, and, in particular, formulas for the local truncation errors are known. By estimating the different terms in these local truncation-error formulas, one can numerically estimate the total truncation error and quantify the local accuracy of the computed solution. By using this information as a criterion for either increasing or decreasing the size of Δt, a computation can be carried out to within a user-specified error tolerance with as large a step size as possible used at each time step. Such a method is called an adaptive time-step method.

Although it is fairly straightforward to program an adaptive stepsize variant of a known ODE method, the task can be daunting to the uninitiated. However, because adaptive algorithms have been popular for some time, very well written and computationally efficient packages that incorporate adaptive methods can be readily obtained. Several examples for the IBM-PC are MATLAB, MATHCAD, PHASPLN, and PLOD, whereas FORTRAN or C source codes of an adaptive version of the fourth-order Runge-Kutta method can be found in the compendium of numerical programs of Press et al. (1986). Such a simple method is discussed in chapter 4. If one is planning to carry out a varied collection of computations of ODE models, it is probably worth the modest extra effort to obtain a program for an adaptive time-step ODE method to use for those computations.

13.2.4   Methods for Stiff Systems

The space-clamped Hodgkin-Huxley ODE model is not particularly stiff; however, it is fairly easy to encounter extremely stiff ODEs that are simply related to eqs. 13.1 and 13.2. If one incorporates the space-clamped Hodgkin-Huxley ODEs into a compartmental model of a neuron, the resulting multicompartment system will generally be stiff, with the stiffness increasing with the number of compartments in the single-neuron model. The reason for this is the correspondence between compartmental models of neurons and the so-called method of lines for the numerical solution of PDE models for the same neurons. This relationship between compartmental models and PDE models will be explained in detail in Appendix 13.A along with an explicit calculation of the stiffness of a compartmental model of a passive dendritic cable. Another example of an ODE model that is stiff is discussed in chapter 4. A model of the bullfrog sympathetic ganglion cell includes ionic currents with the familiar millisecond time scale along with slow currents with time scales in the hundreds of milliseconds.

Appendix 13.A shows us that compartmental models are equivalent to PDE models discretized via the method of lines. Appendix 13.A also demonstrates the stiffness that pervades these types of equations. Thus we see that stiffness is a common property of neuronal models, so we now discuss numerical methods designed for stiff ODEs. A general rule of thumb for stiff ODEs is that explicit finite-difference methods are extremely susceptible to the complications of stiffness, whereas implicit methods behave much better. Thus the implicit versions of the ODE methods mentioned above are viable candidates for integrating our stiff ODEs. One particularly nice class of methods for stiff ODEs is the series of methods due to Gear (Gear 1971b). The Gear methods are predictor-corrector methods based on the Adams linear-multistep methods with explicit prediction and implicit correction. Gear methods are available with first- to seventh-order accuracy. Of particular interest are the adaptive versions of the Gear methods. These adaptive methods combine the predictor-corrector methods of Gear with an adaptive step-size algorithm that provides the user with a reliable method of solving stiff ODEs with a modest amount of computational cost. The adaptive Gear method can be found in many popular ODE packages, and a complete description of these methods can be found in several standard texts on methods for ODEs (Gear 1971a; Lambert 1973). It should be noted that there are alternatives to the Gear methods. Those due to Krough (Krough 1969) offer methods with accuracy ranging from first- to thirteenth-order, as well as versions with automatic step-size control. In some circumstances these methods may be preferable to the Gear methods (Hull et al. 1971); however, the popularity and availability of software incorporating the Gear methods makes these circumstances practically nonexistent.

If one is unsure about the stiffness of a particular ODE system whose numerical solution is required, it may be worthwhile to begin with a low-order explicit method, for example, the second-order Runge-Kutta method, and use it on a test problem where the solution's behavior is known. If the method produces good results, one may not need to look any further for a numerical method; however, if the solution is either obviously wrong or gives unexpected oscillatory behavior, one should suspect stiffness. One should then use an implicit method to recompute the test problem, possibly even to the first-order backward-Euler method (eq. 13.6). If this solution seems more reasonable, then it is safe to assume that stiffness was the original culprit. At this point one should consider Gear's method, especially if long time intervals and repeated computation are foreseen. Otherwise one should choose to compute with another higher-order implicit method.

13.2.5   Boundary Value Problems

Besides the IVP for ODEs, there is another class of mathematical problems that involves ODEs called boundary value problems (BVPs). As an example of a BVP for ODEs, let us consider how one might compute the nonlinear steady-state solution to the Hodgkin-Huxley PDE system. One approach would be to use a numerical method for the PDE system and compute the solution for a long enough time that the PDE settles down to its stable steady-state. This is an acceptable approach, but a conceptually more direct approach is to ask what equation is satisfied by the steady-state solution to eqs. 13.2 and 13.3 and then solve those equations directly. Because we seek the steady-state solution, the time derivative of all the variables in eqs. 13.2 and 13.3 will be zero. Thus we have to solve the following system of ODEs:

$$
\begin{aligned}
\frac{a}{2R}\frac{d^2V}{dx^2} &= \bar{g}_{Na}m_\infty(V)^3 h_\infty(V)(V - E_{Na}) + \\
&\quad \bar{g}_K n_\infty(V)^4(V - E_K) + \bar{g}_{leak}(V - E_{leak}) \\
m_\infty(V) &= \frac{\alpha_m(V)}{\alpha_m(V) + \beta_m(V)} \\
h_\infty(V) &= \frac{\alpha_h(V)}{\alpha_h(V) + \beta_h(V)} \\
n_\infty(V) &= \frac{\alpha_n(V)}{\alpha_n(V) + \beta_n(V)}
\end{aligned}
\tag{13.9}
$$

Here we have renamed the dimensionless variables by adding the ∞ subscript to indicate that they no longer obey differential equations, but are instantaneously defined by the above equations. These equations are obtained from eqs. 13.2 by setting the time derivatives equal to zero and solving the resulting algebraic equations.

As with eqs. 13.1 and 13.2, which required initial conditions to completely specify the problem, the mathematical problem for eq. 13.9 is not yet complete. Boundary conditions are necessary to properly specify this problem. Let us assume that we are interested in the steady-state solution for a Hodgkin-Huxley axon of length L. Then reasonable boundary conditions are

$$V(0) = V^0, \quad V(L) = 0 \qquad (13.10)$$

These boundary conditions demand that the steady-state solution we seek has a voltage value of V^0 at $x = 0$ and a voltage value of zero at $x = L$. This can be accomplished in the laboratory by impaling the squid axon with voltage-clamping electrodes at two points L spatial units away from one another and clamping one electrode to V^0 millivolts and the other to 0 millivolts with respect to the membrane's resting potential.

Equations 13.9 and 13.10 are a properly posed BVP for determining the steady-state behavior of the squid giant axon with two end points having their voltage values clamped. We will discuss two numerical methods for the solution of this BVP. One is called the shooting method, which reduces the problem to an IVP with one unknown initial condition. The other method uses finite differences to solve this problem directly.

Let us begin with the direct approach. If we take eqs. 13.9 and 13.10 and introduce a spatial grid of uniform width $\Delta x = L/N$, and with $x_0 = 0$ and $x_N = L$, and replace the second spatial derivative with the $O((\Delta x)^2)$ accurate finite-difference approximation, these equations become

$$\frac{a}{2R} \frac{V_{i+1} - 2V_i + V_{i-1}}{(\Delta x)^2} = \overline{g}_{Na} m_\infty (V_i)^3 h_\infty (V_i)(V_i - E_{Na}) +$$

$$\overline{g}_K n_\infty (V_i)^4 (V_i - E_K) + \overline{g}_{leak}(V_i - E_{leak})$$

$$V_0 = V^0, \quad V_N = 0 \qquad (13.11)$$

The above equations are no longer differential equations but are merely a nonlinear system of algebraic equations whose solution gives us a finite-difference approximation to the steady-state solution that is $O((\Delta x)^2)$ accurate. We will consider the solution of nonlinear equations of this same form in section 13.3, so here we will only outline a particular solution algorithm.

Equation 13.11 is a nonlinear tridiagonal system of algebraic equations in the sense that the ith equation involves the $i + 1$st, ith, and $i - 1$st unknowns. The Hodgkin-Huxley equations have the fortunate property that if the dimensionless variables m, h, and n are known, the equations reduce to linear equations. Thus, if we guess an initial voltage profile, we can use this to compute the dimensionless variables. These values can then be used to reduce these equations to a linear tridiagonal system, which is readily solved for V_i. This gives us a new voltage profile that can be used to compute new dimensionless variable values, and so on. This iterative method will converge to the steady-state solution, provided we have chosen a reasonable initial guess for V_i and the steady-state solution we seek is analytically a stable solution to eq. 13.11. For the boundary conditions given in eq. 13.10, a good initial guess is the straight line connecting V^0 at $x = 0$ to 0 at $x = L$.

The shooting method for solving this BVP also involves solving nonlinear algebraic equations, but in a very different manner. The second-order ODE for the steady-state BVP (eqs. 13.10 and 13.11) can be thought of as an IVP with $V_0 = V^0$ that happens to pass through $V_N = 0$. Thus, one way to solve this BVP is to solve it as an IVP with initial values given at the $x = 0$ end and try to guess at initial conditions that cause the solution to satisfy the boundary condition at $x = L$. Because eq. 13.11 is a second-order ODE, proper initial conditions are to specify $V(0)$ and $dV(0)/dx$. We know that $V(0) = V^0$, but have no information on what $dV(0)/dx$ should be. If we guess at a value for $dV(0)/dx$, we can solve the IVP up to $x = L$, and if we guess correctly, we will have $V(L) = 0$. Using a numerical method for solving the IVP, a given value for $dV(0)/dx$ will yield a unique value for the solution at $x = L$. Thus the IVP numerical method allows us an unusual way to evaluate the function $V(L; D)$. Here we mean that $V(L; D)$ is the value of the numerical solution at $x = L$, given that the solution starts with $V(0) = V^0$ and $dV(0)/dx = D$. The solution to the BVP is therefore the IVP solution for which the value of D makes $V(L; D) = 0$. We now see why this is called the shooting method. We guess on some initial value at one boundary and shoot the solution to the other boundary, hoping that the solution hits the desired boundary value.

This formulation for the numerical solution of this BVP reduces to solving the single nonlinear equation $V(L; D) = 0$. What do we know about the function $V(L; D)$? We know how to evaluate this function as the solution to an ODE IVP by using a numerical method, and we know that it is a continuous function in the variable D (Coddington and Levinson 1955). Two methods for solving $V(L; D) = 0$ when $V(L; D)$ is known to be continuous are called the bisection and secant methods. For brevity, we will not discuss these well-known methods in this chapter. The reader is instead directed to any elementary numerical analysis text (Conte and de Boor 1980).

The general problem of numerically solving the BVP for ODEs has many complications, which we have avoided in the brief introduction. These complications include problems with singular solutions, finding unstable solutions, and periodic and translational boundary conditions, to mention a few. A good resource for these types of numerical computations is Keller's brief monograph on boundary value problems for ODEs (Keller 1976). Also, Doedel's software package, AUTO, is readily available and can handle these types of BVPs, as well as others related to the existence of periodic solutions and the determination of unstable solutions (Doedel 1981).

13.2.6   Final Comments

We have seen several numerical methods for solving ODEs, as part of both IVPs and BVPs. One set of facts that we have purposely downplayed is the convergence of these numerical methods. The reason for this is that the convergence theory for ODE methods is relatively complete, and the methods presented will converge to well-posed ODE problems provided that we choose the numerical time step Δt sufficiently small. However, this glibness with convergence will not carry over to our discussion of numerical methods for PDEs.

For ODEs, stiffness is the critical factor to consider when choosing between alternative numerical methods. In general, a compartmental model of a neuron will yield a rather stiff system of ODEs, so an implicit method should be used to avoid the numerical instabilities that explicit methods exhibit when used on stiff systems. We have singled out Gear's adaptive time-step method as particularly attractive for stiff systems. In contrast, small systems of ODEs, or a system of ODEs that does not have direct coupling between its domains, may not be that stiff, so it may be computationally cheaper to use an explicit method, such as one of the Runge-Kutta methods. We reiterate that it is usually preferable to use a method that automatically selects its own adaptive step size.

If one is beginning a new series of neuronal computations with ODE models, it is advised that several numerical methods be explored before a decision is made about the method to be used for the extended computations. If one has ready access to computer programs for several different numerical methods, the long-term saving of human and computer time derived by choosing the best method from those available is well worth a few hours of comparative tinkering at the computer terminal.

13.3   Methods for PDEs

In general, numerical methods for PDEs are not as well understood as numerical methods for ODEs. In a large sense, this has to do with the increased mathematical complexity of PDEs over ODEs. In contrast to the numerical methods for ODEs, much of the intuition accumulated for understanding and choosing PDE methods has come from understanding the solution of linear PDEs. For this reason we will begin our discussion not with the example of the Hodgkin-Huxley equations but with its linear counterpart, the passive cable equation from dendritic modeling. This equation is

$$C \frac{\partial V}{\partial t} = \frac{a}{2R} \frac{\partial^2 V}{\partial x^2} - \bar{g}V \tag{13.12}$$

where $\bar{g}$ is the passive membrane conductance per unit area.

13.3.1   Linear PDEs: The Method of Lines

In Appendix 13.A we will see how conceptually close the method of lines for PDEs is to compartmental modeling. Because we will discuss the method of lines in great detail in this Appendix, we will only briefly mention it as the first method for solving PDEs. If we replace the continuous variable x with a uniformly spaced grid of length $\Delta x = x/N$ with $N + 1$ grid points, then the method of lines transforms eq. 13.12 into the following coupled system of ODEs:

$$C \frac{dV_i}{dt} = \frac{a}{2R} \frac{V_{i+1} - 2V_i + V_{i-1}}{(\Delta x)^2} - \bar{g}V_i \tag{13.13}$$

As was mentioned above, this system is stiff, with the stiffness increasing with N. Thus we would like to use an implicit ODE method, most probably Gear's method with automatic and adaptive step-size selection. Equation 13.13 is the example we will use in Appendix 13.A to explicitly compute the numerical stiffness of a simple, compartmental-model ODE formulation. Because eq. 13.13 is a linear system of ODEs, one can readily compute the solution to the equations in analytic form, making this system particularly simple to analyze. It must be stressed that even though it is possible to use the method of lines to reduce all our PDE models to coupled ODE models in the form of compartmental models, this is not a prudent approach for numerical solution. If presented with a PDE model, it is much better both in terms of algorithmic simplicity and computational cost to use one of the PDE methods to be discussed rather than reduce the system to ODEs. In fact, it is my opinion that if one can convert a compartmental model to an equivalent PDE model, this should be done to obtain the benefits of the PDE methods. With this brief observation on the reduction of a PDE model into a (stiff) system of ODEs, we depart the realm of ODE methods.

13.3.2   Defining the PDE Problems

As with ODEs, it is important first to define completely the proper mathematical problem to be solved with PDE models. PDEs are classified as being of the parabolic, hyperbolic, or elliptic type, and the type determines which mathematical problem is correct, or well posed, for that PDE. Elliptic equations describe equilibrium problems, much like the steady-state ODE problem we considered in eq. 13.9, and are solved as BVPs. Hyperbolic equations describe wave propagation, so they are treated as a Cauchy problem. The Cauchy problem for PDEs is the analog of the pure IVP for ODEs (John 1982). Equations of diffusion and dissipation are parabolic equations. The linear cable and the Hodgkin-Huxley cable equations are PDEs of the parabolic type and are related to the equations of heat and diffusion. As such, they are likewise solved as part of a Cauchy problem (John 1982). The particular Cauchy problem most encountered for parabolic equations is the IVP, as parabolic equations are also commonly called evolution equations. This means that parabolic equations describe the evolution in time of some quantity. In our case, we are evolving the membrane potential along a neuronal cable with time.

Recall that PDEs are equations that involve derivatives with respect to more than one independent variable. For neuronal models these independent variables are usually space x and time t. Thus the initial conditions that specify how time evolution is to begin only specify the initial behavior for one of the independent variables, namely t. Boundary conditions are required to deal with how we expect the solution to depend on the variable x. If we are interested in studying an axon or dendrite of infinite length, then there is no need to specify boundary conditions because there are no boundaries. For these cases, it is well known that the pure IVP is the proper mathematical problem (Evans and Shenk 1970).

We are usually interested in computing the solution to a PDE system that corresponds closely to a model of a known neuronal system. Thus we have certain geometrical constraints to the system under study. In particular, we know that the system is not infinite in spatial extent, so the pure initial-value problem is a bit academic at best. Because we like to deal with neuronal models that have spatial boundaries and branching, we must consider imposing boundary conditions on the spatial terminations of our models. Thus for most PDE computations in neuronal modeling, the proper mathematical problem requires imposing both initial and boundary conditions. These types of problems are known as initial-boundary value problems (IBVPs). It has been shown rigorously that the mathematical problem for these types of neuronal PDEs as part of an IBVP is a proper or well-posed mathematical problem (Mascagni 1989). In this case well posed means that this problem has a unique solution that depends continuously on both the initial and boundary conditions and has the property that solution remains bounded above and below for all time. We now consider the mathematical description and biophysical interpretation of several types of boundary conditions encountered in neuronal modeling.

13.3.3   Boundary Conditions

We have already encountered one typical type of boundary condition in our discussion of BVP for ODEs that arise from steady-state computations for PDE problems. Equation 13.10 specifies the voltage at two ends of a neuronal cable. This type of boundary condition, where the solution value is specified at the end points, is called a Dirichlet-type boundary condition. As we will see in the next section, boundary conditions of the Dirichlet type are quite easy to incorporate into finite-difference methods for PDEs.

The second common type of boundary condition is the Neumann boundary condition. Instead of specifying the solution value at the end points, as with the Dirichlet-type boundary conditions, Neumann-type boundary conditions specify the first spatial derivative of the solution at the end points. Neumann-type boundary conditions occur very naturally in neuronal modeling, because $\partial V / \partial x$ is proportional to the longitudinal current through a cable. Thus, specifying Neumann-type boundary conditions for neuronal cable models amounts to specifying the longitudinal current values at the end points. For example, the following Neumann boundary conditions for the Hodgkin-Huxley PDE system, eqs. 13.2 and 13.3,

$$\frac{\partial V(0)}{\partial x} = -\frac{RI}{\pi a^2}, \quad \frac{\partial V(L)}{\partial x} = 0, \qquad (13.14)$$

biophysically correspond to injecting I microamps of current at $x = 0$ and demanding that no current pass out the $x = L$ end. The Neumann-type boundary condition at $x = L$ is commonly called a "no-leak" or "sealed-end" boundary condition in neuronal modeling (Jack, Nobel, and Tsien 1975). Incidentally, open- or killed-end are other names for zero Dirichlet-type boundary conditions. Neumann-type boundary conditions are more complicated than Dirichlet-type boundary conditions to incorporate into finite-difference methods to solve PDE IBVPs, but we will see below that they are only slightly more complicated.

Both the Dirichlet and Neumann boundary conditions are linear boundary conditions, in the sense that linear PDEs with these imposed boundary conditions obey a superposition property with respect to the boundary conditions. A more unusual type of linear boundary condition involves a linear combination of the Dirichlet- and Neumann-type boundary conditions as follows:

$$\alpha_0 \frac{\partial V(0)}{\partial x} + V(0) = \beta_0, \quad \alpha_L \frac{\partial V(L)}{\partial x} + V(L) = \beta_L \qquad (13.15)$$

Because we know that Neumann-type boundary conditions are biophysically statements about the currents at the ends of neuronal cables, it is clear that these mixed-type boundary conditions are merely a statement that the voltage at the end points obeys a linear or ohmic current-voltage relationship. The difficulty of implementing a finite-difference method for a PDE IVBP with these mixed-type boundary conditions is only slightly greater than handling simple Neumann-type boundary conditions. Finally, we mention that by making the coefficients α and β nonlinear functions of the end-point voltages, we can impose a nonlinear current-voltage relationship at the end points. An example of a computation with this type of nonlinear boundary condition is due to Baer and Tier (Baer and Tier 1986). They considered the effects of a Fitzhugh-Nagumo patch that formed the end of a dendritic cylinder as a model of an active membrane site within a passive dendrite.

13.3.4   Finite Difference Methods

Let us now consider methods for solving PDEs. Two popular methods for PDEs are finite-difference and finite-element methods. Although much touted, finite-element methods in many cases reduce to finite-difference methods. This is because finite-element methods reduce differential equations to algebraic equations just as do finite-difference methods. By using particular finite elements, one can derive the same algebraic equations as one would obtain with finite-difference methods, so we will consider only finite-difference methods here. As with finite-difference methods for ODEs, finite-difference methods for PDEs employ finite-difference approximations of the derivatives in the PDEs to reduce the differential equations to algebraic equations. The Hodgkin-Huxley system, as well as the linear cable equation, are PDEs of the parabolic type, and methods we will discuss will also be generally applicable to other parabolic PDEs, such as the heat and diffusion equations.

We will present three finite-difference methods for the numerical solution of these parabolic PDEs. They are called the forward-Euler,
backward-Euler, and Crank-Nicolson methods. We will initially present
them for the linear cable eq. 13.12, and then in a later section we will
discuss the modifications necessary to numerically solve the more complicated Hodgkin-Huxley PDE system from eqs. 13.2 and 13.3.

All three of these finite-difference methods use the $O((\Delta x)^2)$ finite-
difference approximation to the second spatial derivative that we have
previously introduced. The difference between these three methods is
only in the manner in which the time derivative on the left-hand side of
eq. 13.12 is discretized.

Let us now exactly define the computational grid that we plan to use
for all of the finite-difference methods that we will discuss for PDEs. Let
us assume that the spatial domain is L units in length and is divided
into N segments of length $\Delta x = L/N$. The time variable in the PDEs
will be replaced by a discrete set of time values with a uniform spacing
of Δt. The notation we will use to refer to the values of functions
of interest on this computational grid works as follows: V_i^n refers to
$V(i\Delta x, n\Delta t)$. With this notation understood, let us describe these three
finite-difference methods.

The forward-Euler method uses the most naive time discretization to
reduce the PDE from eq. 13.12 to a finite-difference equation

$$C \frac{V_i^{n+1} - V_i^n}{\Delta t} = \frac{a}{2R} \frac{V_{i+1}^n - 2V_i^n + V_{i-1}^n}{(\Delta x)^2} - \overline{g}V_i^n \tag{13.16}$$

If we define the constants $\lambda = a\Delta t/2RC(\Delta x)^2$ and $\gamma = \overline{g}\Delta t/C$, then
this equation can be rewritten as

$$V_i^{n+1} = \lambda V_{i+1}^n + (1 - 2\lambda - \gamma)V_i^n + \lambda V_{i-1}^n \tag{13.17}$$

It is well known that the error in using the forward-Euler method is
$O(\Delta t) + O((\Delta x)^2)$ (Isaacson and Keller 1966).

From eq. 13.17 we see that the forward-Euler method is an explicit
method, because V_i^{n+1} is explicitly defined by the right-hand-side terms,
only involving voltage values at the previous time level. Thus the
forward-Euler method is very easy to implement; however, it has numerical properties that are quite undesirable. The worst of these is the
fact that the forward-Euler method is known to be numerically unstable
for this and similar linear PDEs when $\lambda > 1/2$. Because the definition of λ involves the grid parameters Δt and Δx, the inequality that
must be satisfied for numerical stability, $\lambda \leq 1/2$, can be rewritten as

$\Delta t \leq RC(\Delta x)^2/a$. Thus, if we wish to achieve higher spatial accuracy in our numerical solution by decreasing Δx by a factor Q, we must also decrease Δt by a factor of Q^2 to assure that we maintain numerical stability. Thus the amount of computational work that must be done to obtain the numerical solution to the PDE up to a fixed time multiplied by Q^3 is due to a desire to achieve a factor Q-finer spatial grid. The factor Q^3 comes from having Q times as many spatial grid points and, because of the stability inequality, using a time step that is Q^2 times smaller.

As one might expect, the backward-Euler method for the solution of the PDE in eq. 13.12 is related to the forward-Euler method. If in eq. 13.16 the left-hand-side time difference is set equal to the right-hand side at time value $n + 1$ instead of time value n, we obtain the backward-Euler method

$$C\frac{V_i^{n+1} - V_i^n}{\Delta t} = \frac{a}{2R}\frac{V_{i+1}^{n+1} - 2V_i^{n+1} + V_{i-1}^{n+1}}{(\Delta x)^2} - \overline{g}V_i^{n+1} \qquad (13.18)$$

We can rewrite these equations as

$$-\lambda V_{i+1}^{n+1} + (1 + 2\lambda + \gamma)V_i^{n+1} - \lambda V_{i-1}^{n+1} = V_i^n \qquad (13.19)$$

Unlike eq. 13.17, this equation does not explicitly define the values at that new time step in terms of the values at the old time step. Thus the backward-Euler method is an implicit method, and a linear system of equations must be solved at each time step. The type of linear equation that must be solved is called a tridiagonal linear system, because the left-hand side of eq. 13.19 involves the unknown voltage and its two nearest neighbors on the grid. In a following section we will thoroughly discuss the numerical solution of tridiagonal linear systems of equations, with special emphasis on efficiency.

Even though the backward-Euler method involves the solution of a tridiagonal linear system at each time step, it is considered superior to the forward-Euler method for these types of PDE problems. A reason for this is that one can solve the tridiagonal system that arises at each time step in the backward-Euler method in an $O(N)$ arithmetic operation, which is the same order of complexity as for one time step of the forward-Euler method. More important, the backward-Euler method does not suffer from numerical instability for linear PDEs as does the forward-Euler method. Thus, we can choose the grid parameters Δt and Δx independently and not worry if some combination of these chosen values violates some stability inequality. Also, if the accuracy in one of the variables is insufficient, we may refine that variable without having to readjust the other grid parameter. One of the advantages of this independence in Δt and Δx for the backward-Euler method is the possibility of using a rather large Δt to explore qualitatively the behavior of a system at little computational expense. When interesting behavior is noted, a smaller Δt can be used to reexamine the phenomena of interest with greater numerical accuracy. Finally, we should note that the backward-Euler method has the same numerical accuracy as the forward-Euler method, namely $O(\Delta t) + O((\Delta x)^2)$.

The last method we present is called the Crank-Nicolson method (Crank and Nicolson 1947). The Crank-Nicolson method is related to both the forward- and backward-Euler method in that the right-hand side in the definition of the Crank-Nicolson method is the average of the two Euler right-hand sides

$$
C\frac{V_i^{n+1} - V_i^n}{\Delta t} = \frac{1}{2}\left(\frac{a}{2R}\frac{V_{i+1}^{n+1} - 2V_i^{n+1} + V_{i-1}^{n+1}}{(\Delta x)^2} - \overline{g}V_i^{n+1}\right.
$$
$$
\left. +\frac{a}{2R}\frac{V_{i+1}^n - 2V_i^n + V_{i-1}^n}{(\Delta x)^2} - \overline{g}V_i^n\right) \qquad (13.20)
$$

Unlike the two Euler methods, the Crank-Nicolson method has numerical accuracy that is $O((\Delta t)^2) + O((\Delta x)^2)$. This is due to the fact that setting the time difference equal to the average of the right-hand side at the old and new time levels is equivalent to using the trapezoidal rule of numerical integration to advance the time level, which is a second-order accurate method. Another way to think about this is that forward Euler approximates the time derivative with its value at the beginning of the time step, backward Euler at the end of the time step, and Crank-Nicolson at the midpoint. The two Euler methods are thus only first-order accurate in time, while the Crank-Nicolson method is second-order accurate.

Let us rearrange eq. 13.20 by placing the values at the old time level on the right and the values at the new time level on the left

$$
-\frac{\lambda}{2}V_{i+1}^{n+1} + (1 + \lambda + \frac{\gamma}{2})V_i^{n+1} - \frac{\lambda}{2}V_{i-1}^{n+1} = \qquad (13.21)
$$
$$
\frac{\lambda}{2}V_{i+1}^n + (1 - \lambda - \frac{\gamma}{2})V_i^n + \frac{\lambda}{2}V_{i-1}^n
$$

Here λ and γ are as previously defined. As with the backward-Euler method, this equation implicitly defines the new values as the solution to a tridiagonal system of linear equations. Also, like the backward-Euler method, this method is unconditionally stable in the sense that no numerical instability is encountered for any choice of the grid parameters Δt and Δx. One subtle difference between the backward-Euler method and the Crank-Nicolson method is that the Crank-Nicolson method is in a sense closer to numerical instability than backward Euler. This is observed in numerical solutions obtained via the Crank-Nicolson method in that they often show damped oscillations and over/undershoot where none would be expected when large values of λ are used. The backward-Euler method is much more heavily damping than Crank-Nicolson, so this so-called ringing is almost never observed in backward-Euler numerical solutions.

An interesting implementational detail exploits a useful relationship that exists between the solution to the backward-Euler and the Crank-Nicolson method. If V_i^{n+1} are the solution voltages to the backward-Euler equations (eq. 13.19) starting with voltages V_i^n, then $2V_i^{n+1} - V_i^n$ is the solution to the Crank-Nicolson equations starting with voltages V_i^n (Hines 1984). Thus it is a trivial task to modify a computer program for the solution of these PDEs from an $O(\Delta t)$ backward-Euler solver to an $O((\Delta t)^2)$ Crank-Nicolson solver by modifying a single line of code.

13.3.5   Numerical Boundary Conditions

Now that we have presented three different finite-difference methods for solving our PDE problems, we must comment on how the different BVPs that we have previously discussed may be incorporated into these methods. The Dirichlet-type boundary conditions are the simplest to handle, because they directly prescribe the boundary values. Thus in the forward-Euler method, we use the known end-point values V_0 and V_N in the equations for V_1^{n+1} and V_{N-1}^{n+1}. In the two implicit methods discussed, knowing V_0 and V_N allows us to reduce the number of equations to be solved to $N - 1$. We simply place the terms involving the known boundary values onto the right-hand sides of the equations for V_1^{n+1} and V_{N-1}^{n+1}, and solve the resulting tridiagonal system. For example, in the backward Euler case, the equation for V_1^{n+1} is $-\lambda V_2^{n+1} + (2\lambda + \gamma + 1)V_1^{n+1} - \lambda V_0^{n+1} = V_1^n$. Because V_0^{n+1} is known, we can rewrite this equation as $-\lambda V_2^{n+1} + (2\lambda+\gamma+1)V_1^{n+1} = \lambda V_0^{n+1} + V_1^n$, where everything that is known appears on the right-hand side. We can carry out the same procedure in the equation for V_{N-1}^{n+1}. A similar manipulation can be used to incorporate Dirichlet-type boundary conditions into the equations that result from the Crank-Nicolson method.

It is a bit more difficult to handle Neumann-type boundary conditions because they involve the spatial derivative of the dependent variable. In fact, we would like the manner in which we incorporate the Neumann-type boundary conditions into our finite-difference methods to preserve two properties of numerical methods we have introduced. First, because all of our numerical methods have a spatial accuracy of $O((\Delta x)^2)$, we ask that the boundary condition incorporation be at least this accurate. Second, we ask that the neat tridiagonal form of the linear equations that arise in the implicit methods be maintained. These two requirements are in a sense competing; however, it is possible to achieve both through a fairly elementary construction.

Let us consider the imposition of the Neumann-type boundary conditions from eq. 13.14 for the forward-Euler method. A second-order accurate finite-difference formula for the first derivative that only involves two points is the centered-difference approximation (Dahlquist and Bjorck 1974). If we wish to approximate the first derivative at $x = 0$ using the centered-difference formula, we need to know the value of V at $x = +\Delta x$ and at $x = -\Delta x$, but our computational grid does not include the point at $x = -\Delta x$. If we pretend to have access to V at this point we can include the Neumann boundary conditions into our methods and achieve both of the previous paragraphs' goals (Sod 1985; Cooley and Dodge 1966). If we know both V_1 and V_{-1}, then the centered-difference formula gives us $\frac{V_1 - V_{-1}}{2\Delta x} = \frac{\partial V(0)}{\partial x}$ up to $O((\Delta x)^2)$. Because the Neumann boundary condition specifies the value of $\frac{\partial V(0)}{\partial x}$, the previous expression can be used to express the unknown V_{-1} in terms of the known derivative value and V_1. Thus, the equation for V_0^{n+1} for the forward-Euler method can be rewritten using this new knowledge of the value of V_{-1}^n as

$$V_0^{n+1} = \lambda V_1^n + (1 - 2\lambda - \gamma)V_0^n + \lambda(V_1^n + 2\Delta x \frac{RI}{\pi a^2}) \qquad (13.22)$$

One can follow the same procedure with the equation for V_N^{n+1} with the forward-Euler method to incorporate the $x = L$ Neumann boundary condition into the finite-difference expressions.

Because the implicit methods require the solution of a tridiagonal system of linear equations, we can use this same centered-difference approximation of $\frac{\partial V}{\partial x}$ to incorporate the Neumann-type boundary conditions into the tridiagonal systems. Using the same rationale as above, we can solve for V_{-1}^{n+1} and V_{N+1}^{n+1} using the centered-difference approximation to reexpress the Neumann boundary conditions. We then substitute these expressions into the V_0 and V_N equations. Because we use the centered-difference approximation to the derivative, this construction maintains the tridiagonal structure of the linear equations to be solved at each time step. This is because we incorporate the centered-difference approximation only in equations at the two end points, and so the end points and their nearest neighbors are the only grid-point values that appear in the final equations. If we carry out the algebraic manipulations we have described, the system to be solved for the backward-Euler discretization of the IBVP for eq. 13.12 with Neumann boundary conditions (eqs. 13.14) ends up as

$$(1 + 2\lambda + \gamma)V_0^{n+1} - 2\lambda V_1^{n+1} = V_0^n + \frac{2RI\lambda\Delta x}{\pi a^2}$$

$$-\lambda V_{i+1}^{n+1} + (1 + 2\lambda + \gamma)V_i^{n+1} - \lambda V_{i-1}^{n+1} = V_i^n, \ 1 \le i \le N-1$$

$$-2\lambda V_{N-1}^{n+1} + (1 + 2\lambda + \gamma)V_N^{n+1} = V_N^n \qquad (13.23)$$

Whereas the same problem discretized via the Crank-Nicolson method is

$$(1 + \lambda + \frac{\gamma}{2})V_0^{n+1} - \lambda V_1^{n+1} = (1 - \lambda - \frac{\gamma}{2})V_0^n + \lambda V_1^n$$
$$+ \frac{2RI\lambda\Delta x}{\pi a^2}$$

$$-\frac{\lambda}{2}V_{i+1}^{n+1} + (1 + \lambda + \frac{\gamma}{2})V_i^{n+1} - \frac{\lambda}{2}V_{i-1}^{n+1} = \qquad (13.24)$$

$$\frac{\lambda}{2}V_{i+1}^n + (1 - \lambda - \frac{\gamma}{2})V_i^n + \frac{\lambda}{2}V_{i-1}^n \quad , \quad 1 \le i \le N-1$$

$$-\lambda V_{N-1}^{n+1} + (1 + \lambda + \frac{\gamma}{2})V_N^{n+1} = \lambda V_{N-1}^n + (1 - \lambda - \frac{\gamma}{2})V_N^n$$

Knowing how to incorporate both Dirichlet- and Neumann-type boundary conditions into our three PDE methods, it is relatively easy to combine these techniques to allow mixed-type boundary conditions as in eq. 13.15. Using the two extra grid points, V_{-1} and V_{N+1}, we can discretize eq. 13.15 up to $O((\Delta x)^2)$ as follows:

$$\alpha_0 \left(\frac{V_{-1} - V_1}{2\Delta x} \right) + V_0 = \beta_0, \quad \alpha_L \left(\frac{V_{N-1} - V_{N+1}}{2\Delta x} \right) + V_N = \beta_L \qquad (13.25)$$

We notice that both of these equations involve the grid's end points and their two neighboring points. As with our treatment of the Neumann-type boundary conditions, these equations can be solved for the values at

V_{-1} and V_{N+1}, and the resulting expressions substituted into the equations for V_0 and V_N. This is elementary for the forward-Euler method, and for the two implicit methods it is clear that a linear tridiagonal system of equations is again the final result. Thus the mixed-type boundary conditions lead to finite-difference equations of the same form as Neumann-type boundary conditions.

13.3.6   Spatial Variation

We recall that the Hodgkin-Huxley PDE model was presented for the giant axon of the squid *Loligo*. A basic assumption of this model is that the electronic properties of the squid's neuronal membrane are uniform and do not depend on the longitudinal location along the axon. Although this was a more than adequate assumption for this preparation, one should be able to incorporate spatial variation of the electronic properties in the neuronal membrane into our PDE models as well as into the numerical methods we use to solve them. We will now discuss how to express longitudinal variation in membrane properties in the linear-cable PDE system, as well as how to incorporate this spatial variation into the previously discussed finite-difference methods while preserving the $O((\Delta x)^2)$ spatial accuracy.

In the linear cable-model PDE, one can incorporate spatial variation in both the ionic conductance $\overline{g}$ and the membrane capacitance C in the most trivial way. Simply make them functions of x. The hard part is what to do when the dendritic radius a and the specific axoplasmic resistivity R are functions of x. One cannot make them functions of x in eq. 13.12, because that does not preserve the biophysical meaning of this equation. Equation 13.12 is a statement of the instantaneous conservation of charge along the membrane, and the term $(a/2R)\partial^2 V/\partial x^2$ represents the total membrane current per unit area. This expression was originally obtained by using current conservation for a small slice of dendrite and the differential form of Ohm's law. To see how to rewrite this term when a and R depend on x, we must go back to this derivation and see where the constant and spatially dependent cases differ.

The expression that appears in the two cable eqs. 13.3 and 13.12 for the total membrane current per unit area can be rewritten as

$$\frac{a}{2R}\frac{\partial^2 V}{\partial x^2} = \frac{1}{2\pi a}\frac{\partial}{\partial x}\left(\frac{\pi a^2}{R}\frac{\partial V}{\partial x}\right) \tag{13.26}$$

The term in parentheses is the axial current, and eq. 13.26 means that the divergence of the axial current equals the membrane current. Strictly speaking,   the   total   membrane   current   is   given   by

$I_m = -1/(2\pi a)\partial I_a/\partial x(ds/dx)^{-1}$, where I_a is the axial current and ds/dx is the derivative of the surface area of the membrane as a function of longitudinal distance (Jack, Nobel, and Tsien 1975). However, in most physiological situations $(ds/dx)^{-1}$ is very close to one, and so eq. 13.26 is a very good approximation. The constants in the expression for the total membrane current are to convert the axial current, which is per unit cross-sectional area, into a current per unit membrane area. Using eq. 13.26, we can rewrite the linear cable equation, eq. 13.12, to allow spatial variation in all the cable parameters:

$$C(x)\,\frac{\partial V}{\partial t} = \frac{1}{2\pi a(x)}\frac{\partial}{\partial x}\left(\frac{\pi a^2(x)}{R(x)}\frac{\partial V}{\partial x}\right) - \overline{g}(x)V \qquad (13.27)$$

One performs the analogous substitution with the Hodgkin-Huxley PDE model, eqs. 13.2 and 13.3, to incorporate spatial variation in that case.

Now that we understand how to incorporate spatial variation into neuronal PDE models, we must consider how to take these continuous models and convert them to finite-difference equations with the same level of accuracy that we obtained with constant-coefficient equations. In eq. 13.27, spatial dependence is only problematic when we try to discretize the term for the total membrane current per unit area. This term involves the derivative of a derivative, and so we proceed by discretizing the derivatives one at a time. A first-order approximation to the first derivative is $\partial V/\partial x = (V_{i+1} - V_i)/\Delta x$. Applying this expression twice to the total membrane current term in eq. 13.27 gives us

$$\frac{1}{2\pi a(x)}\frac{\partial}{\partial x}\left(\frac{\pi a^2(x)}{R(x)}\frac{\partial V}{\partial x}\right) \approx \frac{1}{2\pi a_i}\frac{\left(\frac{\pi a^2_{i+1/2}}{R_{i+1/2}}\left(\frac{V_{i+1}-V_i}{\Delta x}\right) - \frac{\pi a^2_{i-1/2}}{R_{i-1/2}}\left(\frac{V_i-V_{i-1}}{\Delta x}\right)\right)}{\Delta x}$$

$$(13.28)$$

The value at grid-point index $i + 1/2$ refers to the numerical value of the indexed function at $x + \Delta x/2$, as $i - 1/2$ refers to $x - \Delta x/2$. Even though the spatial grid does not include these points, it is reasonable to ask for the value of the continuously defined variables $a(x)$ and $R(x)$ at these points. However, if these intermediate values are not available, one can substitute the average of the values at the two flanking grid points in this discretization.

The spatial discretization of the troublesome second-derivative term for the total membrane current given in eq. 13.28 can be shown to yield an $O((\Delta x)^2)$ accurate finite-difference approximation (Cooley and Dodge 1966). Thus one can use this discretization in eq. 13.27 to solve this spatially dependent problem with one of the finite-difference methods we have already described, that is, the forward- and backward-Euler methods and the Crank-Nicolson method, with the same numerical accuracy. These discretizations lead to the same types of equations as in the constant coefficient case. One can incorporate boundary conditions exactly as in the constant coefficient case, so we can think of these spatially dependent coefficient problems as being no more complicated than their constant-coefficient counterparts. Even so, we have yet to describe the solution of tridiagonal linear systems that arise in all our implicit discretizations.

13.3.7 Solving Tridiagonal Linear Systems

We will discuss only one algorithm for the solution of tridiagonal linear systems of equations—Gaussian elimination. Gaussian elimination is also called LU decomposition, as well as forward elimination with back substitution. Gaussian elimination requires $O(M)$ mathematical operations to solve a tridiagonal system with M unknowns. Gaussian elimination has many variants that are specialized for efficiency on specific classes of matrices (Golub and Van Loan 1985). Because all the tridiagonal systems that arise in finite-difference solutions of the PDEs we have discussed share a property called diagonal dominance, we can use the simplest variant of Gaussian elimination that does not involve pivoting to solve these systems.

To say that a matrix is diagonally dominant means that the magnitude of the diagonal dominates the sum of the magnitudes of the off-diagonal elements in each row of the matrix. It is evident from eqs. 13.19 and 13.21 that for the finite-difference PDE approximations we have discussed, the tridiagonal systems that arise are diagonally dominant. In general, finite-difference approximations to well-posed parabolic PDEs will be diagonally dominant. Let us denote our tridiagonal system as

$$L_i V_{i-1} + D_i V_i + U_i V_{i+1} = R_i, \quad 1 \leq i \leq M \tag{13.29}$$

Because the above system is tridiagonal, we have $L_1 = U_M = 0$. Because the system in eq. 13.29 is diagonally dominant, we many proceed with normal Gaussian elimination without pivoting and stably obtain the desired solution (Isaacson and Keller 1966).

The Gaussian elimination algorithm without pivoting proceeds by using adjacent equations in eq. 13.29 to eliminate the subdiagonal unknowns in a step known as forward elimination. One may think of this procedure as sweeping through the equations and redefining the constants L_i, D_i, U_i, and R_i as follows:

$$
\begin{aligned}
D_1 &= D_1, U_1 = U_1/D_1, R_1 = R_1/D_1 \\
D_i &= D_i - L_i U_{i-1}, \quad i = 2, 3, \ldots, M \\
R_i &= (R_i - L_i R_{i-1})/D_i, \quad i = 2, 3, \ldots, M \\
U_i &= U_i/D_i, \quad i = 2, 3, \ldots, M - 1
\end{aligned}
\tag{13.30}
$$

This forward elimination procedure succeeds in reducing the original tridiagonal system into an equivalent bidiagonal system. This bidiagonal system can then be solved by a procedure called backward substitution. We sweep backward through the equations to compute the solution as follows:

$$
\begin{aligned}
V_M &= R_M, \\
V_i &= R_i - U_i V_{i+1}, \quad i = M - 1, M - 2, \ldots, 1
\end{aligned}
\tag{13.31}
$$

We notice that this procedure requires only five arrays of length M, namely, arrays for L, D, U, R, and V. Because we overwrite these arrays in the two-step procedure, the coefficients for the tridiagonal systems that arise in our finite-difference solution must be recomputed each time step. In addition, it is obvious from the definition of the algorithm that this procedure requires $O(M)$ arithmetic operations, as it is defined with several "loops," each with a fixed number of arithmetic operations per iteration and of length no more than M.

13.3.8   Branching

Many of the models we use for individual neurons incorporate anatomical data that lead to PDE models of neuronal cables with branching. We will consider two numerical procedures for solving PDE neuronal models with branching. Both assume that we employ an implicit finite-difference method to the PDEs, so we will really be considering how to solve the tridiagonal-like linear systems that arise from these discretizations. The first method we consider uses a careful numbering of the unknowns on the branching structure to reduce the resulting linear system to what is essentially a single tridiagonal system. The second method uses the technique of domain decomposition to reduce the solution of the single system of equations on the entire branched structure to the solution of many systems of equations each on only a single branch.

Hines (1984) describes an enumeration of the grid points in a branching cable structure that leads to a direct solution of the resulting finite-difference equations that is equivalent to Gaussian elimination without pivoting. Let us describe this enumeration with an example. In fig. 13.1 we have a diagram of a neuronal structure with six branches. We first choose a branch that is connected at only one end and designate this as the "trunk." This trunk will be the highest numbered branch; in our example that is branch 6. The grid points in the trunk are ordered from the branch point towards the free end. We next number the branches that connect to the trunk. Those that are only connected to the trunk receive the largest numbers, and those with two connections are numbered lowest. The grid points in each numbered branch are ordered toward the trunk. Now we designate all branches connected at both ends as new trunks and continue the branch and grid point enumeration recursively.

We have now explained a systematic numbering of unknowns for a branched neuronal structure, and we understand the linear system that arises. Let us discuss the method of solution of this linear system. We can carry out forward elimination on this nearly tridiagonal system without any extra complications provided we eliminate the unknowns in order within the branches and take the branches in a particular order. We start with the first numbered branch and forward eliminate all the unknowns on it. We then forward eliminate all the other branches connected to the first branch's trunk branch; elimination proceeds in the numerical order of the unknowns. We then go to the far end of the trunk and eliminate all the unknowns in the nontrunk branches connected to it via a branch point. Then the trunk unknowns are eliminated in order. This procedure continues recursively with respect to the branches. Forward elimination in the branching case is exactly the same as in the nonbranching case except that we must also eliminate all the off-diagonal elements associated with the several nearest neighbor grid points at a branch point. The order of elimination on the branches is important, because it assures that no new off-diagonal elements are created in the Gaussian elimination. This allows us to store the almost tridiagonal linear system in a statically defined set of three length-M arrays as in the nonbranching case. Thus in our example we would eliminate the unknowns in order on the branches in the following branch order: 1,2,4,5,3,6.

We then proceed to back-substitution, marching backward through the unknowns along the branches. The order of the branches in back-substitution is almost the reverse of their order in forward elimination except that the order of nontrunk nodes is maintained. In our example this means the order for back substitution is 6,3,4,5,1,2. As in forward elimination, we must take into account the nearest neighbors of the branch points. Because this method is a mere reworking of Gaussian

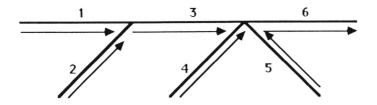

This enumeration yields the following linear equation:

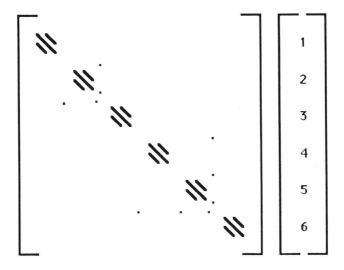

Figure 13.1
Example of branch- and grid-point numbering of a branched neuronal structure
and the resulting linear equation structure that arises with nearest-neighbor finite-
difference discretization. After Hines (1984).

elimination without pivoting, it is obvious that $O(M)$ arithmetic operations are required to solve a branched structure with M grid points.

The second approach to branching is to solve small tridiagonal systems on the individual branches and form the solution on the entire branching structure out of a linear combination of these local solutions. This technique is known generally as domain decomposition, which is the solution of a problem on one domain by solving smaller problems on subdomains and then building up the whole solution from the smaller parts. Because we are solving a linear equation, we can exploit linear superposition. The simplest example of domain decomposition for a branching one-dimensional structure is illustrated in fig. 13.2. Here we take a single cable and assume that an interior grid point is in fact a branch point. If we assume the value of the solution at the branch point V_{Br} is zero, we can solve the tridiagonal systems for the voltages on both branches. We call these solutions $\vec{V}_l^0$ and $\vec{V}_r^0$ for left and right. In general the value at the branch point will not be zero. To take this into account, call $\vec{V}_l^1$ and $\vec{V}_r^1$ the solutions to the tridiagonal systems on each branch with the right-hand side zero except for the contribution from $V_{Br} = 1$. By the principle of superposition, the solution on the left branch is $\vec{V}_l^0 + V_{Br}\vec{V}_l^1$, whereas $\vec{V}_r^0 + V_{Br}\vec{V}_r^1$ gives the solution on the right, where V_{Br} is still unknown. The single equation for V_{Br} involves the nearest neighbors on the left and right branch and so gives us a single equation for V_{Br}. This then gives us the value for V_{Br} that is used to give us the complete solution on each branch via superposition.

In case a branch point is connected to more than two branches, the above procedure still produces the solution on each branch. The only complication is when we have a branch connected at both ends. In this case the solution is a linear combination of three tridiagonal solutions: the solution to the tridiagonal system with a normal right-hand side but with both branch end points is zero; the solution with a zero right-hand side with one branch end point is one. Thus we can use this domain decomposition method to solve the equations on any branching structure. Because we only solve at most three tridiagonal systems per branch to obtain the overall solution, the arithmetic complexity for a structure with M unknowns is still only $O(M)$.

13.3.9   Nonlinear Equations

Up to now we have only considered finite-difference methods for linear PDE models of neuronal activity. As we know, many of the most interesting PDE models in neuroscience are highly nonlinear. The classic example is the PDE model of Hodgkin and Huxley for the giant axon of

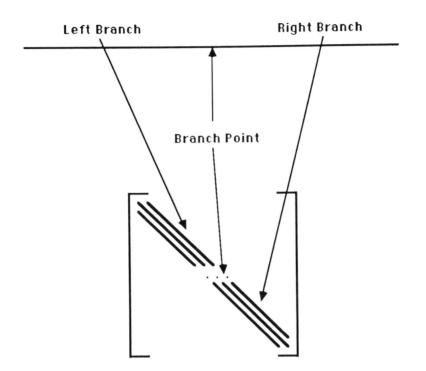

Figure 13.2
An example of domain decomposition for a branching one-dimensional structure using the simplest geometry: Solving a single cable by superimposing right and left branch solutions. We show the geometry and the resulting tridiagonal system.

the squid *Loligo* (eqs. 13.2 and 13.3). We have studied extensively finite-difference methods for the linear cable PDE model (eq. 13.12), and it is possible to incorporate nonlinearities of the Hodgkin-Huxley type into the methods we have already introduced for this linear analog.

It is a trivial matter to use the forward-Euler method on the Hodgkin-Huxley equations. One need only evaluate the nonlinear currents at the old time-step value to do so. This involves the computation of the dimensionless variables at the old time value. The forward-Euler equation for m_i^{n+1} is simply

$$
\begin{aligned}
m_i^{n+1} &= m_i^n + \Delta t \big[(1 - m_i^n)\alpha_m(V_i^n) - m_i^n \beta_m(V_i^n)\big] \qquad (13.32) \\
&= m_i^n \big[1 - \Delta t(\alpha_m(V_i^n) + \beta_m(V_i^n))\big] + \Delta t \alpha_m(V_i^n)
\end{aligned}
$$

The expressions for h_i^{n+1} and n_i^{n+1} are analogous. The finite difference equation for the voltage via the forward-Euler method is then

$$
V_i^{n+1} = \lambda(V_{i+1}^n + V_{i-1}^n) + (1 - 2\lambda - \gamma_i^n)V_i^n + \omega_i^n \qquad (13.33)
$$

Here $\lambda = a\Delta t/2RC(\Delta x)^2$, $\gamma_i^n = (\Delta t/C)\big(\bar{g}_{Na}(m_i^n)^3 h_i^n + \bar{g}_K(n_i^n)^4 + \bar{g}_{leak}\big)$, and $\omega_i^n = (\Delta t/C)\big(\bar{g}_{Na}(m_i^n)^3 h_i^n E_{Na} + \bar{g}_K(n_i^n)^4 E_K + \bar{g}_{leak}E_{leak}\big)$.

Generalizing the two implicit methods we have discussed to nonlinear equations raises much more complicated issues. Because implicit methods require the solution of equations when applied to nonlinear PDEs, nonlinear difference equations arise. The Hodgkin-Huxley equations have a property which considerably simplifies solving these equations, namely that the Hodgkin-Huxley equations are what we will call conditionally linear. Here conditionally linear means that the PDE for the voltage (eq. 13.3) is a linear PDE if the values of the dimensionless variables are known. Similarly, the rate equations for the dimensionless variables (eqs. 13.2) are linear ODEs given the values of V. It is important to point out that this is a fairly generic property of nonlinear neuronal models. The nonlinearities in eq. 13.3 are associated with the nonlinear ionic currents. These nonlinear currents are modeled as the product of a nonlinear ionic conductance and the difference between the membrane potential and the ionic reversal potential. Because the nonlinear ionic conductances are not direct functions of voltage, eq. 13.3 is conditionally linear. Therefore, if we can model our nonlinear ionic currents as the products of the difference between the membrane voltage and the ionic reversal potential and nonlinear ionic conductances that are not direct functions of the membrane conductance, we will have nonlinear PDE models of neurons that are conditionally linear.

What are the computational benefits of conditional linearity? Simply stated, the benefits are the separation of the complicated nonlinear problem into two simpler linear problems. This is expressed in different ways for the backward-Euler and Crank-Nicolson methods. For the backward-Euler method, we will use this separability to give us an algorithm for the iterative solution of the nonlinear-difference equations for each time step, whereas with the Crank-Nicolson method, we will use separability to reduce the nonlinear equations to a single set of linear equations to be solved at each time step.

If we use the backward-Euler method to discretize the Hodgkin-Huxley PDE (eq. 13.3), we arrive at the following system of nonlinear equations:

$$- \lambda V_{i+1}^{n+1} + (1 + 2\lambda + \gamma_i^{n+1})V_i^{n+1} - \lambda V_{i-1}^{n+1} = V_i^n + \omega_i^{n+1} \qquad (13.34)$$

Here the definition of γ_i and ω_i is the same as the above definitions with regard to the forward-Euler method. As opposed to eq. 13.33, these nonlinear-difference equations must be solved for the values of V^{n+1}. To make matters worse, if we use the backward-Euler discretization on the dimensionless variables as well, then eq. 13.34 must be solved in conjunction with the nonlinear-difference equations that arise from this discretization of the dimensionless variables. The equations that arise for m in this situation are

$$m_i^{n+1} = m_i^n + \Delta t\left[(1 - m_i^{n+1})\alpha_m(V_i^{n+1}) - m_i^{n+1}\beta_m(V_i^{n+1})\right] \quad \text{or}$$

$$m_i^{n+1} = \frac{m_i^n}{1 + \Delta t[\alpha_m(V_i^{n+1}) + \beta_m(V_i^{n+1})]} + \qquad (13.35)$$

$$\frac{\Delta t\alpha_m(V_i^{n+1})}{1 + \Delta t[\alpha_m(V_i^{n+1}) + \beta_m(V_i^{n+1})]}$$

The backward-Euler finite-difference equations for h and n are identical in form to eq. 13.35.

The backward-Euler method for the Hodgkin-Huxley system requires the simultaneous solution of eq. 13.34 and three equations of the form of eq. 13.35, one for each of the dimensionless variables, at each time step. The solution of this system of equations is considerably simplified because, as we have already mentioned, the Hodgkin-Huxley PDE system has the property of being conditionally linear. Thus we can hope to solve these nonlinear equations with the following iterative algorithm: (1) Solve eq. 13.34 with the previously known dimensionless-variable values to give new voltage values. (2) Solve the dimensionless-variable equations (eq. 13.35, etc.) using the new voltage values to give new

dimensionless-variable values. (3) Repeat steps 1 and 2 until voltage-
and dimensionless-variable values have converged. The starting values
for this iterative procedure are the values of the unknowns at the previous time step. Because these equations are conditionally separable,
the equations to be solved in steps 1 and 2 will always be linear. The
voltage equations will be a single linear tridiagonal system, and the
equations for the dimensionless variables are reduced to explicit expressions for the new values. This iterative procedure is sometimes called
a Picard, fixed-point, or functional iteration. For the backward-Euler
method applied to the Hodgkin-Huxley equations, this iteration method
has been proved to converge provided that Δt is chosen sufficiently small
(Mascagni 1987a), so this method is a reasonable choice for the solution
of the Hodgkin-Huxley and related equations.

As with the backward-Euler method, the Crank-Nicolson method applied to the Hodgkin-Huxley equations leads to nonlinear equations:

$$-\frac{\lambda}{2}V_{i+1}^{n+1} + (1 + \lambda + \frac{\gamma_i^{n+1}}{2})V_i^{n+1} - \frac{\lambda}{2}V_{i-1}^{n+1} = \qquad (13.36)$$

$$\frac{\lambda}{2}V_{i+1}^n + (1 - \lambda - \frac{\gamma_i^n}{2})V_i^n + \frac{\lambda}{2}V_{i-1}^n + \frac{\omega_i^{n+1} + \omega_i^n}{2}$$

These must be solved concurrently with the difference equations for the
dimensionless variables. If we wish to maintain an overall accuracy of
$O((\Delta t)^2)$, we must use a method of at least second-order accuracy for the
rate equations. The trapezoidal rule is second-order accurate and is the
ODE analog of the Crank-Nicolson method. Applying the trapezoidal
rule to the equation for m gives us

$$m_i^{n+1} = m_i^n + \Delta t[((1 - \frac{m_i^{n+1} + m_i^n}{2})\alpha_m(V_i^{n+1/2})$$

$$-\frac{m_i^{n+1} + m_i^n}{2}\beta_m(V_i^{n+1/2})] \quad \text{or}$$

$$m_i^{n+1} = m_i^n \frac{1 - \Delta t/2[\alpha_m(V_i^{n+1/2}) + \beta_m(V_i^{n+1/2})]}{1 + \Delta t/2[\alpha_m(V_i^{n+1/2}) + \beta_m(V_i^{n+1/2})]} \qquad (13.37)$$

$$+\frac{\Delta t\alpha_m(V_i^{n+1/2})}{1 + \Delta t/2[\alpha_m(V_i^{n+1/2}) + \beta_m(V_i^{n+1/2})]}$$

We have used the values $V_i^{n+1/2}$ in the above expression to simplify the
form of these difference equations while maintaining the desired second-
order accuracy. One can use the average of the voltage at the nth and

$n + 1$st time step to estimate the value at time value $n + 1/2$, or one may use another method, which we will discuss below.

As with the backward-Euler method, eqs. 13.36 and 13.37 and the analogous equations for h and n are a complicated set of simultaneous nonlinear equations. The fact that these equations are conditionally linear can be exploited as with the backward-Euler method to give us an iterative algorithm for their simultaneous solution. There is no rigorous proof for the convergence of this method for the Crank-Nicolson method, but the author believes that the techniques used in the proof of the backward-Euler case can be easily extended to this case. Another approach to these equations, which exploits their conditional linearity and results in no iteration, is to use an implementational detail we have previously mentioned and the second-order accuracy of the midpoint method of numerical integration.

Recall that if one is solving the linear cable equation (eq. 13.12) with the backward-Euler method, then $2V^{n+1} - V^n$, where V^{n+1} is the backward-Euler solution, is a second-order accurate solution. If one uses eq. 13.34 with ω_i^{n+1} replaced with $\omega_i^{n+1/2}$, then $2V^{n+1} - V^n$ gives us a second-order accurate solution to the Hodgkin-Huxley equations. Note that the definition of ω_i^n depends on the time level n only through the dimensionless variables. Thus we need only compute the values $m_i^{n+1/2}$, $h_i^{n+1/2}$, and $n_i^{n+1/2}$ to obtain $\omega_i^{n+1/2}$. This procedure requires values of the dimensionless variables at the midpoints between the usual time levels complementary to the expression for the second-order solution of the dimensionless variables (eq. 13.37) that requires the midpoint values of the voltage. If one were to solve the dimensionless-variable equations at only the midpoint values, and the voltage values at the usual values, then the requirements of the previous sentence would be automatically satisfied. The voltage equations would have access to the dimensionless variables at the time-step midpoints and the dimensionless variables would have access to the voltage values at their time-step midpoints. This staggering of two time grids also simplifies the solution of the difference equations. Because the Hodgkin-Huxley equations are conditionally linear, this grid staggering leads to solving a single tridiagonal system for the voltage equation and evaluating the explicit equations for the dimensionless variables a single time to advance the solution Δt. Thus we maintain second-order accuracy via the midpoint evaluation of terms in each equation and reduce the problem to a linear one via conditional linearity.

The one complication that must be dealt with to reap the benefits of this simplification is the computation of the unknowns on two $\Delta t/2$ staggered time grids. One can accomplish this by starting either the voltage- or dimensionless-variable equations with a $\Delta t/2$-sized time step and then proceeding as normal. A more elegant method for the IVBP, when the initial condition is also the steady-state solution, is to do nothing. This is because at the steady-state nothing is changing, and so if we advance the voltage equation by $\Delta t/2$, we get the same values. Thus from the steady-state initial condition, we can pretend that we have advanced the voltage one-half time step and proceed as normal from that point.

With the backward-Euler and Crank-Nicolson discretizations of the Hodgkin-Huxley equations, we have shown two different ways in which conditional linearity can be exploited to simplify the numerical solution of these nonlinear systems. We should note that the iterative solution method described for the backward-Euler method can be used to solve the nonlinear equations we get with the Crank-Nicolson discretization. In fact, this method was used by Cooley and Dodge (Cooley and Dodge 1966) in a predictor-corrector variant of the method we described to do the first systematic numerical solution of the Hodgkin-Huxley equations. Similarly, one can use the staggering method we presented for the Crank-Nicolson method with the backward-Euler equations; however, because the Crank-Nicolson method had to stagger the voltage- and dimensionless-variable time grids to maintain $O((\Delta t)^2)$ accuracy via the midpoint rule, no such staggering is required with the $O(\Delta t)$ backward-Euler method. Thus the minor complication of the staggered grids for Crank-Nicolson disappears if we are happy with using backward Euler.

Experience in the computation of solutions to the Hodgkin-Huxley PDEs has shown that a majority of the computational time is spent in the evaluation of the α and β rate functions associated with the dimensionless variables. Because of this fact, it is considered prudent to use a look-up table to speed up the repeated evaluation of these functions. If one examines the equations for the advancement of the dimensionless variables (eqs. 13.32, 13.35, and 13.37), one will notice that they are all of the form $m^{n+1} = m^n K_1(V, \Delta t) + K_2(V, \Delta t)$. Thus we need only evaluate the two functions K_1 and K_2 for each dimensionless variable at each time step. The functions K_1 and K_2, which involve combinations of the α and β functions as well as Δt, can be tabulated for the purpose of speed. If one does not plan to change the time-step size Δt during a computation, the functions K_1 and K_2 can be tabulated once for all during the initialization of the computation.

It is most convenient to construct the look-up table over a wide range of possible voltage values using a uniform voltage increment. Experience has shown that the voltage range of -100 millivolts to 150 millivolts with a step of 0.1 millivolt will give sufficient accuracy for the Hodgkin-Huxley equations. If the storage of $6 \times 2{,}500 = 15{,}000$ floating point values for these look-up tables is too large for a particular computer system, one can use an interpolation method to achieve similar accuracy with a smaller table. If one uses a piecewise linear interpolation scheme, a step of 1.0 millivolt is normally sufficient for the purpose of accuracy. With piecewise quadratic interpolation, experience has shown that a step as large as 4.0 millivolts can be used with no degradation in the overall accuracy. Interpolation with equally spaced points in a look-up table is handled quite well in Conte and de Boor (1980).

Unlike linear PDEs, there is no neat Lax equivalence theorem for solving nonlinear PDEs via finite-difference methods. The analysis of finite-difference methods for these nonlinear problems must instead proceed with a case-by-case approach. Fortunately, convergence of the backward-Euler method for the Hodgkin-Huxley equations has been proved (Mascagni 1987a). In addition, there is a considerable body of results on the convergence of the Crank-Nicolson method for many classes of nonlinear parabolic PDEs (Douglass 1956, 1958; Lees 1959; Rose 1956). I believe that, although not proved, the Hodgkin-Huxley equations can be analyzed with similar techniques that will provide for the rigorous convergence of the Crank-Nicolson method. It appears that for both the backward-Euler and Crank-Nicolson methods, no relationship between Δt and Δx must hold for stability; however, it is known for the backward-Euler method and likewise conjectured for the Crank-Nicolson method that convergence occurs for all values of Δt smaller than a certain maximal value (Mascagni 1987a).

In deciding on one of these methods over another, considerations similar to those discussed for choosing finite-difference methods for linear PDEs arise. In general, it takes no more computational work to use an implicit method over an explicit method, so one should use either the backward-Euler or Crank-Nicolson method. The backward-Euler method with iteration has been used with great success for investigating certain problems (Mascagni 1987b), and the observed solutions remain qualitatively correct for rather large values of Δt. The Crank-Nicolson method without iteration was first described in its entirety by Hines (1984). This method has also been used with great success for certain computations (Mascagni 1989b). I have observed that with the Crank-Nicolson method, one cannot use values of Δt as large as with the backward-Euler method due to numerical instabilities. The Crank-Nicolson method is second-order accurate in time, so in circumstances where using a large Δt is necessary and one is willing to sacrifice quantitative accuracy, the backward-Euler method is preferable to the Crank-Nicolson method. However, when accuracy is vital, it is recommended that the second-order accurate method be used, taking care to use Δt small enough to prevent ringing-type numerical instabilities from contaminating the computation.

13.3.10 Networks

Synthesizing the results of the previous six sections gives us the ability to numerically simulate a single arbitrarily branched neuronal model with spatial variation and nonlinear ionic kinetics. This is already a significant capability, however with new developments in computer technology (see chapter 12), it is possible to solve problems of much greater complexity than merely a single neuron. The new technical capabilities provide us with the opportunity to model several hundred very complicated neurons that are synaptically connected to one another. The neuronal modeler should bear these new developments in mind when considering what types of questions to ask and what type of models to build.

The key to modeling a network of neurons is the selection of a model for synaptic conduction that is both biophysically satisfying and is compatible with the finite-difference approach for the numerical solution of the nerve equations. To a large extent this is a matter of personal taste. A general guideline for this selection is that a deterministic model of synaptic conduction is most easily incorporated into a numerical scheme involving finite-difference approximations to nerve equations. For example, such a model might be the initiation of a characteristic postsynaptic conduction change in response to the presynaptic arrival of an action potential. This could be further embellished with a stochastic determination of the shape of the elicited postsynaptic conductance change. The types of models of this general form that cause numerical and implementational difficulties are those in which the repertoire of possible postsynaptic conductance time courses is large. In a computation that has many interacting neuronal elements, the accurate determination of the postsynaptic membrane potential requires the summation over the recent synaptic events. If there are potentially many varied forms in which these synaptic events affect the postsynaptic potential, a considerable amount of computer memory must be used to implement the complicated bookkeeping task underlying the determination of the postsynaptic membrane potential. In a network of p neurons that are totally interconnected, $O(p^2)$ contributions to the postsynaptic potentials must be calculated at each time step. This quadratic scaling with the number of neurons quickly dominates the memory requirements of the computation, and it does so even more quickly when a considerable amount of memory is required to store a single postsynaptic event.

13.4   Computing With Neural Networks

The previous sections have dealt with aspects of numerical computation related to ODE and PDE models in neurobiology. Needless to say, there are a myriad of alternative models for individual neurons that emphasize different aspects of neuronal biophysics. The models are based on the idea of perceptrons, where individual neurons are replaced with interconnected computational elements whose output is a function of the weighted sum of the inputs, and serve as a point of departure for a large class of models that have become particularly popular. The input and output values of these perceptron models are continuously varying quantities whose magnitude is a measure of the activity of the model neuron, much as the instantaneous firing rate might measure the activity of a PDE-modeled neuron. These models do not have any time dynamics, as the output of each unit is an instantaneous function of a linear combination of the instantaneous inputs. Given a set of inputs, there is a unique, explicitly defined output. If the network is a feedforward, multilayered ensemble of these kinds of neuronal models, computing the state of one of these networks is simply an elaborate function evaluation.

A slight complication arises when the network contains feedback as well as feedforward connections. Then instead of being a system where the state can be explicitly computed, the state is only implicitly defined. In fact, the determination of the state of the network is the solution to a system of nonlinear equations. There are several approaches one can take. The simplest approach is to try to find an iterative way to evaluate the output of the units in the hope that the solution to the equations can be approached asymptotically. This amounts to ordering the neural elements in the network and using this ordering to evaluate the output of the elements. One uses the previous iteration values as the input values to the new iteration. One continues this procedure, sweeping through the elements in the hopes that the solution to the nonlinear equations is approached. At best this method is *ad hoc*, yet it is of the same type as the iterative procedures discussed in the context of solving the difference equations associated with implicit discretization of nonlinear PDE models. A more systematic approach is to use a well-known root-solving technique on the nonlinear equations themselves. Once the network is expressed as a system of nonlinear equations, one can use the multi-dimensional Newton's method (Stoer and Bulirsch 1980) to obtain the solution, provided one can compute the first derivative of the nonlinear input/output function. This procedure is more systematic than setting up the iteration method, but is more computationally intensive. If an iterative method can be found, it will most likely be more efficient than Newton's method.

A further complication is when the input/output properties of the neuronal elements incorporate temporal properties as in a simple integrate-and-fire model. Here the output is not an instantaneous function of the inputs but is some weighted sum over the recent past of the inputs, like a convolution. If we call $i(t)$ the input signal, $o(t)$ the output signal, and $m(t)$ the weighting or memory function, then a convolution has the following input/output relationship:

$$o(t) = \int_{-\infty}^{t} i(\tau)m(t-\tau)d\tau \qquad (13.38)$$

This would seem to complicate things substantially; however, if $m(t) = e^{-Kt}$, then this convolution can be reexpressed as a first-order differential equation for $o(t)$,

$$\frac{do(t)}{dt} = i(t) - Ko(t) \qquad (13.39)$$

Thus this type of integrate-and-fire network reduces to a system of coupled first-order ODEs. We have discussed the methods of numerical solution for these systems. We can use high-order numerical methods for the numerical solution, and if we encounter stiffness, we know how to deal numerically with this too. If $m(t)$ is not an exponential function, then, depending on its particular form, it may be possible to convert eq. 13.38 for the given $m(t)$ into a simple and equivalent ODE. This example further emphasizes a major theme of this chapter, namely, the importance and ubiquity of differential equation models in neurobiology.

Last we mention using neuronal elements that are connected to one another with delay lines. Delay lines are simple models for time delays associated with action potential transmission. Here the input/output response of the neuronal elements is a function of certain events that have occurred in the past. There are two general approaches to computing solutions to delay models, the discrete- and continuous-time methods. In the discrete-time approach a Δt is chosen small enough to resolve temporal phenomena of interest, and the equations are advanced Δt at a time. At each time step, one must include the effects of delayed events by maintaining a list of times when delayed events will manifest themselves. If one maintains a master event list, then one can eliminate the use of Δt because one can jump from event to event on the master list without the requirement of a temporal grid. This is the continuous-time method. Between events the network is static, so it is either a network that can be explicitly resolved or a network that requires the solution of nonlinear equations for its resolution. We have discussed these two possibilities briefly above.

This work was supported by a National Institutes of Health/National Research Council Research Associateship grant. Michael V. Mascagni's address is Mathematical Research Branch, N.I.D.D.K., N.I.H., Building 31, Room 4B-54, Bethesda, Maryland 20892. His e-mail address is na.mascagni@na-net.stanford.edu.

Appendix 13.A: Stiffness

Let us consider the PDE model of the squid axon (eqs. 13.2 and 13.3) to illustrate the method of lines and their relationship to compartmental models. In eq. 13.3, the right-hand side has a term involving a second spatial derivative. If we replace the continuous x-axis with a uniform grid of width Δx and replace the term $\partial^2 V/\partial x^2$ with the familiar $O((\Delta x)^2)$ finite-difference approximation $(V_{i+1} - 2V_i + V_{i-1})/(\Delta x)^2$, the PDE is reduced to a system of coupled ODEs. This is the method of lines, where a single PDE is reduced to a system of ODEs by discretizing all but one of the independent variables in the PDE. The resulting method of lines ODE system for the Hodgkin-Huxley PDE model is stiff. This fact is well known from results for the method of lines for the PDE that describes diffusion, $\partial V/\partial t = \partial^2 V/\partial x^2$, which displays the same qualitative stiffness properties.

A compartmental model that uses individual ODE models for each compartment, and where neighboring compartments are resistively coupled, is equivalent to a method of lines discretization of some PDE model. This is easily seen by observing that we can rewrite our difference formula for the second derivative as $((V_{i+1} - V_i)/\Delta x - (V_i - V_{i-1})/\Delta x)/\Delta x$. Now assume that the spatial discretization is no longer uniform. If the distance between grid point $i+1$ and i is denoted by Δx_1, and the distance between grid point i and $i-1$ is called Δx_2, then the second-order accurate approximation to the second derivative on this nonuniform grid is given as $((V_{i+1} - V_i)/\Delta x_1 - (V_i - V_{i-1})/\Delta x_2)/((\Delta x_1 + \Delta x_2)/2)$. This can be rewritten as $LV_{i-1} + DV_1 + UV_{i+1}$, where L, D, and U are constants. This is exactly the form that one encounters in nearest-neighbor, resistively coupled, compartmental-model units, where the ODE at one compartment depends on the voltage values of the central and the two flanking compartments.

We will now perform an elementary calculation that will explicitly compute the stiffness of a linear compartmental-cable model. In our above-mentioned example on the method of lines (eqs. 13.13), we arrived at a system of coupled linear ODEs to describe the time evolution of a linear compartmental model. These ODEs came from a PDE model of a passive cable, so we must impose certain boundary conditions to correctly specify the mathematical problem. For simplicity, let us assume that we desire the solution to eq. 13.13 with zero-Dirichlet-boundary conditions, that is, $V_0 = V_N = 0$. If we define the vector of voltages on the grid to be $\vec{V} = (V_1, V_2, \ldots, V_{N-1})$, we can rewrite eq. 13.13 as the following linear system of ODEs:

$$\frac{d\vec{V}}{dt} = \mathbf{A}\vec{V} \tag{13.40}$$

The matrix $\mathbf{A}$ is a tridiagonal matrix with the additional property that $\mathbf{A}$ is Toeplitz. A Toeplitz matrix has constant diagonals. Thus if the elements of $\mathbf{A}$ are denoted as a_{ij}, then $a_{ij} = K_d$ whenever $i - j = d$ for $\mathbf{A}$ Toeplitz. Therefore our Toeplitz tridiagonal $\mathbf{A}$ has $a/2RC$ on both off-diagonals and $-(a/RC + \bar{g})$ along the main diagonal. Because eq. 13.40 is a linear system of ODEs, the general solution to this system can be expressed as a linear combination of exponential functions of the form $e^{\lambda t}$, where λ is an eigenvalue of the matrix $\mathbf{A}$. Because we are interested in computing the stiffness of this system, which, we recall, is the ratio of the largest to smallest time scale in the problem, we need only compute λ_{N-1}/λ_1, which is the ratio of the largest to the smallest eigenvalue of $\mathbf{A}$. It should be noted that this ratio of eigenvalues is exactly the l_2-norm condition number of this matrix (Stoer and Bulirsch 1980).

The eigenvalues of the tridiagonal Toeplitz matrix $\mathbf{A}$ are known to be (Isaacson and Keller 1966)

$$\lambda_k = \frac{a}{2RC}\left(-4\sin^2(\frac{k\pi}{2N}) + \rho\right), \quad 1 \le k \le N - 1 \tag{13.41}$$

where $\rho = 2RC\bar{g}/a$. Thus the numerical stiffness is given by

$$\frac{\sin^2(\frac{(N-1)\pi}{2N}) + \rho}{\sin^2(\frac{\pi}{2N}) + \rho} \tag{13.42}$$

The constant ρ is a parameter that measures the dissipation of this particular cable model in terms of the membrane time constant RC. Large values of ρ mean the system relaxes due to this dissipation much faster than does the membrane time constant.

With this explicit formula for the stiffness, we can ask what happens to the stiffness of this system as we vary certain parameters, namely ρ and N. Because $0 \le \sin^2(x) \le 1$, if ρ is large, then eq. 13.42 has a numerical value close to 1, so the system is in fact not very stiff. Thus, if the system is very dissipative, it is numerically well behaved. On the other hand, if ρ is small, then the stiffness is approximately the ratio of the sine terms in eq. 13.42. It can be shown that $\sin^2(\frac{(N-1)\pi}{2N})/\sin^2(\frac{\pi}{2N}) = O(N^2)$ as N gets large. Thus for small values of ρ, the stiffness gets extremely large as we increase the number of compartments in our cable model. In fact, it grows as the square of the number of compartments in our models.

Thus we see that compartmental models can be very stiff when there is little dissipation via the membrane conductance. Paradoxically this stiffness increases as we use smaller and smaller compartments to better resolve spatial details. This relationship of stiffness to the number of compartments is related to the inequality that must be satisfied for numerical stability of the forward-Euler method for these PDEs (Lambert 1973).

Bibliography

Adams, P.R. and Brown, D.A. (1982) Pharmacological inhibition of the M-current. *J. Physiol. (London)* **332**: 263–272.

Adams, P.R., Brown, D.A., and Constanti, A. (1982a) M-currents and other potassium currents in bullfrog sympathetic neurones. *J. Physiol. (London)* **330**: 537–572.

Adams, P.R., Brown, D.A., and Constanti, A. (1982b) Voltage clamp analysis of membrane currents underlying repetitive firing of bullfrog sympathetic neurons. In: *Physiology and Pharmacology of Epileptogenic Phenomena*, Klee, M.R. *et al.* (eds.), Raven Press, New York, pp. 175–187.

Adams, D.J., Smith, S.J., and Thompson, S.H. (1980) Ionic currents in molluscan soma. *Ann. Rev. Neurosci.* **3**: 141–167.

Adams, P.R., Jones, S.W., Pennefather, P., Brown, D.A., Koch, C,. and Lancaster, B. (1986) Slow synaptic transmission in frog sympathetic ganglia. *J. Exp. Biol.* **124**: 259–285.

Adrian, E.D. (1950) The electrical activity of the mammalian olfactory bulb. *Electroenceph. clin. Neurophysiol.* **2**: 377–388.

Albus, A. (1975) Quantitative study of the projection area of the central and the paracentral visual field in Area 17 of the cat. I. The Precision of the Topography. *Exp. Brain Res.* **24**: 159–179.

Alkon, D.L. (1984) Calcium-mediated reduction of ionic currents – a biophysical memory trace. *Science* **226**: 1037–1045.

Amari, S.-I. (1972) Learning patterns and pattern sequences by self-organizing nets of threshold elements. *IEEE Trans. Comp.* **21**: 1197–1206.

Amit, D.J. (1988) Neural networks counting chimes. *Proc. Nat. Acad. Sci. USA* **85**: 2141–2145.

Amit, D.J., Gutfreund, H., and Sompolinsky, H. (1985a) Spin-glass models of neural networks. *Phys. Rev. A* **2**: 1007–1018.

Amit, D.J., Gutfreund, H., and Sompolinsky, H. (1985b) Storing infinite numbers of patterns in a spin-glass model of neural networks. *Phys. Rev. Lett.* **55**: 1530–1533.

Andrews, B.W. and Pollen, D.A. (1979) Relationship between spatial frequency selectivity and receptive field profile of simple cells. *J. Physiol. (London)* **287**: 163–167.

Atwater, I. and Rinzel, J. (1986) The β-cell bursting pattern and intracellular calcium. In: *Ionic Channels in Cells and Model Systems*, Latorre, R. (ed.), Plenum Press, New York.

Baer, S.M. and Tier, C. (1986) An analysis of a dendritic neuron model with an active membrane site. *J. Math. Biol.* **23:** 137–161.

Baird, B. (1986) Nonlinear dynamics of pattern formation and pattern recognition in the rabbit olfactory bulb. *Physica D* **22:** 150–175.

Barchi, R.L. (1987) Sodium channel diversity: subtle variations on a complex theme. *Trends Neurosci.* **10:** 221–223.

Barrett, J.N. and Crill, W.E. (1974) Influence of dendritic location and membrane properties on the effectiveness of synapses on cat motoneurones. *J. Physiol. (London)* **293:** 325–345.

Barron, I.M., Cavill, P., May, D. and Wilson, P. (1983) The transputer. *Electronics*, Nov. 17: 109.

Barto, A.G. and Sutton, R.S. (1982) Simulation of anticipatory responses in classical conditioning by a neuron-like adaptive element. *Behav. Brain. Sci.* **4:** 221–235.

Beaulieu, C. and Colonnier, M. (1983) The number of neurons in the different laminae of the binocular and monocular regions of Area 17 in the Cat. *J. Comp. Neurol.* **217:** 337–344.

Benevento, L.A., Creutzfeldt, O.D. and Kuhnt, U. (1972) Significance of intracortical inhibition in the visual cortex. *Nature New Biol.* **238:** 124–126.

Biedenbach, M.A. and Stevens, C.F. (1969a) Electrical activity in cat olfactory cortex produced by synchronous orthodromic volleys. *J. Neurophysiol.* **32:** 193–203.

Biedenbach, M.A. and Stevens, C.F. (1969b) Synaptic organization of the cat olfactory cortex as revealed by intracellular recording. *J. Neurophysiol.* **32:** 204–214.

Bishop, P.O., Coombs J.S., and Henry, G.H. (1971) Interaction effects of visual contours on the discharge frequency of simple striate neurones. *J. Physiol. (London)* **219:** 659–687.

Bishop, P.O., Kozak, W. and Vakkur, G.J. (1962) Some quantitative aspects of the cat's eye: axis and plane of reference, visual field coordinates and optics. *J. Physiol. (London)* **163:** 466–502.

Bloomfield, S.A., Hamos, J.E., and Sherman, S.M. (1987) Passive cable properties and morphological correlates of neurones in the lateral geniculate nucleus of the cat. *J. Physiol. (London)* **383:** 653–692.

Bolanowski, S.L. (1987) Contourless stimuli produce binocular brightness summation. *Vis. Res.* **27:** 1943–1951.

Boltz, J. and Gilbert, C. D. (1986). Generation of end-inhibiton in the visual cortex via interlaminar connections. *Nature* **320:** 362–365.

Borg-Graham, L.J. (1988) Simulations suggest information processing roles for the diverse currents in hippocampal neurons. In: *Neural*

Information Processsing Systems, Dana Z. Anderson (ed.), American Institute of Physics, New York.

Bower, J.M. and Rao, M. (1986) The modulation of synaptic facilitation in synapses associated with different fiber systems in piriform (olfactory) cortex of the rat. *Soc. Neurosci. Abst.* **12:** 27.

Bowler, K.C., Bruce, A.D., Kenway, R.D., Pawley, G.S., and Wallace, D.J. (1987) Exploiting highly concurrent computers for physics. *Physics Today*, October.

Boycott, B.B. and Wässle, H.(1974) The morphological types of ganglion cells of the domestic cat's retina. *J. Physiol. (London)* **240:** 307–410.

Braitenberg, V. and Braitenberg, C. (1979) Geometry of orientation columns in the visual cortex. *Biol. Cybern.* **33:** 179–186.

Brazier, M.A.B. (1959) The historical development of neurophysiology. In: *Handbook of Physiology, Neurophysiology, Sec. 1, Vol. 1*, Field, Magoun, and Hall (eds.), American Physiology Society, Washington, D.C., pp. 1–58.

Brown, T.H., Fricke, R.A., and Perkel, D.H. (1981) Passive electrical constants in three classes of hippocampal neurons. *J. Neurophysiol.* **46:** 812–827.

Bruce, A.D., Gardner, E.J., and Wallace, D.J. (1986) Static and dynamic properties of the Hopfield model. University of Edinburgh preprint 86/387.

Buhmann, J. and Schulten, K. (1987) Noise-driven temporal association in neural networks. *Europhys. Lett.* **4:** 1205–1209.

Bullier, J. and Norton, T.T. (1979) X and Y relay cells in cat lateral geniculate nucleus: quantitative analysis of receptive—field properties and classification. *J. Neurophysiol.* **42:** 244–291.

Bunow, B., Segev, I., and Fleshman, J.W. (1985) Modeling the electrical properties of anatomically complex neurons using a network analysis program: excitable membrane. *Biol. Cyber.* **53:** 41–56.

Burke, R.E. and ten Bruggencate, G. (1971) Electrotonic characteristics of α-motoneurones of varying size. *J. Physiol. (London)* **21;** 1–20.

Butz, E.G. and Cowan, J.D. (1974) Transient potentials in dendritic systems of arbitrary geometry. *Biophys. J.* **14:** 661–689.

Cannon, S., Robinson, D., and Shamma, S. (1983) A proposed neural network for the integrator of the oculomotor system. *Biol. Cybern.* **49:** 127.

Carbone, E. and Lux, H.D. (1984) A low voltage activated fully inactivating Ca-channel in vertebrate sensory neurones. *Nature* **310:** 501–502.

Carnevale, N.T., and Lebeda, F.J. (1987) Numerical analysis of electrotonus in multicompartmental neuron models. *J. Neurosci. Meth.*
19: 69–87.

Chay, T.R. and Keizer, J.E. (1983) Minimal model for membrane oscillations in the pancreatic β-cell. *Biophys. J.* **42:** 181–190.

Chomsky, N. (1965) *Aspects of the Theory of Syntax*, MIT Press, Cambridge.

Churchland, P.S., Koch. C., and Sejnowski, T.J. (1989) What is computational neuroscience? In: *Computational Neuroscience*, E. Schwartz
(ed.), MIT Press, Cambridge.

Clay, J.R. and DeFelice, L.J. (1983) The relationship between membrane
excitability and single channel open-close kinetics. *Biophys. J.* **42:**
151–157.

Cleland, B.G. and Levick, W.R. (1974) Properties of rarely encountered
types of ganglion cells in the cat's retina and an overall classification.
J. Physiol. (London) **240:** 457–492.

Cleland, B.G., Dubin, M.W., and Levick, W.R. (1971) Sustained and
transient neurones in the cat's retina and lateral geniculate nucleus.
J. Physiol. (London) **217:** 473–496.

Clements, J.D. and Redman, S.J. (1989) Cable properties of cat spinal
motoneurones measured by combining voltage clamp, current clamp
and intracellular staining. *J. Physiol. (London)*, in press.

Coddington, E. and Levinson, N. (1955) *Theory of Ordinary Differential
Equations*, McGraw-Hill Book Company, New York.

Cohen, M.A. and Grossberg, S. (1983) Absolute stability of global pattern formation and parallel memory storage by competitive networks. *IEEE Trans. Sys. Man Cybern.* **13:** 815–826.

Cohen, A.H., Rossignol, S., and Grillner, S., eds. (1986) *Neural Control
of Rhythmic Movements*, John Wiley, New York.

Cole, K.S. (1968) *Membranes, Ions and Impulses: A Chapter of Classical
Biophysics*, University of California Press, Berkeley.

Cole, K.S., Guttman, R., and Bezanilla, F. (1970) Nerve excitation without threshold. *Proc. Nat. Acad. Sci.* **65:** 884–891.

Cole, A.E. and Nicoll, R. (1984) Characterization of a slow choliner-
gic post-synaptic potential recorded in vitro from rat hippocampal
pyramidal cells. *J. Physiol. (London)* **352:** 173–188.

Collatz, L. (1960) *The Numerical Treatment of Differential Equations*,
Third Edition, Springer-Verlag, New York, Heidelberg, Berlin.

Connor, J.A. and Stevens, C.F. (1971a) Voltage clamp analysis of a
transient outward membrane current in gastropod neural somata.
J. Physiol. (London) **213:** 21–30.

Connor, J.A. and Stevens, C.F. (1971b) Inward and delayed outward membrane currents in isolated neural somata under voltage clamp. *J. Physiol. (London)* **213**: 31–53.

Connor, J.A., Walter, D., and McKown, R. (1977) Neural repetitive firing: modifications of the Hodgkin-Huxley axon suggested by experimental results from crustacean axons. *Biophys. J.* **18**: 81–102.

Connors, B.W. and Kriegstein, A.R. (1986) Cellular physiology of the turtle visual cortex: distinctive properties of pyramidal and stellate neurons. *J. Neurosci.* **6**: 164–177.

Conradi, S., Kellerth, J.-O., Berthold, C.-H. and Hammarberg, C. (1979) Electron microscopic studies of serially sectioned cat spinal α-motoneurons. IV. Motoneurons innervating slow-twitch (type S) units of the soleus muscle. *J. Comp. Neurol.* **184**: 769–782.

Conte, S.D. and de Boor, C. (1980), *Elementary Numerical Analysis: An Algorithmic Approach*, Third edition, McGraw-Hill Book Company, New York.

Cooley, J.W. and Dodge, F.A. (1966) Digital computer solutions for excitation and propagation of the nerve impulse. *Biophys. J.* **6**: 583–599.

Coombs, J.S., Eccles, J.C., and Fatt, P. (1955a) The electrical properties of the motoneurone membrane. *J. Physiol. (London)* **130**: 291–325.

Coombs, J.S., Eccles, J.C., and Fatt, P. (1955b) The specific ionic conductances and the ionic movements across the motoneurone membrane that produce the inhibitory post-sysnaptic potential. *J. Physiol. (London)* **130**: 326–373.

Crank, J. (1975) *The Mathematics of Diffusion*, Second edition, Clarendon Press, Oxford.

Crank, J. and Nicolson, P. (1947) A practical method for numerical evaluation of solutions of partial differential equations of the heat conduction type. *Proc. Camb. Phil. Soc.* **43**: 50–67.

Crick, F. (1984) The function of the thalamic reticular complex: the searchlight hypothesis. *Proc. Natl. Acad. Sci. USA* **81**: 4586–4590.

Crisanti, A., Amit, D.J., and Gutfreund, H. (1986) Saturation level of the Hopfield model for neural network. *Europhys. Lett.* **2**: 337–341.

Crunelli, V., Kelly, J.S., Leresheche N. and Pirchio, M. (1987) The ventral and dorsal lateral geniculate nucleus of the cat: intracellular recording in vitro. *J. Physiol. (London)* **384**: 587–601.

Cooley, J.W. and Dodge, F.A. (1966) Digital computer solution for excitation and propagation of the nerve impulse. *Biophys. J.* **6**: 583–599.

Courant, R. and Hilbert, D. (1962) *Methods of Mathematical Physics*, Vols. 1 and 2, Interscience Publishers, New York.

Cullheim, S., Fleshman, J.W., Glenn, L.L. and Burke, R.E. (1987) Membrane area and dendritic structure in type-identified triceps surae alpha-motoneurons. *J. Comp. Neurol.* **255:** 68–81.

Dahlquist, G. and Bjorck, A. (1974) *Numerical Methods*, Prentice-Hall, Englewood Cliffs, New Jersey.

Daugman, J.G. (1985) Uncertainty relation for resolution in space, spatial frequency, and orientation optimized by two-dimensional visual cortical filters. *J. Opt. Soc. Am.* **2:** 1160–1169.

Davis, L., Jr. and Lorente de Nó, R. (1947) Contribution to the mathematical theory of the electrotonus. *Studies from the Rockefeller Institute for Medical Research* **131:** 442–496.

Dawis, S., Shapley, R., Kaplan, E., and Tranchina, D. (1984) The receptive field organization of X-cells in the cat: spatiotemporal coupling and asymmetry. *Vision Res.* **24:** 549–564.

DeFelice, L.J. and Clay, J.R. (1983) Membrane current and membrane potential from single-channel kinetics. In: *Single-Channel Recording*, Sakmann, B. and Neher, E. (eds.), Plenum Press, New York, pp. 323–342.

DeFelipe, J., Hendry, S.H.C., and Jones, E.G. (1986) A correlative electron microscopic study of basket cells and large gabaergic neurons in the monkey sensory-motor cortex. *Neuroscience* **17:** 991–1009.

Dehaene, S., Changeux, J.-P., and Nadal, J.-P. (1987) Neural networks that learn temporal sequences by selection. *Proc. Natl. Acad. Sci. USA* **84:** 2727–2731.

Dekin, M.S., Getting, P.A., and Johnson, S.M. (1987) *In vitro* characterization of neurons in the ventral part of the nucleus tractus solitarius. I. Identification of neuronal types and repetitive firing properties. *J. Neurophysiol.* **58:** 195–214.

Delcomyn, F. (1980) Neural basis of rhythmic behavior in animals. *Science* **210:** 492–498.

Delgutte, B. (1984) Speech coding in the auditory nerve: II. Processing schemes for vowel-like sounds. *J. Acoust. Soc. Am.* **75:** 879–886.

Deng, L., Geisler. C.D., and Greenberg, S. (1987) A composite auditory model for processing speech sounds. *J. Acoust. Soc.* **82:** 2001-2012.

Denker, J.S. (1986a) Neural network models of learning and adaptation. *Physica D* **22:** 216–232.

Denker, J.S. (1986b) Neural network refinements and extensions. In: *Neural Networks for Computing*, Denker, J.S. (ed.), American Institute of Physics, New York.

De Schutter, E. (1986) Alternative equations for molluscan ion currents described by Connor and Stevens. *Brain Res.* **382:** 134–138.

De Schutter, E. (1988) Computer software for development and simulation of compartmental models of neurons. *Comput. Biol. Med.*, in press.

DeValois, K.K, DeValois, R.K., and Yund, E.W. (1979) Responses of striate cortical cells to grating and checkerboard patterns. *J. Physiol. (London)* **291**: 483–505.

Devor, M. (1976) Fiber trajectories of olfactory bulb afferents in hamster. *J. Comp. Neurol.* **166**: 31–48.

Devor, M. (1977) Central processing of odor signals: lessons from adult and neonatal olfactory tract lesions. In: *Chemical Signals in Vertebrates*, Muller-Schwartz, D. and Mozell, M. (eds.), Plenum, New York.

Diederich, S. and Opper, M. (1987) Learning of correlated patterns in spin-glass networks by local learning rules. *Phys. Rev. Lett.* **58**: 949–952.

DiFrancesco, D. and Noble, D. (1985) A model of cardiac electrical activity incorporating ionic pumps and concentration changes. *Phil. Trans. R. Soc. Lond. B* **307**: 353–398.

Dionne, V.E. (1984) Synaptic noise. In: *Membranes, Channels, and Noise*, Eisenberg, R.S., Frank, M., and Stevens, C.F. (eds.), Plenum Press, New York.

DiPolo, R. and Beauge, L. (1983) The calcium pump and sodium-calcium exchange in squid axons. *Ann. Rev. Physiol.* **45**: 313.

Dodge, F.A. and Frankenhaeuser, B. (1958) Membrane currents in isolated frog nerve fibres under voltage clamp conditions. *J. Physiol. (London)* **143**: 76–90.

Doedel, E.J. (1981) AUTO: A program for the automatic bifurcation and analysis of autonomous systems. *Cong. Num.* **30**: 265–284.

Dongarra, J.J. (1987a) *Experimental Parallel Computing Architectures*, Dongarra, J.J. (ed.), North-Holland, Amsterdam.

Dongarra, J.J. (1987b) The LINPAK benchmark: an explanation. In: *Proceedings of ICS87, International Conference on Supercomputers*, published as *A Lecture Note in Computer Science*, Polychronoupolos, C. (ed.), Springer Verlag, New York, pp. 456–474.

Douglas, J., Jr. (1956) On the numerical integration of quasi-linear parabolic differential equations. *Pacific J. Math.* **6**: 35–42.

Douglas, J., Jr. (1958) The application of stability analysis in the numerical solution of quasi-linear parabolic differential equations. *Trans. Am. Math. Soc.* **89**: 484–518.

Durand, D. (1984) The somatic shunt cable model for neurons. *Biophys. J.* **46**: 645–653.

Durand, D., Carlen, P.L., Gurevich, N., Ho A. and Kunov, H. (1983) Measurements of the passive electrotonic parameters of granule cells in the rat hippocampus using HRP staining and short current pulse. *J. Neurophysiol.* **50:** 1080–1096.

Eckert, R. and Chad, J.E. (1984) Inactivation of calcium channels. *Prog. Biophys. Molec. Biol.* **44:** 215–267.

Edelstein-Keshet, L. (1988) *Mathematical Models in Biology*, Random House, New York.

Edwards, D.H. and Mulloney, B. (1984) Compartmental models of electrotonic structure and synaptic integration in an identified neurone. *J. Physiol. (London)* **348:** 89–113.

Eichenbaum, H., Shedlack, K.J., and Eckmann, K.W. (1980) Thalamocortical mechanisms in odor-guided behavior. I. Effects of lesions of the mediodorsal thalamic nucleus and frontal cortex on olfactory discrimination in the rat. *Brain Behav. Evol.* **17:** 255–275

Enroth-Cugell, C. and Robson, J.G. (1966) The contrast sensitivity of retinal ganglion cells of the cat. *J. Physiol. (London)* **187:** 517–552.

Enroth-Cugell, C., Robson, J.G., Schweizer-Tong, D.E., and Watson, A.B. (1983) Spatio-temporal interactions in cat retinal ganglion cells showing linear spatial summation. *J. Physiol. (London)* **341:** 279–307.

Ermentrout, G.B. (1981) n:m phase-locking of weakly coupled oscillators. *J. Math. Biol.* **12:** 327–342.

Ermentrout, G.B. and Cowan, J.D. (1980) Large scale spatially organized activity in neural nets. *SIAM J. Appl. Math.* **38:** 1–21.

Ermentrout, G.B. and Kopell, N. (1984) Frequency plateaus in a chain of weakly coupled oscillators, I. *SIAM J. Math. Analysis* **15:** 215–237.

Evans, J. and Shenk, N. (1970) Solutions to axon equations. *Biophys. J.* **6:** 583–599.

Fatt, P. and Katz, B. (1953) The effect of inhibitory nerve impulses on a crustacean muscle fibre. *J. Physiol. (London)* **121:** 374–389.

Fenwick, E.M., Marty, A., and Neher, E. (1982) Sodium and potassium channels in bovine chromaffin cells. *J. Physiol. (London)* **331:** 599–635.

Ferster, D. (1986) Orientation selectivity of the synaptic potentials in neurons of cat primary visual cortex. *J. Neurosci.* **6:** 1284–1301.

Ferster, D. (1988) Spatially opponent excitation and inhibition in simple cells of the cat visual cortex. *J. Neurosci.* **8:** 1172–1180.

Ferster, D. and Koch, C. (1987) Neuronal connections underlying orientation selectivity in cat visual cortex. *Trends Neurosci.* **10:** 487–492.

Fifkova, E., Markham, J.A., and Delay, R.J. (1983) Calcium in the spine apparatus of the dendritic spines in the dentate molecular layer *Brain Res. (London)* **266:** 163–168.

Finkel, A.S. and Redman, S.J. (1983) The synaptic current evoked in cat spinal motoneurons by impulse in single group Ia axons. *J. Physiol. (London)* **342:** 615–632.

Fischer, B. (1973) Overlap of receptive field centers and representation of the visual field in the opic tract, *Vision Res.* **13:** 2113–2120.

FitzHugh, R. (1960) Thresholds and plateaus in the Hodgkin-Huxley nerve equations. *J. Gen. Physiol.* **43:** 867–896.

FitzHugh, R. (1961) Impulses and physiological states in models of nerve membrane. *Biophys. J.* **1:** 445–466.

FitzHugh, R. (1969) Mathematical models for excitation and propagation in nerve. In: *Biological Engineering*, Schwan, H.P. (ed.), Mc-Graw Hill, New York.

Fitzpatrick, D., Penny, G.R., and Schmechel, D.E. (1984) Glutamic acid decarboxylase immunoreactive neurons and terminals in the lateral geniculate nucleus of the cat. *J. Neurosci.* **4:** 1809–1829.

Flach, K., Carnevale, N.T. and Sussman-Fort, S.E. (1987) Neuron simulations using SABER. *Soc. Neurosci. Abst.* **13:** 45.19

Fleshman, J.W., Segev, I., and Burke, R.E. (1988) Electrotonic architecture of type- identified α-motoneurons in the cat spinal cord. *J. Neurophysiol.* **60:** 60–85.

Fox, G.C. (1987) A graphical approach to load balancing and sparse matrix vector multiplication on the hypercube. In: *Numerical Algorithms for Modern Parallel Computer Architectures*, Springer Verlag, New York.

Fox, S.E. and Chan, C.Y. (1985) Location of membrane conductance changes by analysis of the input impedance of neurons. II. Implementation. *J. Neurophysiol.* **54:** 1594–1606.

Fox, G.C. and Furmanski, W. (1987) Hypercube communication for neural network algorithms. Caltech report, $C^3P - 405$.

Fox, G.C. and Furmanski, W. (1988a) Load balancing loosely synchronous problems with a neural network. In: *Proceeding of the Third Conference on Hypercube Concurrent Computers and Applications*, Fox, G.C. (ed.), ACM, New York.

Fox, G.C. and Furmanski, W. (1988b) Optimal Communication Algorithms for Regular Decompositions on the Hypercube. In: *Proceeding of the Third Conference on Hypercube Concurrent Computers and Applications*, Fox, G.C. (ed.), ACM, New York.

Fox, G.C., Johnson, M.A., Lyzenga, G.A., Otto, S.W., Salmon, J.K. and Walker, D.W. (1988) *Solving Problems On Concurrent Processors*, Prentice Hall, New Jersey.

Fox, G.C. and Messina, P.C. (1987) Advanced Computer Architectures. *Sci. Am.* **256:** 66–77.

Fox, G.C. and Walker, D. (1988) Concurrent supercomputers in science. Proceedings of the conference on *Use of Computers in Physics*, North Carolina.

Frank, K. and Fuortes, M.G.F. (1956) Stimulation of spinal motoneurones with intracellular electrodes. *J. Physiol. (London)* **134:** 451–470.

Frankenhaeuser, B. (1963) A quantitative description of potassium currents in mylenated nerve fibres of *Xenopus laevin. J. Physiol. (London)* **169:** 424–430.

Frankenhaeuser, B. and Hodgkin, A.L. (1956) The after effects of impulses in the giant nerve fibres of *Loligo. J. Physiol. (London)* **131:** 341–376.

Frankenhaeuser, B. and Huxley, A.F. (1964) Action potential in mylenated nerve fibre of *Xenopus laevis* as computed on the basis of voltage clamp data. *J. Physiol. (London)* **171:** 302–315.

Freeman, W.J. (1959) Distribution in time and space of prepyriform electrical activity. *J. Neurophysiol.* **22:** 664–665.

Freeman, W.J. (1960) Correlation of electrical activity of prepyriform cortex and behavior in cat. *J. Neurophysiol.* **23:** 111–131.

Freeman, W.J. (1968) Relation between unit activity and evoked potentials in prepiriform cortex of cats. *J. Neurophysiol.* **31:** 337–348.

Freeman, W.J. (1975) *Mass Action in the Nervous System*, Academic Press, New York.

Freeman, W.J. (1979a) Nonlinear gain mediating cortical stimulus response relations. *Biol. Cybern.* **33:** 237–247.

Freeman, W.J. (1979b) Nonlinear dynamics of paleocortex manifested in the olfactory EEG. *Biol. Cybern.* **35:** 21–37.

Freeman, W.J. (1983) The physiological basis of mental images. *Biol. Psychol.* **18:** 1107–1125.

Freund, T.F., Martin, K.A.C., and Whitteridge, D. (1985a) Innervation of cat visual areas 17 and 18 by physiologically identified X- and Y-type thalamic afferents. I. Arborization patterns and quantitative distribution of postsynaptic elements. *J. Comp. Neurol.* **242:** 263–274.

Freund, T.F., Martin, K.A.C., Somogyi, P., and Whitteridge, D. (1985b) Innervation of cat visual areas 17 and 18 by physiologically identified

X- and Y-type thalamic afferents. II. Identification of postsynaptic targets by GABA immunocytochemistry and Golgi impregnation. *J. Comp. Neurol.* **242**: 275–291.

Fuortes, M.G.F. and Mantegazzini, F. (1962) Interpretation of the repetitive firing of nerve cells. *J. Gen. Physiol.* **45**: 1163–1179.

Fukushima, K. (1973) A model of associative memory in the brain. *Kybern.* **12**: 58–63.

Galvan, M., Grafe, P., and Bruggencate, G. (1982) Convulsant actions of 4-aminopyridine on the guinea-pig olfactory cortex slice. *Brain Res.* **241**: 75–86.

Gamble, E. and Koch, C. (1987) The dynamics of free calcium in dendritic spines in response to repetitive input. *Science* **236**: 1311–1315.

Gardner, E. (1988) The space of interactions in neural network models. *J. Phys. A* **21**: 257–270.

Gault, F.P. and Leaton, R.N. (1963) Nasal air flow and rhinencephalic activity. *Electroenceph. clin. Neurophysiol* **18**: 617–624.

Gault, F.P. and Coustan, D.R. (1965) Electrical activity of the olfactory system. *Electroenceph. clin. Neurophysiol.* **15**: 229–304.

Gear, C.W. (1971a) *Numerical Initial Value Problems in Ordinary Differential Equations*, Prentice-Hall, Englewood Cliffs, New Jersey.

Gear, C. W. (1971b) The automatic integration of ordinary differential equations. *Comm. ACM* **14**: 176–179.

Gelperin, A., Hopfield, J.J., and Tank, D.W. (1985) The logic of *Limax* learning. In: *Model Neural Networks and Behavior*, Selverston, A.I. (ed.), Plenum Press, New York.

Georgopoulos, A.P., Schwartz, A.B., and Kettner, R.E. (1986) Neuronal population coding of movement direction. *Science* **233**: 1416–1419.

Getting, P.A. (1977) Neuronal organization of escape swimming in *Tritonia*. *J. Comp. Physiol.* **121**: 325–342.

Getting, P.A. (1981) Mechanisms of pattern generation underlying swimming in *Tritonia*. I. Network formed by monosynaptic connections. *J. Neurophysiol.* **46**: 65–79.

Getting, P.A. (1983a) Mechanisms of pattern generation underlying swimming in *Tritonia*. II. Network recostruction. *J. Neurophysiol.* **49**: 1017–1035.

Getting, P.A. (1983b) Mechanisms of pattern generation underlying swimming in *Tritonia*. III. Intrinsic and cellular mechanisms of delayed excitation. *J. Neurophysiol.* **49**: 1036–1050.

Getting, P.A. (1983c) Neural control of swimming in *Tritonia*. In: *Neural Origin of Rhythmic Movements*, Roberts, A. and Roberts, B.L.

(eds.), Cambridge University Press, London and New York, pp. 89-128.

Getting, P.A. (1988) Comparative analysis of invertebrate central pattern generators. In: *Neural Control of Rhythmic Movements in Vertebrates*, Cohen, A.H., Rossignol, S., and Grillner, S. (eds.), John Wiley and Sons, Inc., New York, pp. 101-128.

Getting, P.A. (1989) Emerging principles governing the operation of neural networks. *Ann. Rev. Neurosci.*, in press.

Getting, P.A. and Dekin, M.S. (1985a) Mechanisms of pattern generation underlying swimming in *Tritonia*. IV. Gating of a central pattern generator. *J. Neurophysiol.* **53:** 466–480.

Getting, P.A. and Dekin, M.S. (1985b) *Tritonia* swimming: a model system for integration within rhythmic motor systems. In: *Model Neural Networks and Behavior*, Selverston, A.I. (ed.), Plenum Publishing, New York, pp. 3–20.

Getting, P.A., Lennard, P.R., and Hume, R.I. (1980) Central pattern generator mediating swimming in *Tritonia*. I. Identification and synaptic interactions. *J. Neurophysiol.* 44: 151–164.

Gilbert, C. (1977) Laminar differences in receptive field properties of cells in cat primary visual cortex. *J. Physiol. (London)* **268:** 391–421.

Gilbert, C.D. (1983) Microcircuitry of the visual cortex. *Ann. Rev. Neurosci.* **6:** 217–247.

Glass, L. and Mackey, M.C. (1988) *From Clocks to Chaos: The Rhythms of Life*, Princeton University Press, Princeton.

Glass, L. and Young, R.E. (1979) Structure and dynamics of neural network oscillators. *Brain. Res.* **179:** 208–218.

Glasser, S., Miller, J, Xuong, N.G. and Selverston, A. (1977) Computer reconstruction of invertebrate nerve cells. In: *Computer Analysis of Neuronal Structure*, Lindsay, R.D. (ed.), Plenum Publishing, New York, pp. 21–58.

Goldman, D.E. (1943) Potential, impedance, and rectification in membranes *J. Gen. Phys.* **27:**37–60.

Goldstein, S.S. and Rall, W. (1974) Changes in action potential shape and velocity for changing core conductor geometry. *Biophys. J.* **14:** 731–757.

Golub, G. H, and Van Loan, C. F. (1985) *Matrix Computations*, Johns Hopkins University Press, Baltimore.

Grasman, J. (1987) *Asymptotic Methods for Relaxation Oscillations and Applications.* Applied Mathematical Sciences **83**, Springer-Verlag, Heidelberg.

Gray, E.G. (1959) Axo-somatic and axo-dendritic synapses of the cerebral cortex: an electron microspcope study. *J. Anat.* **93:** 420–433.

Gregory. R.L. (1966) *Eye and Brain: The Psychology of Seeing*, McGraw-Hill, New York.

Gremillion, M., Mandell, A., and Travis, B. (1987) Neural nets with complex structure: a model of the visual system. In *IEEE 1st Intl. Conf. Neural Networks*, Vol. 4, Institute of Electrical and Electronics Engineers, San Diego, pp. 235–246.

Grillner, S. (1975) Locomotion in vertebrates. Central mechanisms and reflex interaction. *Physiol. Rev.* **55:** 247–304.

Grinvald, A. (1985) Real-time optical mapping of neural activity: from single growth cones to the mammalian brain. *Ann. Rev. Neurosci.* **8:** 263–305.

Grossberg, S. (1976) Adaptive pattern classification and universal recoding. I. Parallel development and coding of neural feature detectors. *Biol. Cybern.* **23:** 121–134.

Gurney, A.M., Tsien, R.Y., and Lester, H.A. (1987) Activation of a potassium current by rapid photochemically generated step increases of intracellular calcium in rat sympathetic neurons. *Proc. Natl. Acad. Sci. U.S.A.* **84(10):** 3496–3500.

Gutfreund, H. and Mézard, M. (1988) Processing temporal sequences in neural networks. *Phys. Rev. Lett.* **61:** 235–238.

Guthrie, P.B. and Westbrook, G.L. (1984) Non-uniform distribution of membrane resistivity in cultured mouse ventral horn neurons. *Soc. Neurosci. Abst.* **10:** 242.

Guttman, R., Lewis, S., and Rinzel, J. (1980) Control of repetitive firing in squid axon membrane as a model for a neuroneoscillator. *J. Physiol. (London)* **305:** 377–395.

Guyon, I., Personnaz, L., Nadal, J.P., and Dreyfus, G. (1988) Storage and retrieval of complex sequences in neural networks. *Phys. Rev. A* **38:** 6365–6372.

Haberly, L.B. (1973a) Unitary analysis of opossum prepyriform cortex. *J. Neurophysiol.* **36:** 762–774.

Haberly, L.B. (1973b) Summed potentials evoked in opossum prepyriform cortex. *J. Neurophysiol.* **36:** 775–788.

Haberly, L.B. (1978) Application of collision testing to investigate properties of multiple association axons originating from single cells in the piriform cortex of the rat. *Soc. Neurosci. Abst.* **4:** 75.

Haberly, L.B. (1983) Structure of the piriform cortex of the opossum. I. Description of neuron types with Golgi methods. *J. Comp. Neurol.* **213:** 163–187.

Haberly, L.B. (1985) Neuronal circuitry in olfactory cortex: anatomy and functional implications. *Chem. Senses* **10:** 219–238.

Haberly, L.B. and Behan, M. (1984) Structure of the piriform cortex of the opossum. III. Ultrastructural characterization of synaptic terminals of association and olfactory bulb afferent fibers. *J. Comp. Neurol.* **219:** 448–460.

Haberly, L.B. and Bower, J.M. (1984) Analysis of association fiber system in piriform cortex with intracellular recording and staining techniques. *J. Neurophys.* **51:** 90–112.

Haberly, L.B. and Presto, S. (1986) Ultrastructural analysis of synaptic relationships of intracellular stained pyramidal cell axons in piriform cortex. *J. Comp. Neurol.* **248:** 464–474.

Haberly, L.B. and Price, J.L. (1977) The axonal projection patterns of the mitral and tufted cells of the olfactory bulb in the rat. *Brain Res.* **129:** 152–157.

Haberly, L.B. and Price, J.L. (1978) Association and commissural fiber system of the olfactory cortex of the rat. I. System originating in the piriform cortex and adjacent areas. *J. Comp. Neurol.* **178:** 711–740.

Haberly, L.B. and Shepherd, G.M. (1973) Current density analysis of opossum prepyriform cortex. *J. Neurophysiol.* **36:** 789–802.

Hagiwara, S. and Ohmari, H. (1982) Studies of calcium channels in rat clonal pituitary cells with patch electrode voltage clamp. *J. Physiol. (London)* **331:** 231–252.

Halliwell, J. and Adams, P.R. (1982) Voltage clamp analysis of muscarinic excitation in hippocampal neurons. *Brain Res.* **250:** 71–92.

Harmon, L.D. (1964) Neuromimes: action of a reciprocally inhibitory pair. *Science* **146:** 1323–1325.

Harris-Warrick, R.M. (1988) Chemical modulation of central pattern generators. In: *Neural Control of Rhythmic Movements in Vertebrates*, Cohen, A.H., Rossignol, S., and Grillner, S. (eds.), John Wiley and Sons, Inc., New York.

Harth, E., Lewis, N.S., and Csermely, T.J. (1975) Escape of *Tritonia:* dynamics of neuromuscular control mechanisms. *J. Theor. Biol.* **55:** 210–228.

Hartline, H.K. (1974) *Studies on Excitation and Inhibition in the Retina*, Ratliff, E. (ed.), Rockefeller University Press, New York.

Hartline, D.K. and Gassie Jr., D.V. (1979) Pattern generation in the lobster (*Panulirus*) stomatogastric ganglion. I. Pyloric neuron kinetics and synaptic interactions. *Biol. Cyber.* **33:** 209–222.

Hartline, D.K. (1979) Pattern generation in the lobster (*Panulirus*) stomatogastric ganglion. II. Pyloric network simulation. *Biol. Cyber.* **33**: 223–236.

Hearon, J.Z. (1963) Theorems on linear systems. *Ann. N. Y. Acad. Sci.* **108**: 36–68.

Hebb, D.O. (1948) *The Organization of Behavior: A Neuropsychological Theory*, John Wiley, New York.

Heggelund, P. (1981) Receptive field organization of simple cells in cat striate cortex. *Exp. Brain Res.* **42**: 89–98.

Heggelund, P. (1986) Quantitative studies of the discharge fields of single cells in cat striate cortex. *J. Physiol. (London)* **373**: 272–292.

Heimer, L. (1968) Synaptic distribution of centripetal and centrifugal nerve fibers in the olfactory system of the rat: an experimental anatomical study. *J. Anat.* **102**: 413–432.

Hendry, S.H.C., Schwark, H.D., Jones, E.G., and Yan. J. (1987) Numbers and proportions of GABA- immunoreactive neurons in different areas of monkey cerebral cortex. *J. Neurosci.* **7**: 1503-1519.

Henrici, P. (1962) *Discrete Variable Methods in Ordinary Differential Equations*, John Wiley and Sons, Inc., New York.

Hille, B. (1984) *Ionic Channels of Excitable Membranes*, Sinauer, Sunderland, Massachusetts.

Hillis, W.D. (1985) *The Connection Machine*, MIT Press, Cambridge, Massachusetts.

Hillis, W.D. (1987) The Connection Machine. *Sci. Am.* **256**: 108–117.

Hines, M. (1984) Efficient computation of branched nerve equations. *Int. J. Bio-Med. Comp.* **15**: 69–76.

Hinton, G.E., McClelland, J.L., and Rumelhart, D.E. (1986) Distributed representations. In: *Parallel Distributed Processing: Explorations in the Microstructure of Cognition. Vol. 1: Foundations*, Rumelhart, D.E. and McClelland, J.L. (eds.), MIT Press, Cambridge.

Hodgkin, A.L. (1948) The local electric changes associated with repetitive action in a non-medullated axon. *J. Physiol. (London)* **107**: 165–181.

Hodgkin, A.L. and Huxley, A.F. (1952) A quantitative description of membrane current and its application to conduction and excitation in nerve. *J. Physiol. (London)* **117**: 500–544.

Hodgkin, A.L. and Katz, B. (1949) The effect of sodium ions on the electrical activity of the giant axon of the squid. *J. Physiol. (London)* **108**: 37–77.

Hodgkin, A.L. and Keynes, R.D. (1957) Movements of labelled calcium in squid giant axon. *J. Physiol. (London)* **138**: 253–281.

Hodgkin, A.L. and Rushton, W.A.H. (1946) The electrical constants of a crustacean nerve fibre. *Proc. Roy. Soc. London B* **133**: 444–479.

Hoffman, K.P., Stone, J., and Sherman, S.M. (1972) Relay of receptive-field properties in dorsal lateral geniculate nucleus of cat. *J. Neurophys.* **35**: 518–531.

Holmes, W.R. (1986) A continuous cable method for determining the transient potential in passive trees of known geometry. *Biol. Cyber.* **55**: 115–124.

Holmes, M.H. and Cole, J.D. (1984) Cochlear mechanics: analysis for a pure tone. *J. Acoust. Soc. Am.* **76**: 767–778.

Honma, S. (1984) Functional differentiation in SB and SC neurons of toad sympathetic ganglia. *Jap. J. Physiol.* **20**: 281.

Hopfield, J.J. (1982) Neural networks and physical systems with emergent collective computational abilities. *Proc. Nat. Acad. Sci. USA* **79**: 2554–2558.

Hopfield, J.J. (1984) Neurons with graded response have collective computational properties like those of two-state neurons. *Proc. Nat. Acad. Sci. USA* **81**: 3088–3092.

Hopfield, J.J. and Tank, D.W. (1985) "Neural" computation of decisions in optimization problems. *Biol. Cyber.* **52**: 141–152.

Hopfield, J.J. and Tank, D.W. (1986) Computing with neural circuits: a model. *Science* **233**: 625–632.

Horn, B.K.P. (1986) *Robot Vision*, MIT Press, Cambridge.

Horwitz, B. (1981) An analytical method for investigating transient potentials in neurons with branching dendritic trees. *Biophys. J.* **36**: 155–192.

Horwitz, B. (1983) Unequal diameters and their effect on time-varying voltages in branched neuron. *Biophys. J.* **41**: 51–66.

Hubel, D.H. and Wiesel, T.N. (1961) Integrative action in the cat's lateral geniculate body. *J. Physiol.(London)* **155**: 385–398.

Hubel, D.H. and Wiesel, T.N. (1962) Receptive fields, binocular interactions, and functional architecture in the cat's visual cortex. *J. Physiol. (London)* **160**: 106–154.

Hubel, D.H. and Wiesel, T.N. (1963) Shape and arrangement of columns in cat's striate cortex. *J. Physiol. (London)* **165**: 559–568.

Hubel, D.H. and Wiesel, T.N. (1965) Receptive fields and the functional architecture in two non-striate visual areas (18 and 19) of the cat. *J. Neurophysiol.* **28**: 229–289.

Hull, T. E., Enright, W. H., Fellen, B. M., and Sedgewick, A. E. (1971) Comparing numerical methods for ordinary differential equations.

University of Toronto, Department of Computer Science Technical Report No. 29, Toronto, Canada.

Hume, R.I. and Getting, P.A. (1982) Motor organization of *Tritonia* swimming. II. Synaptic drive to flexion neurons from premotor interneurons. *J. Neurophysiol.* **47**: 75–90.

Humphrey, A.L., Sur, M., Uhlrich D.J., and Sherman, S.M. (1985) Projection patterns of individual X- and Y-cell axons from the lateral geniculate nucleus to cortical area 17 in the cat. *J. Comp. Neurol.* **233**: 159–189.

Ikeuchi, K. and Horn, B.K.P. (1981) Numerical shape from shading and occluding boundaries. *Artif. Intell.* **17**: 141–184.

Irvine, D. F. (1986) *The Auditory Brainstem: Sensory Physiology*, Springer Verlag, Berlin.

Isaacson, E. and Keller, H.B. (1966) *Analysis of Numerical Methods*, John Wiley and Sons, Inc., New York.

Jack, J.J.B., Noble, D., and Tsien, R.W. (1975) *Electrical Current Flow in Excitable Cells*, Second edition, Clarendon Press, Oxford.

Jack, J.J.B. and Redman, S.J. (1971) The propagation of transient potentials in some linear cable structures. *J. Physiol. (London)* **215**: 283–320.

Jack, J.J.B. and Redman, S.J. (1971b) An electrical description of the motonerone and its application to the analysis of synaptic potentials. *J. Physiol. (London)* **215**: 321–352.

Jahnsen, H. (1986) Responses of neurons in isolated preparations of the mammalian central nervous system. *Prog. Neurobiol.* **27**: 351–372.

Jahnsen, H. and Llinas, R. (1984) Electrophysiological properties of guinea pig thalamic neurones: an *in vitro* study. *J. Physiol. (London)* **349**: 205–226.

Jahr, C.E. and Stevens, C.F. (1987) Glutamate activates multiple single channel conductances in hippocampal neurons. *Nature* **325**: 522–525.

Jan, L.Y. and Jan, Y.N. (1982) Peptidergic transmission in sympathetic ganglion of the frog. *J. Physiol. (London)* **327**: 219–246.

Jeffrey, W. and Rosner, R. (1986) Optimization algorithms: simulated annealing and neural network processing. *Astrophys. J.* **310**: 473–481.

Jennings, D.M., Landweber, L.H., Fuchs, I.H., Farber, D.J., and Adrion, W.R. (1986) Computer networking for scientists. *Science* **231**: 943–950.

John, F. (1952) On integration of parabolic differential equations by difference methods. *Comm. Pure Appl. Math.* **5**: 155–211.

John, F. (1965) *Ordinary Differential Equations*, Courant Institute of
    Mathematical Sciences Lecture Notes, New York University, New
    York.
John, F. (1982) *Partial Differential Equations*, Fourth edition, Springer-
    Verlag, Heidelberg.
Jones, S.W. (1987) Sodium currents in dissociated bullfrog sympathetic
    neurons *J. Physiol. (London)* **389**:605–627.
Jones, J.P. and Palmer, L.A. (1987) An evaluation of the two-dimensional
    gabor filter model of simple receptive fields in cat striate cortex. *J.
    Neurophysiol.* **58**: 1233–1258.
Jones, E.G., Hendry, S.H.C., and DeFelipe, J. (1987) GABA-peptide
    neurons of the primate cerebral cortex: a limited cell class. In: *Cere-
    bral Cortex*, Jones, E.G. and Peters, A. (eds.), Plenum Press, New
    York, pp. 237–266.
Jones, J.P., Stepnoski, A., and Palmer, L.A. (1987) The two-dimensional
    spectral structure of simple receptive fields in cat striate cortex, *J.
    Neurophys.* **58**: 1212–1232.
Joyner, R.W., Westerfield, M., and Moore, J.W. (1980) Effects of cellu-
    lar geometry on current flow during a propagated action potential.
    Biophys. J. **31**: 183–194.
Julesz, B. (1971) *Foundations of Cyclopean Vision*, University of Chicago
    Press, Chicago.
Kaczmarek, L.K. and Levitan, I.B., eds. (1987) *Neuromodulation*, Ox-
    ford Univ. Press, New York.
Kandel, E.R. (1981) Calcium and the control of synaptic strength by
    learning. *Nature* **293**: 697–700.
Kaneko, C.R.S., Merickel, M., and Kater, S.B. (1978) Centrally pro-
    grammed feeding in *Helisoma*: identification and characteristics of
    an electrically coupled premotor neuron network. *Brain Res.* **126**:
    1–21.
Kanter, I. and Sompolinsky, H. (1987) Associative recall of memory with-
    out errors. *Phys. Rev. A* **35**: 380–392.
Kawato, M. (1984) Cable properties of a neuron model with non-uniform
    membrane resistivity. *J. Theoret. Biol.* **111**: 149–169.
Keeler, J.D. (1988) Comparison between Kanerva's SDM and Hopfield-
    type neural network models. *J. Cognitive Sci.* **12**: 299–329.
Kehoe, J. and Marty, A. (1980) Certain slow synaptic responses: their
    properties and possible underlying mechanisms. *Ann. Rev. Biophys.
    Bioeng.* **9**: 437–465.

Keller, H.B. (1976) *Numerical Solution of Two Point Boundary Problems*, CMBS-NSF Regional Conference Series in Applied Mathematics, number 24, SIAM, Philadelphia.

Kellerth, J.-O., Berthold, C.-H. and Conradi, S. (1979) Electron microscopic studies of serially sectioned cat spinal α-motoneurons. III. Motoneurons innervating fast-twitch (type FR) units of the gastrocnemius muscle. *J. Comp. Neurol.* **184:** 755–767.

Kennedy, D., Evoy, W.H., and Hanawaly, J.T. (1966) Release of coordinated behavior in crayfish by single central neurons. *Science* **154:** 917–919.

Kisvarday, Z.F., Martin, K.A.C., Whitteridge, D., and Somogyi, P. (1985) Synaptic connections of intracellularly filled clutch cells: a type of small basket cell in the visual cortex of the cat. *J. Comp. Neurol.* **241:** 111–137.

Klee, C.B. and Haiech, J. (1980) Concerted role of calmodulin and calcineurin in calcium regulation. *Ann. NY Acad. Sci.* **356:** 43–54.

Klee, M. and Rall, W. (1977) Computed potentials of cortically arranged populations of neurons. *J. Neurophysiol.* **40:** 647–666.

Kleinfeld, D. (1986) Sequential state generation by model neural networks. *Proc. Nat. Acad. Sci. USA* **83:** 9469–9473.

Kleinfeld, D. and Sompolinsky, H. (1988) Associative neural network model for the generation of temporal patterns: theory and application to central pattern generators. *Biophys. J.* **54:** 1039–1051.

Kling, U. and Szekély, G. (1968) Simulation of rhythmic activities. I. Function of networks with cyclic inhibitions. *Kybern.* **5:** 89–103.

Klopf, A.H. (1987) A drive-reinforcement model of single neuron function: an alternative to the Hebbian neuronal model. Air Force Wright Aeronautical Laboratories preprint.

Koch, C. (1987) The action of the corticofugal pathway on sensory thalamic nuclei: a hypothesis. *Neurosci.* **23:** 399–406.

Koch, C. (1987) A network model for cortical orientation selectivity in cat striate cortex. *Invest. Ophthalmol. Vis. Sci.* **28:** 126.

Koch, C. and Adams, P.R. (1984) Computer simulation of bullfrog sympathetic ganglion cell excitability. *Soc. Neurosci. Abst.* **11:** 48.7.

Koch, C. and Poggio, T. (1985) A simple algorithm for solving the cable equation in dendritic trees of arbitrary geometry. *J. Neurosci. Meth.* **12:** 303–315.

Koch, C. and Poggio, T. (1986) Computations in the vertebrate retina: motion discrimination, gain enhancement and differentiation. *Trends Neurosci.* **9:** 204–211.

Koch, C. and Poggio, T. (1987) Biophysics of computation: neurons, synapses, and membranes. In: *Synaptic Function*, Edelman, G.M., Gall, W.E., and Cowan, W.M. (eds.), Wiley, New York, pp. 637–698.

Koch, C., Marroquin, J., and Yuille, A. (1986) Analog "neuronal" networks in early vision. *Proc. Nat. Acad. Sci. USA 83:* 4263–4267.

Koch, C., Poggio, T., and Torre, V. (1982) Retinal ganglion cells: a functional interpretation of dendritic morphology. *Phil. Trans. R. Soc. Lond. (Biol.)* **298:** 227–264.

Koch, C., Poggio, T., and Torre, V. (1983) Nonlinear interactions in a dendritic tree: localization, timing, and role in information processing. *Proc. Natl. Avad. Sci. USA* **80:** 2799–2802.

Koenderink, J.J. and van Doorn, A.J. (1980) Photometric invariants related to solid shape. *Optica Acta* **27:** 981–996.

Kohonen, T. (1980) *Content-Addressable Memories*, Springer Verlag, New York.

Kohonen, T. and Ruohonen, M. (1973) Representation of associated data by matrix operators. *IEEE Trans. Comput.* **22:** 701–702.

Kopell, N. (1986) Coupled oscillators and locomotion by fish. In: Lect. Notes Biomath. 66, *Oscillations in Chemistry and Biology*, Othmer, H. (ed.), Springer Verlag, New York.

Kopell, N. 1988 Toward a theory of modelling central pattern generators. In: *Neural Control of Rhythmic Movements in Vertebrates*, Cohen, A.H., Rossignol, S., and Grillner, S. (eds.), John Wiley, New York.

Kristan Jr., W.B. (1980) Generation of rhythmic motor patterns. In: *Information Processing in the Nervous System*, Pinsker, H.M. and Willis Jr., W.D. (eds.), Raven Press, New York.

Krough, F. T. (1969) Variable order integrators for the numerical solution of ordinary differential equations. Jet Propulsion Laboratory Technical Memorandum, Pasadena, California.

Kuba, K. and Nishi, S. (1979) Characteristics of fast excitatory postsynaptic current in bullfrog sympathetic ganglion cells—effects of membrane potential, temperature and Ca ions. *Pflueger's Arch.* **378:** 205–212.

Kuffler, S.W. and Sejnowski, T.J. (1983) Peptidergic and muscarinic excitation at amphibian sympathetic synapses. *J. Physiol. (London)* **341:** 257–278.

Kulikowski, J.J. and Bishop, P.O. (1981) Linear analysis of the responses of simple cells in the cat visual cortex. *Exp. Brain Res.* **44:** 386–400.

Kupfermann, I. and Weiss, K.R. (1978) The command neuron concept. *Behav. Brain Sci.* **1:** 3–39.

Lambert, J.D. (1973) *Computational Methods in Ordinary Differential Equations*, John Wiley and Sons, Inc., New York.

Lancaster, B. and Adams, P.R. (1986) Calcium dependent current generating the afterhyperpolarization of hippocampal neurons. *J. Neurophysiol.* **55**: 1268–1282.

Lancaster, B. and Pennefather, P. (1987) Potassium currents evoked by brief depolarizations in bull-frog sympathetic gangliopn cells. *J. Physiol. (London)* **387**: 519–548.

Lax, P. D. and Richtmeyer, R. D. (1956) Survey of the stability of linear finite difference equations. *Comm. Pure Appl. Math.* **9**: 267–293.

Le Cun, Y. (1985) Une procedure d'apprentissage pour reseau a seuil assymetrique. In: *Proceedings of Cognitiva* June, 1985, Paris.

Lee, B.B., Cleland, B.G., and Creutzfeldt, O.D. (1977) The retinal input to cells in area 17 of the cat's cortex. *Exp. Brain Res.* **30**: 527–538.

Lees, M. (1959) Approximate solution of parabolic equations. *J. SIAM* **7**: 167–183.

Lehky, S.R. (1983) A model of binocular brightness and binaural loudness perception in humans with general applications to nonlinear summation of sensory inputs. *Biol. Cybern.* **49**: 89–97.

Lehky, S.R. (1988) An astable multivibrator model of binocular rivalry. *Perception* **17**: 215–228.

Lehky, S.R. and Sejnowski, T.J. (1988) Network model of shape from shading: neural function arises from both receptive and projective fields. *Nature* **333**: 452–454.

Lennard, P.R., Getting, P.A., and Hume, R.I. (1980) Central pattern generator mediating swimming in *Tritonia*. II. Initiation, maintenance and termination. *J. Neurophysiol.* **44**: 165–173.

LeVay, S. (1986) Synaptic organization of claustral and geniculate afferents to the visual cortex of the cat. *J. Neurosci.* **6**: 3564–3575.

Linsenmeier, R.A., Frishman, L.J., Jakiela, H.G., and Enroth-Cugell, C. (1982) Receptive field properties of X and Y cells in the cat retina derived from contrast sensitivity measurements. *Vision Res.* **22**: 1173–1183.

Little, W.A. (1974) The existence of persistent states in the brain. *Math. Biosci.* **19**: 101–120.

Lorenz, K. (1970) *Studies in Animal and Human Behavior*, Harvard University Press, Cambridge.

Luskin, M.B and Price, J.L. (1983a) The topographic organization of associational fibers of the olfactory system in the rat, including centrifugal fibers to the olfactory bulb. *J. Comp. Neurol.* **216**: 264–291.

Luskin, M.B and Price, J.L. (1983b) The laminar distribution of intra-cortical fibers originating in the olfactory cortex of the rat. *J. Comp. Neurol.* **216:** 292–302.

Lux, H.-D. (1967) Eigenschafen eines Neuron Modells mit Dendriten begrenzter Länge. *Pflueger's Arch. Ges. Physiol.* **297:** 238–255.

Lux, H.-D., Schubert, P., and Kreutzberg, G.W. (1970) Direct matching of morphological and electrophysiological data in cat spinal mo-toneurons. In: *Excitatory Synaptic Mechanisms*, Andersen, P. and Jansen, J.K.S. (eds.), Universitetsforlaget, Oslo, pp. 189–198.

MacGregor, R.J. (1987) *Neural and Brain Modeling*, Academic Press, New York.

Macrides, F. (1982) Temporal relationship between sniffing and the lim-bic theta rhythm during odor discrimination reversal learning. *J. Neurosci.* **2:** 1705–1717.

Madison, D.V. and Nicoll, R.A. (1984) Control of repetitive discharges of rat CA1 pyramidal neurons *in vitro*. *J. Physiol. (London)* **354:** 319–331.

Marder, E. and Hooper, S.L. (1985) Neurotransmitter modulation of the stomatogastric ganglion of decapod crustaceans. In: *Model Neural Networks and Behavior*, Selverston, A.I. (ed.), Plenum, New York.

Marr, D. (1982) *Vision: A computational investigation into the human representation and processnig of visual information*, Freeman, San Francisco.

Marr, D. and Hildreth, E. (1980) Theory of edge detection. *Proc. R. Soc. Lond. B* **207:** 187–127.

Marr, D. and Poggio, T. (1976) Cooperative computation of stereo dis-parity. *Science* **194:** 283–287.

Martin, K.A., Somogyi, P., and Whitteridge, D. (1983) Physiological and morphological properties of identified basket cells in the cat's visual cortex. *Exp. Brain Res.* **50:** 193–200.

Mascagni, M. (1987a) *Negative Feedback in Neural Networks*, Doctoral Dissertation in Mathematics, Courant Institute of Mathematical Sciences, New York University.

Mascagni, M. (1987b) Computer simulation of negative feedback in neu-rons. *Soc. Neurosci. Abstr.* **13:** 375.4.

Mascagni, M. (1989a) An initial-boundary value problem of physiological significance for equations of nerve conduction. *Comm. Pure Appl. Math.*, in press.

Mascagni, M. (1989b) Animation's role in modeling the nervous system, *Iris Universe*. In press.

Matsuoka, K. (1984) The dynamic model of binocular rivalry. *Biol. Cybern.* **49:** 201–208.

Matsuoka, K. (1985) Sustained oscillations generated by mutually inhibiting neurons with adaptation. *Biol. Cybern.* **52:** 367–376.

Matteson, D.R. and Armstrong, C.M. (1984) Na and Ca channels in a transformed line of anterior-pituitary cells. *J. Gen. Physiol.* **83:** 371–394.

Mayer, M.L., Westbrook, G.L. and Guthrie, P.B. (1984) Voltage dependent block by Mg^{2+} of NMDA response in spinal cord neurones. *Nature* **309:** 261–263.

McBurney, R.N. and Neering, I.R. (1987) Neuronal calcium homeostasis. *Trends Neurosci.* **10:** 164–169.

McClelland, J.L. and Rumelhart, D.E. (1986) *Parallel Distributed Processing: Explorations in the Microstructure of Cognition.* MIT Press, Cambridge, Massachusetts.

McClelland, J.L. and Rumelhart, D.E. (1988) *Explorations in Parallel Distributed Processing: a Handbook of Models, Programs, and Exercises.*, MIT Press, Cambridge, Massachusetts.

McCormick, D.A., Connors, B.W., Lighthall, J.W., and Prince, D.A. (1985) Comparative electrophysiology of pyramidal and sparsely spiny stellate neurons of the neocortex. *J. Neurophysiol.* **54:** 782–806.

McCulloch, W.S. and Pitts, W. (1943) A logical calculus of the ideas immanent in nervous activity. *Bull. Math. Biophys.* **5:** 115–133.

Mead, C. (1989) *Analog VLSI and Neural Systems*, Addison-Wesley, Reading, Massachusetts.

Meech, R.W. (1978) Calcium-dependent potassium activation in nervous tissues. *Ann. Rev. Biophys. and Bioeng.* **7:** 1–18.

Messina, P.C. (1987) Emerging Supercomputer Architectures. In: *A report to the Federal Coordinating Council on Science, Engineering and Technology on The U.S. Supercomputer Industry*, DOE/ER-0362, December 1987.

Miller, R.F. and Bloomfield, S.A. (1983) Electroanatomy of a unique amacrine cell in the rabbit retina. *Proc. Natl. Acad. Sci. A.* **80:** 3069–3073.

Miller, M.I. and Sachs, M.B. (1983) Representation of stop consonants in the discharge patterns of auditory-nerve fibers. *J. Acoust. Soc. Am.* **74:** 502–517.

Mingolla, E. and Todd, J.T. (1986) Perception of solid shape from shading. *Biol. Cybern.* **53:** 137–151.

Minsky, M. and Papert, S. (1969) *Perceptrons*, MIT Press, Cambridge.

Miranker, W.L. (1975) The computational theory of stiff differential equations, Istituto per le Applicazioni del Calcolo, Series 3, Number 102, Consiglio Nazionale delle Ricerche, Rome.

Moczydlowski, E. and Latorre, R. (1983) Gating kinetics of Ca^{2+} activated K^+ channels from rat muscle incorporated into planar lipid bilayers: evidence for two voltage-dependant Ca^{2+} binding reactions. *J. Gen. Physiol.* **82:** 511–542.

Moore, J.W. and Ramon, F. (1974) On numerical integration of the Hodgkin and Huxley equations for a membrane action potential. *J. theor. Biol.* **45:** 249–273.

Morishita, I. and Yajima, A. (1972) Analysis and simulation of networks of mutually inhibiting neurons. *Kybern.* **11:** 154–165.

Morris, C. and Lecar, H. (1981) Voltage oscillations in the barnacle giant muscle fiber. *Biophys. J.* **35:** 193–213.

Morrone, M.C., Burr, D.C., and Maffei, L. (1982) Functional implications of cross-orientation inhibition of cortical visual cells. I. Neurophysiological evidence. *Proc. R. Soc. Lond. B* **216:** 335–354.

Nagumo, J.S., Arimoto, S., and Yoshizawa, S. (1962) An active pulse transmission line simulating a nerve axon. *Proc. IRE* **50:** 2061–2070.

Neher, E. and Sakmann,B. (1983) *Single Channel Recording*, Plenum Press, New York.

Nelson, P.G. and and Lux, H.-D. (1970) Some electrical measurements of motoneuron parameters. *Biophys. J.* **10:** 55-73.

Nunez, P.L. (1981) *Electric Fields of the Brain*, Oxford University Press, New York.

Nowycky, M.C., Fox, A.P., and Tsien, R.W. (1983) Three types of neuronal calcium channels with different calcium agonist sensitivity. *Nature* **316:** 440–443.

O'Donnell, P., Koch, C., and Poggio, T. (1985) Demonstrating the nonlinear interaction between excitation and inhibition in dendritic trees using computer-generated color graphics: a film. *Soc. Neurosci. Abst.* **11:** 142.1.

Ogutzoreli, M.N. (1979) Activity analysis of neural networks. *Biol. Cybern.* **34:** 159–169.

O'Keefe, J. (1983) Spatial memory within and without the hippocampal system. In: *Neurobiology of the Hippocampus*, Seifert, W. (ed.), Academic Press, New York.

Oppenheim, A. and Schafer, R. (1976) *Digital Signal Processing*, Prentice-Hall, New Jersey.

Orban, G.A. (1984) *Neuronal Operations in the Visual Cortex*, Springer, Berlin.

Orban, G.A., Gulyas, B., and Vogels, R. (1987) Influence of moving textured background on direction selectivity of cat striate cortex. *J. Neurophysiol.* **57:** 1792–1812.

O'Shea, R. (1983) *Spatial and Temporal Aspects of Binocular Contour Rivalry*, Ph.D. dissertation, Department of Physiology, University of Queensland, Brisbane, Australia.

Palmer, J. (1986) The NCUBE: A VLSI parallel supercomputer. *Hypercube Multiprocessors*, Heath, M.T. (ed.), SIAM, Philadelphia.

Palmer, L.A. and Davis, T.L. (1981) Receptive-field structure in cat striate cortex. *J. Neurophysiol.* **46:** 260–276.

Parker, D.B. (1985) *Learning Logic*, MIT Center for Computational Research in Economics and Management Science Technical Report TR-47.

Parnas, I. and Segev, I. (1979) A mathematical model for the conduction of action potentials along bifurcating axons. *J. Physiol. (London)* **295:** 323–343.

Peichl, L. and Wässle, H. (1979) Size, scatter and coverage of ganglion cell receptive field centres in the cat retina. *J. Physiol. (London)* **291:** 117–141.

Pellionisz, A., Llinas, R., and Perkel, D.H. (1977) A computer model of the cerebellar cortex of the frog. *Neuroscience* **2:** 19–35.

Pennefather, P., Lancaster, B., Adams, P.R., and Nicoll, R.A. (1985a) Two distinct Ca-dependent K currents in bullfrog sympathetic ganglion cells. *Proc. Natl. Acad. Sci. USA* **82:** 3040–3044.

Pennefather, P., Jones, S.W., and Adams, P.R. (1985b) Modulation of repetitive firing in bullfrog sympathetic ganglion cells by two distinct K^+ currents, I_{AHP} and I_M. *Soc. Neurosci. Abst.* **11:** 48.6.

Pentland, A.P. (1984) Local shading analysis. *IEEE Trans. Patt. Anal. Mach. Intell.* **6:** 170–187.

Pentland, A.P. (1986) Perceptual organization and the representation of natural form. *Artif. Intell.* **28:** 293–331.

Pentland, A.P. (1988) On the extraction of shape information from shading. *Proc. Am. Ass. A.I. 7th Natl. Conf. on AI*, August 21-26, 1988; St. Paul, Minnesota.

Peretto, P. (1984) Collective properties of neural networks: a statistical physics approach. *Biol. Cyber.* **50:** 51–62.

Peretto, P. and Niez, J.J. (1986) Collective properties of neural networks. In: *Disordered Systems and Biological Organization*, Bienenstock, E., Fogelman, F., and Weisbuch, G. (eds.), Springer Verlag, Berlin.

Perkel, D.H. (1965) Applications of a digital computer simulation of a neural network. In *Biophysics and Cybernetic Systems*, Maxfield, M., Callahan, A., and Fogel, L.J. (eds.), Spartan Books, Washington, D.C.

Perkel, D.H. and Mulloney, B. (1978a) Electrotonic properties of neurons: steady-state compartmental model. *J. Neurophysiol.* **41:** 627–639.

Perkel, D.H. and Mulloney, B. (1978b) Calibrating compartmental models of neurons. *Am. J. Physiol.* **235:** R93–R98.

Perkel, D.H., Mulloney, B., and Budelli, R.W. (1981) Quantitative methods for predicting neuronal behavior. *Neuroscience* **6:** 823–837.

Perkel, D.H., Schulman, J.H., Bullock, T.H., Moore, G.P., and Segundo, J.P. (1964) Pacemaker neurons: effects of regularly spaced synaptic input. *Science* **145:** 61–63.

Personnaz, L., Guyon, I., and Dreyfus, G. (1986) Information storage and retrieval in spin-glass like neural networks. *J. Phys. Lett.* **46:** 359–365.

Peskin, C. (1976) *Partial Differential Equations in Biology*, Courant Institute of Mathematical Sciences Lecture Notes, New York University, New York.

Peters, A. and Jones, E.G. (1984) *Cerebral Cortex*, Vols. 1 and 6, Plenum Press, New York.

Pineda, F.J. (1987) Generalization of back-propagation to recurrent neural networks. *Phys. Rev. Lett.* **59:** 2229–2232.

Pinsker, H.M. and Ayers, J. (1983) Neuronal oscillators. In: *The Clinical Neurosciences*, Eillis, W.D. (ed.), Churchill Livingston, New York.

Poggio, G.F. and Poggio, T. (1984) The analysis of stereopsis. *Ann. Rev. Neurosci.* **7:** 379–412.

Poggio, T. and Torre, V. (1977) A new approach to synaptic interactions. In: *Lecture Notes in Biomathematics. Theoretical Approaches to Computer Systems, Vol. 21*, Heim., H. and Palm, G. (eds.), pp. 89–115, Springer, Berlin, Heidelberg, New York.

Poggio, T., Torre, V., and Koch. C. (1985) Computational vision and regularization theory. *Nature* **317:** 314–317.

Poznanski, R.R. (1987) Techniques for obtaining analytical solutions for the somatic shunt cable model. *Math. Biosci.* **85:** 13–35.

Press, W.H., Flannery, B.P., Teukolsky, S.A., and Vetterling, W.T. (1986) *Numerical Recipes: The Art of Scientific Computing*, Cambridge University Press, Cambridge.

Price, J.L. (1973) An autoradiographic study of complementary laminar patterns of termination of afferent fibers to the olfactory cortex. *J. Comp. Neurol.* **150**: 87–108.

Qian, N., Sejnowski, T. (1986) Electro-diffusion model of electrical conduction in neuronal processes. *Proc. Intl. Un. Physiol. Sciences, Satellite Symposium on "Cellular Mechanisms of Conditioning and Behavioral Plasticity"* July 9-12, 1986, Seattle, Washington.

Rall, W. (1957) Membrane time constant of motoneurons. *Science* **126**: 454.

Rall, W. (1959) Branching dendritic trees and motoneuron membrane resistivity. *Exp. Neurol.* **2**: 503–532.

Rall, W. (1960) Membrane potential transients and membrane time constant of motoneurons. *Expt. Neurol.* **2**: 503–532.

Rall, W. (1962a) Theory of physiological properties of dendrites. *Ann. N.Y. Acad. Sci.* **96**: 1071–1092.

Rall, W. (1962b) Electrophysiology of a dendritic neuron model. *Biophys. J.* **2(2)**: 145–167.

Rall, W. (1964) Theoretical significance of dendritic tree for input-output relation. In: *Neural Theory and Modeling*, Reiss, R.F. (ed.), Stanford University Press, Stanford, pp. 73–97.

Rall, W. (1967) Distinguishing theoretical synaptic potentials computed for different soma-dendritic distributions of synaptic inputs. *J. Neurophys.* **30**: 1138–1168.

Rall, W. (1969a) Time constant and electrotonic length of membrane cylinders and neurons. *Biophys. J.* **9**: 1483–1168.

Rall, W. (1969b) Distributions of potential in cylindrical coordinates and time constants for a membrane cylinder. *Biophys. J.* **9**: 1509–1541.

Rall, W. (1970) Dendritic neuron theory and dendrodendritic synapses in a simple cortical system. In: *The Neurosciences: Second Study Program*, Schmitt, F.O. (ed.), Rockefeller University Press, New York.

Rall, W. (1977) Core conductor theory and cable properties of neurons. In: *Handbook of Physiology: The Nervous System, Vol. 1*, Kandel, E.R., Brookhardt, J.M., and Mountcastle, V.B. (eds.), Williams and Wilkins, Co., Baltimore, Maryland, pp. 39-98.

Rall, W. (1980) Functional aspects of neuronal geometry. In: *Neurons Without Impulses*, Roberts, A., and Bush, B.M.H. (eds.), Cambridge University Press, Cambridge.

Rall, W. (1982) Theoretical models which increase R_m with dendritic distance help fit lower value for C_m. *Soc. Neurosci. Abst.* **8**: 414.

Rall, W. (1989) Perspectives on neuron modeling. In: *The Segmental Motor System*, Binder M.D. and Mendell, L.M. (eds.), Oxford Press, Oxford, in preparation.

Rall, W. and Rinzel J. (1973) Branch input resistance and steady attenuation for input to one branch of a dendritic neuron model. *Biophys. J.* **13**: 648-688.

Rall, W. and Segev, I. (1985) Space-clamp problems when voltage clamping branched neurons with intracellular microelectrodes. In: *Voltage and Patch Clamping With Microelectrodes*, Smith, T.G., Jr., Lecar, H., Redman, S.J., and Gage, P.W. (eds.), Am. Physiol. Soc., Bethesda, Maryland, pp. 191–215.

Rall, W. and Segev, I. (1987) Functional possibilities for synapses on dendrites and on dendritic spines. In: *Synaptic Function*, Edelman., G.M., Gall, E.E., and Cowan, W.M. (eds.), New York, Wiley, pp. 605–636.

Rall, W. and Shepherd, G.M. (1968) Theoretical reconstruction of field potentials and dendrodendritic synaptic interactions in olfactory bulb. *J. Neurophysiol.* **31**: 884–915.

Rall, W., Burke, R.E., Smith, T.G., Nelson, P.G., and Frank, K. (1967) Dendritic location of synapses and possible mechanism for the monosynaptic EPSP in motoneurons. *J. Neurophysiol.* **30**: 1169–1193.

Rall, W., Shepherd, G.M., Reese, T.S., and Brightman, M.W. (1966) Dendro-dendritic synaptic pathway for inhibition in the olfactory bulb. *Exptl. Neurol.* **14**: 44–56.

Ramachandran, V.S. (1988a) Perceiving shape from shading. *Scientific American* **259**: 76–83.

Ramachandran, V.S. (1988b) Perception of shape from shading. *Nature* **331**: 163–165.

Ramoa, A.S., Shadlen, M., Skottun, B.C., and Freeman, R.D. (1986) A comparison of inhibition in orientation and spatial frequency selectivity of cat visual cortex. *Nature* **321**: 237–239.

Rand, R.H. and Armbruster, D. (1987) *Perturbation Methods, Bifurcation Theory, and Computer Algebra*, Applied Mathematical Sciences **65**, Springer Verlag, Heidelberg.

Ratliff, F. (1974) *Studies on Excitation and Inhibition in the Retina*, Rockefeller University Press, New York.

Redman, S., and Walmsley, B. (1983) The time course of synaptic potentials evoked in cat spinal motoneurones at identified group Ia synapses. *J. Physiol. (London)* **343**: 117–133.

Reiss, R.F. (1964) A theory of resonant networks. In: *Neural Theory and Modeling*, Reiss, R.F. (ed.), Stanford University Press, California.

Richter, J. and Ullman, S. (1982) A model for the temporal organization of X- and Y-type receptive fields in the primate retina. *Biol. Cybern.* **43**: 127–145.

Richtmeyer, R. D. and Morton, K. W. (1967) *Difference Methods for Initial-Value Problems*, Second edition, Interscience Publishers, division of John Wiley and Sons, Inc., New York.

Rinzel, J. (1977) Repetitive nerve impulse propagation: numerical results and methods. In: *Research Notes in Mathematics—Nonlinear Diffusion*, Fitzgibbon, W.E. and Walker, H.F. (eds.), Pitman Publishing Ltd., London, pp. 186–212.

Rinzel, J. (1978) On repetitive activity in nerve. *Fed. Proc.* **37**: 2793–2802.

Rinzel, J. (1985) Excitation dynamics: insights from simplified membrane models. *Fed. Proc.* **44**: 2944–2946.

Rinzel, J. and Lee, Y.S. (1987) Dissection of a model for neuronal parabolic bursting. *J. Math. Biol.* **25**: 653–675.

Rinzel, J. and Rall, W. (1974) Transient response in a dendritic neuron model for current injected at one branch. *Biophys. J.* **14**: 759–790.

Roberts, A. and Roberts, B.L., eds. (1983) *Neural Origin of Rhythmic Movements*, Cambridge University Press, Cambridge.

Robertson, M. and Pearson, K.G. (1985) Neural circuits in the flight system of the locust. *J. Neurophysiol.* **53**: 110–128.

Rodieck, R. (1965) Quantitative analysis of cat retinal ganglion cell response to visual stimuli. *Vision Res.* **5**: 583–601.

Rodieck, R. (1979) Visual pathways. *Ann. Rev. Neurosci.* **2**: 193–225.

Rose, M.E. (1976) On the integration of nonlinear parabolic equations by implicit methods. *Quart. Appl. Math.* **15**: 237–248.

Ross, W.N. and Werman, R. (1987) Mapping calcium transients in the dendrites of Purkinje cells from the guinea-pig cerebellum in vitro. *J. Physiol. (London)* **389**: 319–336.

Rumelhart, D.E., Hinton, G.E., and Williams, R.J. (1986) Learning internal representations by error propagation. In: *Parallel Distributed Processing: Explorations in the Microstructure of Cognition, Vol. 1: Foundations*, Rumelhart, D.E. and McClelland, J.L. (eds.), MIT Press, Cambridge.

Sachs, M.B. and Young, E.D. (1979) Encoding of steady state vowels in the auditory-nerve: representation in terms of discharge rate. *J. Acoust. Soc. Am.* **66**: 470–479.

Sanderson, K.J. (1971) Visual field projection columns and magnification factors in the lateral geniculate nucleus of the cat. *Exp. Brain Res.* **13**: 159-177.

Sargent, P.B. (1983) The number of synaptic boutons terminating on *Xenopus* cardiac ganglion cells is directly correlated with cell size. *J. Physiol. (London)* **343:** 85–104.

Satou, M., Mori, K., Tazawa, Y., and Takagi, S.F. (1982) Long lasting disinhibition in pyriform cortex of the rabbit. *J. Neurophysiol.* **48:** 1157–1163.

Schierwagen, A. (1986) Segmental cable modelling of electrotonic transfer properties of deep superior culliculus neurons in the cat. *J. Hirnforsch* **27:** 679–690.

Schmid-Antomarchi, H., Hugues, M., and Lazdunski, M. (1986) Properties of the apamine sensitive Ca^{2+}-activated K^+ channels in PC12 pheochromocytoma cells which hyper-produce the apamin receptor. *J. Biol. Chem.* **261:** 8633–8637.

Schmidt, G.E. (1987) The Butterfly parallel processor. In: *Proceedings of the Second International Conference on Supercomputing*, St. Petersburg, Florida.

Scholfield, C.N. (1978) A depolarizing inhibitory potential in neurones of the olfactory cortex in vitro. *J. Physiol. (London)* **279:** 547–557.

Schwartz, E.L. (1980) Computational anatomy and functional architecture of striate cortex: a spatial mapping approach to perceptual coding. *Vision Res.* **20:** 645–669.

Schwob, J.E. and Price, J.L. (1978) The cortical projections of the olfactory bulb: development in fetal and neonatal rats correlated with quantitative variations in adult rats. *Brain Res.* **151:** 369–374.

Segev, I. and Parnas, I. (1977) Computer-model analysis of possible mechanisms underlying differetial channeling of information at bifurcating axons *Isr. J. Med. Sci.* **13:** 1145.

Segev, I. and Parnas, I. (1983) Synaptic integration mechanisms: a theoretical and experimental investigation of temporal postsynaptic interactions between excitatory and inhibitory inputs. *Biophys. J.* **41:** 41–50.

Segev, I. and Rall, W. (1983) Theoretical analysis of neuron models with dendrites of unequal electrical lengths. *Soc. Neurosci. Abst.* **9:** 102.20.

Segev, I., Fleshman, J.W., Miller, J.P., and Bunow, B. (1985) Modeling the electrical properties of anatomically complex neurons using a network analysis program: passive membrane. *Biol. Cyber.* **53:** 27–40.

Sejnowski, T. (1977) Storing Covariance with Nonlinearly Interacting Neurons. *J. Math. Biol.* **4:** 303–321.

Sejnowski, T.J. (1988) Neural populations revealed. *Nature* **332**: 308.

Sejnowski, T., Koch, C., and Churchland, P. (1988) Computational neuroscience. *Science*, **241**: 1299-1306.

Sellami, L. (1988) *Vowel Recognition in Adaptive Neural Networks*, Master's Thesis, Department of Electrical Engineering, University of Maryland, College Park.

Selverston, A.I. (1980) Are central pattern generators understandable? *Behav. Brain Sci.* **3**: 535–571.

Selverston, A.I., ed. (1985) *Model Neural Networks and Behavior*, Plenum Publishing, New York.

Selverston, A.I. and Moulins, M. (1986) *The Crustacean Stomatogastic System*, Springer Verlag, New York.

Seneff, S. (1984) Pitch and spectral estimation of speech based on auditory synchrony model. *Working Papers on Linguistics, MIT* **4**: 44.

Shamma, S. (1985a) Speech processing in the auditory system. I: Representation of speech sounds in the responses of the auditory-nerve. *J. Acoust. Soc. Am.* **78**: 1612–1621.

Shamma, S. (1985b) Speech processing in the auditory system. II: Lateral inhibition and the processing of speech evoked activity in the auditory-nerve. *J. Acoust. Soc. Am.* **78**: 1622–1632.

Shamma, S. (1986) Encoding the acoustic spectrum in the spatio-temporal responses of the auditory-nerve. In: *Auditory Frequency Selectivity*, Moore, B.C.J. and Patterson, R. (eds.), Plenum Press, Cambridge, pp. 289-298.

Shamma, S.A., Chadwick, R., Wilbur, J., Rinzel, J., and Moorish, K. (1986) A biophysical model of cochlear processing: intensity dependence of pure tone responses. *J. Acoust. Soc. Am.* **80(1)**:133-145.

Shapley, R. and Enroth-Cugell, C. (1984) Visual adaptation and retinal gain control. *Prog. Retinal Res.* **3**: 263–346.

Shapley, R.M. and Lennie, P. (1985) Spatial frequency analysis in the visual system. *Ann. Rev. Neurosci.* **8**: 547–583.

Shapley, R.M. and Victor, J.D. (1978) The effect of contrast on the transfer properties of cat retinal ganglion cells. *J. Physiol. (London)* **285**: 275–298.

Shelton, D.P. (1985) Membrane resistivity estimated for the Purkinje neuron by means of a passive computer model. *Neuroscience* **14**: 41–50.

Shepherd, G.M. (1979) *The Synaptic Organization of the Brain*, Oxford University Press, New York.

Shepherd, G.M. and Brayton, R.K. (1979) Computer simulation of a dendro-dendritic synaptic circuit for self- and lateral-inhibition in the olfactory bulb. *Brain Res.* **175**: 377–382.

Shepherd, G.M., Carnevale, N.T., and Woolf, T.B. (1988) Comparisons between computational operations generated by active responses in dendritic branches and spines, using SABER. *Soc. Neurosci. Abstr.* **14**: 252.6.

Sherman, M. (1985) Functional organization of the W-, X- and Y-cell pathways: a review and hypothesis. In: *Progress in Psychobiology and Physiological Psychology*, Vol. 11, Sprague. J.M. and Epstein, A.N. (eds.), Academic Press, New York, pp. 233-314.

Sherman, S.M. and Koch, C. (1986) The control of retinogeniculate transmission in the mammalian lateral geniculate nucleus. *Exp. Brain Res.* **63**: 1–20.

Siebert, W.M. (1970) Frequency discrimination in the auditory system: place or periodicity mechanisms? *Proc. IEEE* **58**: 723–730.

Siegelbaum, S.A. and Tsien, R.W. (1983) Modulation of gated ion channels as a mode of transmitter activity. *Trends Neurosci.* **6**: 307–313.

Sillito, A.M. (1975) The contribution of inhibitory mechanisms to the receptive field properties of neurons in the striate cortex of the cat. *J. Physiol. (London)* **250**: 305–322.

Sillito, A.M., Kemp, J.A., Milson, J.A., and Berardi, N. (1980) A re-evaluation of the mechanisms underlying simple cell orientation selectivity. *Brain Res.* **194**: 517–520.

Simon, S.M. and Llinas, R. (1985) Compartmentalization of the submembrane calcium activity during calcium influx and its significance in transmitter release. *Biophys. J.* **48**: 485–498.

Sinex, D.G. and Geisler, C.D. (1983) Responses of auditory-nerve fibers to consonent-vowel syllables. *J. Acoust. Soc. Am.* **73**: 602–615.

Singer, W. and Creutzfeldt, O.D. (1970) Reciprocal lateral inhibition of on- and off-center neurones in the lateral geniculate body of the cat. *Exp. Brain Res.* **10**: 311–330.

Skottun, B., Bradley, A., Sclar, G., Ohzawa, I., and Freeman, R. (1987) The effects on contrast on visual orientation and spatial frequency discrimination: a comparison of single cells and behaviour. *J. Neurophys.* **57**: 773–786.

Smith, G.D. (1985) *Numerical Solutions of Partial Differential Equations: Finite Difference Methods*, Third edition, Clarendon Press, Oxford.

Smith, S.J. (1987) Progress on LTP at hippocampal synapses: a post-synaptic Ca^{2+} trigger for memory storage? *Trends Neurosci.* **10:** 142–144.

Smith, T.G., Wuerker, R.B., and Frank, K. (1967) Membrane impedance changes during synaptic transmission in cat spinal motoneurons. *J. Neurophysiol.* **30:** 1072–1096.

Snyder, D.L. (1975) *Random Point Processes,* Wiley, New York.

Sod, G.A. (1985) *Numerical Methods in Fluid Dynamics: Initial and Initial Boundary-Value Problems,* Cambridge University Press, Cambridge.

Sompolinsky, H. and Kanter, I. (1986) Temporal association in asymmetric neural networks. *Phys. Rev. Lett.* **57:** 2861–2864.

Spray, D.C., Spira, M.E., and Bennett, M.V.L. (1980) Synaptic connections of buccal mechanosensory neurons in the opisthobranch mollusc, *Navanax inermis. Brain Res.* **182:** 271–286.

Stein, P.S.G., Camp, A.W., Robertson, G.A., and Mortin, L.I. (1986) Blends of rostral and caudal scratch reflex motor patters elicited by simultaneous stimulation of two sites in the spinal turtle. *J. Neurosci.* **6:** 2259–2266.

Stein, R.B., Leung, K.V., Oguztoreli, M.N., and Williams, D.W. (1974) Properties of small neural networks. *Kybern.* **14:** 223–230.

Stent, G.S., Kristan Jr., W.B., Friesen, W.O., Ort, C.A., Poon, M., and Calabrese, R.L. (1978) Neuronal generation of the leech swimming movement. *Science* **200:** 1348–1356.

Stoer, J. and Bulirsch, R. (1980) *Introduction to Numerical Analysis,* Springer Verlag, Heidelberg.

Stone, J. (1983) *Parallel Processing in the Visual System,* Plenum Press, New York.

Stone, J. and Dreher, B. (1973) Projection of X- and Y-cells of the cat's lateral geniculate nucleus to areas 17 and 18 of visual cortex. *J. Neurophysiol.* **36:** 551–567.

Tanabe, T., Iino, M. and Takagi, S.F. (1975) Discrimination of odors in olfactory bulb, amygdaloid areas, and orbitofrontal cortex of monkey. *J. Neurophysiol.* **38:** 1284–1296.

Tanaka, K. (1983) Cross-correlation analysis of geniculostriate neuronal relationships in cats. *J. Neurophysiol.* **49:** 1303–1318.

Tank, D.W. and Hopfield, J.J. (1987) Neural computation by time compression. *Proc. Nat. Acad. Sci. USA* **84:** 1896–1900.

Taxi, J. (1976) In: *Frog Neurobiology,* Llinas, R. and Precht, W. (eds.), Springer Verlag, Heidelberg, pp. 95–150.

Taylor, R.E. (1963) Cable theory. In: *Physical Techniques in Biological Research, Vol. 6*, Nastuk, W.L. (ed.), Academic Press, New York, pp. 219–262.

Tesauro, G.J. (1986) Simple neural models of classical conditioning. *Biol. Cybern.* **55:** 187–200.

Thompson, R.S. (1982) A model for basic pattern generating mechanisms in the lobster stomatogastric ganglion. *Biol. Cybern.* **43:** 71–78.

Tömböl, T. (1974) An electron microscopic study of the neurons of the visual cortex. *J. Neurocytol.* **3:** 525-531.

Tootel, R.B., Silverman, M.S., and DeValois, R.L. (1982) De-oxyglucose analysis of retinotopic organization in primate striate cortex. *Science* **218:** 902–904.

Traub, R.D. and Wong, R.K.S. (1983) Synchronized burst discharge in the disinhibited hippocampal slice. II. Model of the cellular mechanism. *J. Neurophysiol.* **49:** 459–471.

Tseng, G.F. and Haberly, L.B. (1986) A synaptically mediated K+ potential in olfactory cortex: characterization and evidence for interneuronal origin. *Soc. Neurosci. Abst.* **12:** 667.

Ts'o, D.Y., Gilbert, C.D., and Wiesel T.N. (1986) Relationships between horizontal interactions and functional architecture in cat striate cortex as revealed by cross-correlation analysis. *J. Neurosci.* **6:** 1160–1170.

Turner, D.A. and Schwartzkroin, P.A. (1984) Passive electrotonic structure and dendritic properties of hippocampal neurons. In: *Brain Slices*, Dingledine, G. (ed.), Plenum Press, New York.

Tusa, R.J., Palmer, L.A., and Rosenquist, A.C. (1978) The retinotopic organization of area 17 (striate cortex) in the cat. *J. Comp. Neur.* **177:** 213-236.

Ulfhake B. and Kellerth J.-O. (1981) A quantitative light microscopic study of the dendrites of cat spinal α-motoneurons after intracellular staining with horseradish peroxidase. *J. Comp. Neurol.* **202:** 571–583.

van Hateren, J.H. (1986) An efficient algorithm for cable theory, applied to blowfly photoreceptor cells and LMCs. *Biol. Cybern.* **54:** 301–311.

Varela, F. and Singer, W. (1987) Neuronal dynamics in the visual cortico-thalamic pathway revealed through binocular rivalry. *Exp. Brain Res.* **66:** 10–20.

Victor, J.D. (1987) The dynamics of the cat retinal X cell centre. *J. Physiol. (London)* **386:** 219–246.

Vidyasagar, T.R. and Heide, W. (1984) Geniculate orientation biases seen with moving sine wave gratings: implications for a model of simple cell afferent connectivity. *Exp. Brain Res.* **57**: 196–200.

Vladimirescu, A., Zhang, K., Newton, A.R., Pederson, D.O., and Sangiovani-Vincentelli, A. (1981) *SPICE Version 2G User's Guide*, EECS Dept., University of California, Berkeley.

Wässle, H., Boycott, B.B., and Illing, R.-B. (1981) Morphology and mosaic of on- and off-beta cells in the cat retina and some functional considerations. *Proc. R. Soc. Lond. B* **212**: 177–195.

Wässle, H., Peichl, L., and Boycott, B.B. (1983) A spatial analysis of on- and off- ganglion cells in the cat retina. *Vision Res.* **10**: 1151–1160.

Wallace, D.J. (1987) Scientific Computation on SIMD and MIMD Machines. Edinburgh preprint 87/429, Invited Talk at Royal Society Discussion Meeting, London, Dec. 9–10.

Waltman, P. (1986) *A Second Course in Elementary Differential Equations*, Academic Press, New York.

Wang, H.T., Mathur, B. and Koch, C. (1989) Computing optical flow in the primate visual system, *Neural Computation*, in press.

Watkins, D.W. and Berkley, M.A. (1974) The orientation selectivity of single neurons in cat striate cortex. *Exp. Brain Res.* **19**: 433–446.

Waxman, S.G. and Ritchie, J.M. (1985) Organization of ion channels in the myelinated nerve fiber. *Science* **228**: 1502–1507.

Weeks, J.C. (1981) Neuronal basis of leech swimming: separation of swim initiation, pattern generation, and intersegmental coordination by selective lesions. *J. Neurophys.* **45**: 698–723.

Weight, F.F. and Votava, J. (1970) Inactivation of potassium conductance in slow postsynaptic excitation. *Science* **170**: 755–758.

Werbos, P.J. (1987) Building and understanding adaptive systems: a statistical-numerical approach to factory automation and brain research. *IEEE Trans. Systems, Man & Cybern.* **17**: 7–20.

Westerman, L.A. and Smith, R.L. (1984) Rapid and short term adaptation in auditory nerve responses. *Hear. Res.* **15**: 249–260.

White, E.L. and Rock, M.P. (1980) Three dimensional aspects and synaptic relationships of a Golgi impregnated spiny stellate cell reconstructed from serial thin sections. *J. Neurocytol.* **9**: 615–636.

Willows, A.D.O. (1967) Behavioral acts elicited by stimulation of single, identifiable brain cells. *Science* **157**: 570–574.

Willows, A.D.O. and Hoyle, G. (1969) Neuronal network triggering of fixed action pattern. *Science* **166**: 1549–1551.

Wilson, C.J. (1984) Passive cable properties of dendritic spines and spiny neurons. *J. Neurosci.* **4**: 281–297.

Wilson, D.M. (1961) The central nervous control of flight in a locust. *J. Exp. Biol.* **38:** 471–490.

Wilson, D.M. and Waldron, I. (1968) Models for the generation of the motor output pattern in flying locusts. *Proc. IEEE* **56:** 1058–1064.

Wilson, H.R. and Cowan, J.D. (1972) Excitatory and inhibitory interactions in localized populations of model neurons. *Biophys. J.* **12:** 1–24.

Wilson, J. and Sherman, S. (1976) Receptive field characteristics of neurones in cat striate cortex: changes with visual field eccentricity. *J. Neurophysiol.* **39:** 512–533.

Wilson, M.A. and Bower, J.M. (1987) A computer simulation of a three-dimensional model of piriform cortex with functional implications for storage and recognition of spatial and temporal olfactory patterns. *Soc. Neurosci. Abst.* **13:** 1401

Wilson, M.A. and Bower, J.M. (1988) A computer simulation of olfactory cortex with functional implications for storage and retrieval of olfactory information. *Proceedings of the Conference on Neural Information Processing Systems*, Anderson, D.(ed.), AIP Press, New York, pp. 114–126.

Wilson, M.A., Bower, J.M., Chover, J., and Haberly, L.B. (1986) A computer simulation of piriform cortex. *Soc. Neurosci. Abst.* **12:** 1358.

Winfield, D.A., Gatter, K.C., and Powell, T.P.S. (1980) An electron microscopic study of the types and proportions of neurons in the cortex of the motor and visual areas of the cat and rat. *Brain* **103:** 245–258.

Winfree, A.T. (1980) The geometry of biological time. In: *Biomathematics* **8**, Springer Verlag, Heidelberg.

Wong, R.K.S. and Traub, R.D. (1983) Synchronized burst discharge in disinhibited hippocampal slice. I. Initiation in CA2-CA3 region. *J. Neurophys.* **49:** 442–458.

Yamada, W., Koch, C., and Adams, P.R. (1988) Modelling electrical excitability in the cell body and axon of type B bullfrog sympathetic ganglion cells. *Soc. Neurosci. Abst.* **14:** 118.11.

Young, E.D. and Sachs, M.B. (1979) Representation of steady state vowels in the temporal aspects of the discharge patterns of populations of auditory-nerve fibers. *J. Acoust. Soc. Am.* **66:** 1381–1403.

Zipser, D. and Andersen, R.A. (1988) A back-propagation programmed network that simulates response properties of a subset of posterior parietal neurons. *Nature* **331:** 679–684.

Index